National Cancer Institute

18

Greater Than the Sum

Systems Thinking in Tobacco Control

Edited by
Allan Best, Ph.D.
Pamela I. Clark, Ph.D.
Scott J. Leischow, Ph.D.
William M. K. Trochim, Ph.D.

U.S. DEPARTMENT OF HEALTH AND HUMAN SERVICES
National Institutes of Health

Other NCI Tobacco Control Monographs

Strategies to Control Tobacco Use in the United States: A Blueprint for Public Health Action in the 1990's. Smoking and Tobacco Control Monograph No. 1. NIH Pub. No. 92-3316, December 1991.

Smokeless Tobacco or Health: An International Perspective. Smoking and Tobacco Control Monograph No. 2. NIH Pub. No. 92-3461, September 1992.

Major Local Tobacco Control Ordinances in the United States. Smoking and Tobacco Control Monograph No. 3. NIH Pub. No. 93-3532, May 1993.

Respiratory Health Effects of Passive Smoking: Lung Cancer and Other Disorders. Smoking and Tobacco Control Monograph No. 4. NIH Pub. No. 93-3605, August 1993.

Tobacco and the Clinician: Interventions for Medical and Dental Practice. Smoking and Tobacco Control Monograph No. 5. NIH Pub. No. 94-3693, January 1994.

Community-based Interventions for Smokers: The COMMIT Field Experience. Smoking and Tobacco Control Monograph No. 6. NIH Pub. No. 95-4028, August 1995.

The FTC Cigarette Test Method for Determining Tar, Nicotine, and Carbon Monoxide Yields of U.S. Cigarettes. Report of the NCI Expert Committee. Smoking and Tobacco Control Monograph No. 7. NIH Pub. No. 96-4028, August 1996.

Changes in Cigarette-Related Disease Risks and Their Implications for Prevention and Control. Smoking and Tobacco Control Monograph No. 8. NIH Pub. No. 97-4213, February 1997.

Cigars: Health Effects and Trends. Smoking and Tobacco Control Monograph No. 9. NIH Pub. No. 98-4302, February 1998.

Health Effects of Exposure to Environmental Tobacco Smoke. Smoking and Tobacco Control Monograph No. 10. NIH Pub. No. 99-4645, August 1999.

State and Local Legislative Action to Reduce Tobacco Use. Smoking and Tobacco Control Monograph No. 11. NIH Pub. No. 00-4804, August 2000.

Population Based Smoking Cessation. Smoking and Tobacco Control Monograph No. 12. NIH Pub. No. 00-4892, November 2000.

Risks Associated with Smoking Cigarettes with Low Machine-Measured Yields of Tar and Nicotine. Smoking and Tobacco Control Monograph No. 13. NIH Pub. No. 02-5047, October 2001.

Changing Adolescent Smoking Prevalence. Smoking and Tobacco Control Monograph No. 14. NIH Pub. No. 02-5086, November 2001.

Those Who Continue to Smoke. Smoking and Tobacco Control Monograph No. 15. NIH Pub. No. 03-5370, September 2003.

ASSIST: Shaping the Future of Tobacco Prevention and Control. Tobacco Control Monograph No. 16. NIH Pub. No. 05-5645, May 2005.

Evaluating ASSIST: A Blueprint for Understanding State-level Tobacco Control. Tobacco Control Monograph No. 17. NIH Pub. No. 06-6058, October 2006.

Note, when citing this monograph in other works, please use the following format:

National Cancer Institute. *Greater Than the Sum: Systems Thinking in Tobacco Control.* Tobacco Control Monograph No. 18. Bethesda, MD: U.S. Department of Health and Human Services, National Institutes of Health, National Cancer Institute. NIH Pub. No. 06-6085, April 2007.

Contents

Illustrations

Tables

Figures

Foreword

As we have come to see time and time again, complexity is the hobgoblin of health policy. This is of course no surprise to biologists. During a time in the mid-twentieth century when penicillin was driving pneumonia and wound infection into retreat, and when vaccine was beginning to stop the polio epidemic in its tracks, the biologist Ludwig von Bertalanffy was proposing what came to be called "systems theory." In some respects a direct reaction to the reductionist single organ system or "silver bullet" notions of disease and its control, systems theory emphasizes that the behavior of any entity—be it an organization, an individual, a human body—can only be truly understood not by focusing on the properties of its component parts, but by examining and characterizing the collective nature of the positions and relationships among the parts.

Tobacco—and the control of its use and impact—offers a splendid model for using a systems perspective to advantage and gleaning insights about potentially broader applications in health. We have for some time known that health status is the product of the dynamics at play within several domains of influence: our genetic predispositions, our social circumstances, the physical environments within which we live, the behavior patterns we choose, and the medical care we receive. We are also learning that often more important than what happens *within* any given domain is what happens *between* and *among* domains. How does the interplay of our genetic predispositions with our physical environments or behavior choices influence our risk for disease? How do social circumstances affect the medical care we receive and our responses to it? How are our behavioral choices influenced by our social and physical environments?

In tobacco, some of the answers to these questions are coming into closer focus—certainly that is the case for a stronger appreciation of the complexity. We are long past the time that tobacco use is purely a matter of "individual choice" and its control dependent on a strategy of "one-person-at-a-time." Tax policy, school interventions, clean indoor air regulations, agricultural initiatives, advertising campaigns, medical care initiatives, community mobilization, and political action are all among the elements at work to reduce the use of tobacco among Americans. The results have been impressive, deriving from the loosely coordinated contributions of often disparate players. The challenge now is to better understand how these efforts work best in concert under different circumstances. If, through accurate characterization of the nature of the relationships at work, we can develop testable hypotheses about the circumstances in which elements of tobacco control are more, or less, effective, we can accelerate the push to the next level of tobacco control.

The Initiative on the Study and Implementation of Systems (ISIS), a four-year project sponsored by the National Cancer Institute (NCI), represents an innovative and potentially important contribution in that respect. Through ISIS, NCI has supported a careful exploration of four elements of systems approaches to improving tobacco control: systems organizing, system dynamics, system networks, and systems knowledge. This monograph reflects the first two years of the project. Beginning with the identification of key stakeholder groups—practitioners, leaders, advocates, and researchers—ISIS has carefully worked to identify characteristics, apparent and subtle, that shape, and are shaped by, the characteristics of the interactions and networks both within and among stakeholder groups; the structure of the feedback loops involved in fostering synergy; and the role of learning as an integral feature of the systems at play. The lessons of that exploration are presented in this monograph as potential insights for the ways organization, management, adaptation, and learning might be enhanced for tobacco control and, by reflection, for work in other areas.

The possibilities for application to a broad range of public health challenges are clear. Complexity is simply the central feature to be addressed in the terms of effective engagement for any public health initiative. What we used to think of as the products of personal behavior—diet, physical activity, obesity, substance abuse, teen pregnancy, violence—we now know to be the dynamic results of complex physiologic, social, and environmental influences. Whereas we formerly thought of social circumstances as simply shaping exposures to health risks and complicating the ability to defend against them, we are now beginning to understand that they may in fact be integral components in the etiology of disease and disability. And rapidly occurring climate changes that interact with urbanization and population growth to accelerate altered ecological equilibrium, with potentially dramatic and irreversible implications for human health, underscore the necessity to better understand not only the system dynamics, but also the urgency of the mandate.

As important as are the issues presented in this monograph, equally compelling is the need to keep the concepts accessible and to guard against the creation of a new guild of systems theorists. The ISIS project has performed an important service by giving emphasis and structure to the reality, embodied in both physics and philosophy, that entities and actions interrelate, and that true understanding derives from understanding the nature of the relationships. This is a notion so fundamental that it must be a central feature of problem analysis, strategy formulation, program development, and research design in every social endeavor—not cordoned off as the province of those who have access to the credentials and the thesaurus.

The times are different now from when elements of systems theory were initially advanced. Now we have the tools from epidemiology, statistics, large-scale databases, and computational science that allow more structured exploration of the dynamics. But an impedance to progress when various academic disciplines were beginning to explore systems theory in the 1960s may have been the inclination—typical of many academic pursuits of the time—to construct structures and terms that defined its separateness and limited its accessibility. The irony is obvious for a concept rooted in commonality.

Laudably, the ISIS project and this monograph give emphasis to the importance of translation, linkages, synergies, and common perspectives, as work proceeds. We should be grateful to NCI and the ISIS leadership for this insightful contribution.

J. Michael McGinnis, M.D., M.P.P.
Senior Scholar
Institute of Medicine
National Academy of Sciences

Message from the Series Editor

The evolution of the Tobacco Control Monograph Series underscores its growing importance as a resource for researchers, practitioners, and policy makers in tobacco control as well as in other areas of public health. Lessons learned from tobacco prevention and control can be applied to a variety of public health issues, including physical activity, diet and nutrition, overweight and obesity, and substance abuse. The National Cancer Institute (NCI) is committed to disseminating this cross-cutting knowledge to the widest possible audience so that others can benefit from the experience of the tobacco prevention and control community. By so doing, NCI is increasing the evidence base for effective public health interventions and improving the translation of research to practice and policy.

In 1991, NCI published the first monograph in a series designed to address cutting-edge issues and research on tobacco control. That monograph, *Strategies to Control Tobacco Use in the United States: A Blueprint for Public Health Action in the 1990's,* was visionary in its scope and focus: not only did it acknowledge that tobacco use was a complex problem that demanded new ways of thinking and acting, but it also encouraged expanded exploration of tobacco use issues by the tobacco control community. The three-axis model for the American Stop Smoking Intervention Study for Cancer Prevention (ASSIST), described in Monograph 1, was designed to address the complex interplay of varied target populations, critical channels for intervening (e.g., health care, schools, worksites, and community groups), and intervention types (e.g., mass media, program services, and policy). (See Monograph 16: *ASSIST: Shaping the Future of Tobacco Prevention and Control* and Monograph 17: *Evaluating ASSIST: A Blueprint for Understanding State-level Tobacco Control* for more details.)

Although it did not adopt the "systems" nomenclature, Monograph 1 laid the foundation for this monograph (Monograph 18), which provides a new and expanded vision of tobacco control as a complex adaptive system. This new model encourages the tobacco control community to (1) collect and use vast arrays of data more effectively; (2) develop and optimize networks to enable the community to more efficiently address varied populations, critical channels for intervention, and intervention types; and (3) support the analysis of complex systems so that more effective strategic decisions are made. Monograph 18 builds on the foundation laid by Monograph 1 by explicitly encouraging (1) the development of informatics infrastructures and collaborative networks, (2) analysis of complex interacting variables, and (3) adoption of new interventions that can speed research to practice (and practice to research). Monograph 18, as the conceptual heir to Monograph 1, provides a new framework for thinking about and acting on the complex relationships among causal factors of public health threats, and it challenges us to consider not just whether we can more effectively use our knowledge of informatics and information management, networks, and complex systems, but whether we will use those essential tools to more rapidly benefit the public's health.

Stephen E. Marcus, Ph.D.
Monograph Series Editor
April 2007

Preface

> *There is always an easy solution to every human problem—neat, plausible, and wrong.*
>
> —H. L. Mencken (1880–1956)

The world of tobacco control has become increasingly complex over the past several decades. It involves more extensive collaborations; new structures and configurations for coordinating efforts; and multilevel social, professional, and knowledge networks to improve information sharing for public health. Given such complexity, there has been a corresponding increased need to address tobacco control issues using a systems perspective that enables one to better understand and navigate the dynamic and evolving nature of the terrain to achieve the next generation of improved health outcomes.

This monograph describes the results of the initial two years of the Initiative on the Study and Implementation of Systems (ISIS), a four-year project. This initiative is one of the first major coordinated efforts to study and implement a systems thinking perspective using several systems approaches and methodologies that appeared to be promising for tobacco control in itself and as an exemplar for other complex issues in today's public health environment. In the ancient, revered Egyptian myth, the goddess Isis breathed clean air into her late husband Osiris to restore him to life. In analogous fashion, the ISIS project hopes to contemporize the myth in a tobacco control context and encourage systems perspectives that have the potential to help people breathe cleaner air and be restored to a smoke-free life.

Although this work is aimed at the efforts of the tobacco control community, the word "tobacco" intentionally appears only in the subtitle of this monograph. That is because ISIS was a research effort that focused on the tobacco control environment to examine how to apply systems approaches to issues that have become endemic throughout public health, including the need for

- Better understanding of outcomes, including the unintended consequences of complex interventions and events

- Effective capture, dissemination, and management of knowledge throughout the multilayered public health system

- More efficient organization and linkage of the efforts of multiple, diverse stakeholders

- Adoption of evidence-based practices that inform practice and improve outcomes

- Strengthening of collaborative networks of scientists, policy makers, government and foundation managers, practitioners, and the public

This work was undertaken to help address some of the fundamental organizational issues in tobacco control and, by corollary, much of public health. The goal was to investigate the potential of integrated, systems-based approaches to facilitate the efforts of all stakeholders to make substantive changes in public health outcomes. The lack of such linkages poses a particularly serious challenge to the public health system. For example, a 2001 Institute of Medicine report, *Crossing the Quality Chasm,* points to "a health care system that frequently falls short in its ability to translate knowledge into practice…"*[(p3)] In this view, the lack of progress is due to (1) a system that fosters research that does not always translate directly into outcomes in patients and (2) practitioners who do not often have a voice in this research community. These types of disconnections illustrate the need for more synergistic teamwork, within a system of systems, that has the potential to dramatically improve public health outcomes.

In ISIS, the term *systems* plays a central role. However, its definition remains elusive. The term has multiple manifestations and meanings in the world of tobacco control, encompassing everything from the structure of organizations, to the arrangement of networks, to the dynamics of change, to the patterning of information. The evolution of this project puts it squarely in the trajectory of some of the key trends in contemporary public health, all of which can be viewed as essentially "systems" issues:

- **There is a growing macro-level focus in tobacco control and public health.** A review of the history of tobacco control efforts shows that the earliest initiatives were aimed at the individual and cessation; intermediate efforts increasingly focused on the community level and collaborative interventions; and subsequent efforts emphasized larger population groups and more broad-based interventions, such as legislative changes, taxation, and media advocacy. A systems-level focus on tobacco control is a logical next step in understanding and managing the complex nature of tobacco use, as both an epidemiological and a personal health issue.

- **There is a growing need to better integrate research and practice.** The core concerns of putting evidence-based knowledge about tobacco control into practice and giving practitioners a voice in the research agenda point to a need to re-examine the basic paradigms of science, how it interfaces with society, and how society's investment in research and development is understood.

- **The tobacco control environment has, in and of itself, become a system of systems.** Understanding and navigating a landscape that includes national organizations, community-based advocacy groups, health practitioners, public health officials, researchers, funding sources, and the community itself have become the next major challenge in creating and implementing evidence-based practice that changes public health outcomes.

- **The systems of systems that now characterize tobacco control are embedded within a larger public health context with important focal outcomes such as reduced morbidity and mortality.** Tobacco control has had tremendous successes in reducing

---

*Committee on Quality of Health Care in America, Institute of Medicine. 2001. *Crossing the quality chasm: A new health system for the 21st century. Executive summary.* Washington, DC: National Academies Press. http://books.nap.edu/execsumm_pdf/10027.pdf.

consumption, prevalence, morbidity, and mortality. Universally applying what we know would have a tremendous impact on tobacco control and disease reduction. Being able to do so and reaching the next level of achievements in outcomes, however, require a better understanding of the complex interrelationships and dynamics of the tobacco control system, its connections to both the public health system and the public, and its dynamic relationships with the industry that continues to generate both products and profits.

These trends, at many levels, reflect the evolution of public health itself—from treatment of specific diseases, to prevention, to social and policy movements, to the study of interrelated factors and beyond. This monograph is the result of that evolution; its aim is to contribute to continued evolution by encouraging consideration and use of systems thinking in tobacco control and potentially in public health in general.

Acknowledgments

This monograph was developed by the National Cancer Institute under the editorial direction of **Stephen E. Marcus,** Monograph Series Editor, and Senior Scientific Editors **Allan Best, Pamela I. Clark, Scott J. Leischow,** and **William M. K. Trochim.** Individual chapters of this monograph and the entire volume were subjected to extensive peer review and revision.

Editors

Allan Best, Ph.D.
Principal Investigator
Senior Scientist
Centre for Clinical Epidemiology and
    Evaluation
Vancouver Coastal Health Research Institute
Clinical Professor, Health Care and
    Epidemiology
University of British Columbia
Professional Staff
British Columbia Cancer Agency
Vancouver, British Columbia, Canada

Pamela I. Clark, Ph.D.
Principal Investigator
Co-lead, Chapter 2
Senior Health Research Scientist
Battelle Centers for Public Health Research
    & Evaluation
Baltimore, MD

Scott J. Leischow, Ph.D.
Principal Investigator
Co-lead, Chapter 2
Professor, Department of Family and
    Community Medicine
Deputy Director for Strategic Partnerships
    and Policy
Arizona Cancer Center
The University of Arizona
Tucson, AZ

Stephen E. Marcus, Ph.D.
Monograph Series Editor
Epidemiologist
Tobacco Control Research Branch
Behavioral Research Program
Division of Cancer Control and Population
    Sciences
National Cancer Institute
Bethesda, MD

William M. K. Trochim, Ph.D.
Principal Investigator
Co-lead, Chapter 3
Co-lead, Chapter 4
Professor
Policy Analysis and Management
Cornell University
Ithaca, NY

Authors

Gabriele Bammer, Ph.D.
Co-lead, Chapter 3
Co-lead, Chapter 5
Professor
National Centre for Epidemiology and
    Population Health
College of Medicine and Health Sciences
The Australian National University
Canberra, Australia
Hauser Center for Nonprofit Organizations
Harvard University
Cambridge, MA

Alex Berland, R.N., M.Sc.
President
A. Berland Inc.
Adjunct Professor
Department of Healthcare and Epidemiology
University of British Columbia
Vancouver, British Columbia, Canada

Derek Cabrera, Ph.D.
Co-lead, Chapter 3
Co-lead, Chapter 4
National Science Foundation Post Doctoral
    Associate in Human Ecology
National Science Foundation/IGERT Fellow
    in Nonlinear Systems
Cornell University
Ithaca, NY

Noshir Contractor, Ph.D.
Co-lead, Chapter 6
Professor
Departments of Speech Communication
    and Psychology
University of Illinois at Urbana-Champaign
Urbana, IL

William C. Horrace, Ph.D.
Associate Professor
Department of Economics and Center for
    Policy Research
Syracuse University
Syracuse, NY

Timothy Huerta, Ph.D.
Scientist
Child and Family Research Institute and
Provincial Health Research Authority
Vancouver, British Columbia, Canada
Assistant Professor
Rawls College of Business
Texas Tech University
Lubbock, TX

Francis Lau, Ph.D.
Lead, Chapter 7
Associate Professor
School of Health Information Science
University of Victoria
Vancouver, British Columbia, Canada

Douglas A. Luke, Ph.D.
Director
Center for Tobacco Policy Research
Saint Louis University School of Public
    Health
St. Louis, MO

Bobby Milstein, Ph.D., M.P.H.
Behavioral Scientist
Syndemics Prevention Network
Centers for Disease Control and Prevention
Atlanta, GA

Keith Provan, Ph.D.
Co-lead, Chapter 6
McClelland Professor of Public
    Administration and Policy
Director of the SPAP Ph.D. Program
School of Public Administration and Policy
Eller College of Management
University of Arizona
Tucson, AZ

George P. Richardson, Ph.D.
Co-lead, Chapter 5
Chair
Department of Public Administration
    and Policy
Nelson A. Rockefeller College of Public
    Affairs and Policy
University at Albany
State University of New York
Albany, NY

James W. Shaw, Ph.D., Pharm.D., M.P.H.
Assistant Professor
Department of Pharmacy Administration
    and Center for Pharmacoeconomic
    Research
College of Pharmacy
University of Illinois at Chicago
Chicago, IL

Ramkrishnan (Ram) V. Tenkasi, Ph.D.
Professor of Organizational Change
Ph.D. Program in Organization
  Development and Change
Department of Management and
  Organizational Behavior
Benedictine University
Lisle, IL

Reviewers

Michele Bloch, M.D., Ph.D.
Medical Officer
Tobacco Control Research Branch
Behavioral Research Program
Division of Cancer Control and Population
  Sciences
National Cancer Institute
Bethesda, MD

Jonathan P. Caulkins, Ph.D.
Professor of Operations Research and Public
  Policy
Qatar Campus, H. John Heinz School of
  Public Policy and Management
Carnegie Mellon University
Doha, Qatar

Tom Cummings, Ph.D.
Department Chair
Management and Organization Department
Marshall School of Business
University of Southern California
Los Angeles, CA

Susan J. Curry, Ph.D.
Director
Institute for Health Research and Policy
Professor
Health Policy and Administration
School of Public Health
University of Illinois, Chicago
Chicago, IL

Samuel R. Friedman, Ph.D.
Senior Research Fellow
Director, Social Theory Core
Center for Drug Use and HIV Research
National Development and Research
  Institutes, Inc.
New York, NY

Russell E. Glasgow, Ph.D.
Senior Scientist
Clinical Research Unit
Kaiser Permanente
Aurora, CO

Linda M. Harris, Ph.D.
Senior Health Communication Scientist
Health Communication and Informatics
  Research Branch
Behavioral Research Program
Division of Cancer Control and Population
  Sciences
National Cancer Institute
Rockville, MD

William S. (Bill) Harris Jr.
Principal
Facilitated Systems
Everett, WA

Jack B. Homer, Ph.D.
Homer Consulting
Voorhees, NJ

Corinne Husten, M.D., M.P.H.
Acting Director
Office on Smoking and Health
Centers for Disease Control and Prevention
Atlanta, GA

David M. Introcaso, Ph.D.
Health Policy Analyst
Office of Health Policy Research and Planning
Office of the Assistant Secretary for Planning
  and Evaluation
U.S. Department of Health and Human
  Services
Washington, DC

Brick Lancaster, M.A., CHES
Chief
Program Services Branch
Office on Smoking and Health
Centers for Disease Control and Prevention
Atlanta, GA

Ken McLeroy, Ph.D.
Associate Dean for Academic Affairs
School of Rural Public Health
Texas A&M Health Science Center
College Station, TX

Gerald Midgley, Ph.D.
Professor
Institute of Environmental Science
and Research
Christchurch Science Centre
Christchurch, New Zealand

John Millar, M.D.
Executive Director
Population Health Surveillance & Disease
Control Planning
Provincial Health Services Authority
Vancouver, British Columbia, Canada

Jonathan A. Morell, Ph.D.
Senior Policy Analyst
NewVectors
Ann Arbor, MI

David Mowat, M.B.Ch.B., M.P.H., F.R.C.P.C.
Deputy Chief Public Health Officer
Public Health Practice and Regional
Operations
Public Health Agency of Canada
Ottawa, Ontario, Canada

Diana Newman, Ed.D., R.N.
Professor
School of Nursing
Massachusetts College of Pharmacy and
Health Sciences
Boston, MA

Brian Oldenburg, Ph.D.
Professor and Chair
International Public Health
Department of Epidemiology and
Preventive Medicine
Monash University
Melbourne, Australia

C. Tracy Orleans, Ph.D.
Senior Scientist and Distinguished Fellow
Robert Wood Johnson Foundation
Princeton, NJ

William A. Pasmore, Ph.D.
Partner
Mercer Delta Organizational Consulting
New York, NY

Peter Robertson, Ph.D.
Associate Professor
School of Policy, Planning, and Development
University of Southern California
Los Angeles, CA

Khalid Saeed, Ph.D.
Professor of Economics
Department Head
Social Science and Policy Studies
Worcester Polytechnic Institute
Worcester, MA

Gregory J. Sherman, Ph.D.
Senior Health Architect
Science and Research Advisory Unit
Office of Public Health Practice
Public Health Agency of Canada
Ottawa, Ontario, Canada

Glorian Sorensen, Ph.D., M.P.H.
Professor
Harvard School of Public Health
Director
Center for Community Based Research
Dana-Farber Cancer Institute
Boston, MA

Stephen Taplin, M.D., M.P.H.
Senior Scientist
Applied Research Program
Division of Cancer Control and Population
  Sciences
National Cancer Institute
Bethesda, MD

Thomas W. Valente, Ph.D.
Associate Professor and Director
Master of Public Health Program
Department of Preventive Medicine
School of Medicine
University of Southern California
Alhambra, CA

K. Viswanath, Ph.D.
Associate Professor
Department of Medical Oncology
Dana-Farber Cancer Institute
Associate Professor
Department of Society, Human
  Development, and Health
Harvard School of Public Health
Harvard University
Boston, MA

Saul Weingart, M.D., Ph.D.
Vice President for Patient Safety
Dana-Farber Cancer Institute
Boston, MA

Bob Williams
Wellington
Aotearoa, New Zealand

Derek Yach, M.B.Ch.B., M.P.H.
Director
Health Equity
The Rockefeller Foundation
New York, NY

*The editors wish to acknowledge the
contributions of the following individuals
to the ISIS project:*

Lawrence W. Green, Dr.P.H.
Adjunct Professor
Department of Epidemiology and
  Biostatistics
Co-Leader
Society, Diversity and Disparities Program
Comprehensive Cancer Center
University of California at San Francisco
San Francisco, CA

Jack Henningfield, Ph.D.
Vice President for Research and Policy
Pinney Associates
Professor
Behavioral Biology
Johns Hopkins School of Medicine
Baltimore, MD

Peter Robertson, Ph.D.
Associate Professor
School of Policy, Planning, and Development
University of Southern California
Los Angeles, CA

Carol L. Schmitt, Ph.D.
Senior Health Research Scientist
Battelle Centers for Public Health Research
  & Evaluation
Baltimore, MD

Frances A. Stillman, Ed.D.
Co-Director
Institute for Global Tobacco Control
Associate Professor
Department of Epidemiology
Bloomberg School of Public Health
Johns Hopkins University
Baltimore, MD

The editors would like to acknowledge the contributions of the following staff who provided technical and editorial assistance in the preparation of this monograph:

Jennifer S. Brown, M.A.
Ph.D. Candidate
Department of Human Development
Cornell University
Ithaca, NY

Richard S. Gallagher
Chief Science Writer
R.S. Gallagher and Associates
Newfield, NY

Snjezana Huerta-Kralj
Project Coordinator and Research Assistant
Department of Psychology
Simon Fraser University
Burnaby, British Columbia, Canada

Gregg Moor
Project Coordinator
UBC Institute for Health Promotion
   Research
Centre for Clinical Epidemiology &
   Evaluation
Vancouver Coastal Health Research Institute
Vancouver, British Columbia, Canada

April Roggio
Research Assistant
Department of Public Administration and
   Policy
Nelson A. Rockefeller College of Public
   Affairs and Policy
University at Albany
State University of New York
Albany, NY

In addition, the editors wish to acknowledge and thank those who participated in the brainstorming and planning process leading to the ISIS project as well as the many others who shared their insights with the ISIS project.

Last, the editors would like to acknowledge the publication support services provided for this monograph:

American Institutes for Research
Margot Raphael, Project Director
Elizabeth Bruce, Monograph Editor
Michael Rollins and Matthew Mowczko,
   Production Artists

Cygnus Corporation
Terry Kelly, Publications Manager
Ruth Christie, Copyeditor
Mary Bedford, Proofreader

Acronyms

4P-KMT	Four P-knowledge management and translation
ACS	American Cancer Society
ALA	American Lung Association
ASSIST	American Stop Smoking Intervention Study for Cancer Prevention
caBIG	Cancer Biomedical Informatics Grid
CAS	complex adaptive systems
CBPR	community-based participatory research
CDC	Centers for Disease Control and Prevention
CHP	Consumer Health Profiles
CISNET	Cancer Intervention and Surveillance Modeling Network
COMMIT	Community Intervention Trial for Smoking Cessation
DHHS	U.S. Department of Health and Human Services
FCTC	Framework Convention on Tobacco Control
FY	fiscal year
GTRN	Global Tobacco Research Network
ISIS	Initiative on the Study and Implementation of Systems
KMT	knowledge management and translation
KTNs	knowledge-translation networks
LGIs	large-group interventions
MDS	multidimensional scaling
MSA	Master Settlement Agreement and Amendments
NCI	National Cancer Institute
NIH	National Institutes of Health
PLANET	Plan, Link, Act, Network with Evidence-based Tools
SEER	Surveillance, Epidemiology, and End Results
SES	socioeconomic status
SoTC	Strength of Tobacco Control
TTURC	Transdisciplinary Tobacco Use Research Center

1

Overview

Tobacco control and public health have evolved into a complex set of interconnected and largely self-organizing systems. Their components include international, national, and local governmental agencies; individual advocacy groups; policy makers; health care professionals; nonprofit foundations; and the general population itself. The issues require the exploration of approaches and methodologies that speak to the evolving, dynamic nature of this systems environment.

This monograph focuses on the first two years of the Initiative on the Study and Implementation of Systems (ISIS), which was funded by the National Cancer Institute to examine the potential for systems thinking in tobacco control and public health. ISIS explored the general idea of a systems thinking rubric encompassing a great variety of systems-oriented methodologies and approaches. Four approaches have particular promise for their applicability to tobacco control and public health and thus were chosen as areas for initial investigation: (1) organizing and managing as a system, (2) system dynamics and how to model those dynamics, (3) system networks and their analysis, and (4) systems knowledge and its management and translation.

As a transdisciplinary effort that linked both tobacco control stakeholders and systems experts, ISIS combined a number of exploratory projects and case studies within these four approaches with a detailed examination of the potential for systems thinking in tobacco control. Its end product was a set of expert consensus guidelines for the future implementation of systems thinking and systems perspectives for tobacco control and public health.

Introduction

Tobacco use remains a leading cause of preventable death. Even though reductions in the prevalence of tobacco use and cigarette consumption over the past four decades have been substantial, tobacco use continues to be a major challenge for public health.[1-3] With the recent development of clear, evidence-based best practices in tobacco control, along with funding new research to better understand the complex and changing tobacco environment, the potential exists to improve public health outcomes substantially in the future.

However, the promise of implementing demonstrably effective tobacco control initiatives to achieve greater gains in health outcomes remains only partly realized. Strong scientific evidence exists for effective tobacco control practices. Nonetheless, desired outcomes remain at levels far lower than what is achievable in areas such as the prevalence of tobacco use and product consumption and related morbidity and mortality.[2,4] This situation is attributable to numerous factors, ranging from multiple diverse stakeholders, to declining funding, to the systematic efforts of the tobacco industry to undermine the efforts of the tobacco control community.

It is increasingly apparent that the implementation and, more important, the integration of systems approaches (e.g., systems organization, system dynamics, system networks, and systems knowledge) have the potential to significantly enhance the efforts of groups of tobacco control stakeholders to improve outcomes associated with tobacco control initiatives (e.g., increased smoking cessation, reduced initiation to tobacco use, and above all, reduced morbidity and mortality associated with smoking).[5] These efforts, applied to tobacco control practices, can be an essential foundation for creating a new, scientifically credible framework for future public health efforts.

The ISIS project was undertaken to examine the value and potential impact of systems thinking for tobacco control, both to improve its outcomes and as a template for strategies to apply these methods to other public health issues. This monograph describes the findings of the first two years of this project and their potential implications for tobacco control and public health. The monograph examines the synthesis of four key systems approaches applied to the fundamental problems of tobacco control (figure 1.1):

1. **Systems organizing** to understand and foster the development of participatory, complex, and adaptive collaborative systems in tobacco control; ensure their effective facilitation and management; and encourage productive system action and learning

2. **System dynamics** to understand and model the complex dynamic interactions involved in the tobacco control system and among the factors influencing tobacco use, including political actions such as taxes and legislation, research advances, tobacco control activities, industry forces, and social and cultural factors

3. **System networks** to understand and analyze effective collaborative relationships among stakeholders, improve collaboration strategies, and help reduce duplication of effort

4. **Systems knowledge** to develop and manage the knowledge infrastructure required for effective dissemination and evolution of scientifically credible, evidence-based practices, together with an effective strategy to package, deliver, and maintain this knowledge

Most important, integration of these systems approaches promises to help in the creation

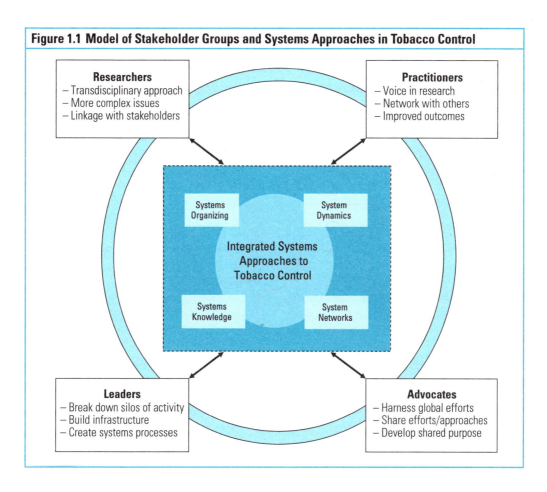

Figure 1.1 Model of Stakeholder Groups and Systems Approaches in Tobacco Control

of a more consistent and adaptive research-based infrastructure for effective tobacco control and, by corollary, for public health in general. The ISIS project is an important step in bringing such an environment to fruition and, in turn, changing the practice of tobacco control to take the next step to improve health outcomes.

Monograph Framework

This monograph is structured as a discussion of the core issues in systems thinking for tobacco control, followed by detailed consideration of specific systems approaches and their potential synthesis, together with consensus guidelines for future systems efforts in tobacco control and public health. The monograph's core areas include

- An overview of the state of tobacco control and the potential for using systems thinking approaches to address future tobacco control issues;

- A detailed examination of four initial systems thinking approaches chosen for potential applicability to tobacco control and public health: systems organizing and management, system dynamics and its modeling, system network analysis, and systems knowledge management and translation; and

- A look at the potential areas of synthesis among these and other systems approaches and methods. The general rubric of systems thinking is used, together with guidelines for exploring how a future systems thinking environment for tobacco control can affect each of the major stakeholders in tobacco control and potentially improve public health outcomes.

Chapter 2, "Tobacco Control at a Crossroads," examines the state of tobacco control, the immediate context for exploring systems thinking within this area, and the evolution of tobacco control efforts. It tracks the development of current views of tobacco use and discusses systems approaches as the logical next step in addressing tobacco use.

Chapter 3, "Systems Thinking: Potential to Transform Tobacco Control," then lays out the case for the four broad systems thinking approaches examined within this project. The chapter summarizes the value of systems thinking, the approaches and issues that drive systems thinking, and the potential of systems thinking to change outcomes in tobacco control. In the process, the chapter examines the research underpinnings of a variety of systems thinking methods, including system dynamics modeling, network analysis, knowledge management, systems organizing and management, and the synthesis of these and other approaches.

Chapter 4, "How to Organize: Systems Organizing," examines the management, operational, and logistic aspects of working in a diverse systems environment involving multiple stakeholders. This section explores the view that systems thinking is becoming an integral feature of contemporary management. It presents a model for systems organizing that encompasses and extends the traditional management model around a systems framework of vision, structure, action, and learning. It also examines current thinking in cross-organizational systems, including the use of participatory mixed methods for planning and evaluation that integrate with a systems approach, together with the concept of effective complex adaptive systems for tobacco control and public health, illustrating systems organizing principles with several empirical case studies.

Chapter 5, "How to Anticipate Change in Tobacco Control Systems," follows this organization framework with a look at the specifics of modeling public health issues as a system to better understand them and plan more effective interventions. This chapter focuses on understanding the nature of system dynamics, including the development of dynamic models that include feedback processes and the use of system dynamics modeling as a technology for understanding tobacco control outcomes, together with results from a study developing a system dynamics representation of tobacco control variables and simulation of the aging chain of smokers.

Chapter 6, "Understanding and Managing Stakeholder Networks," explores system network theory and methods, examining the question of "who works with whom" in a system and how organizations are brought together based on concepts of network analysis and related approaches. It also examines applications of network analysis to improve community and public health collaboration, including a case study of network analysis for evaluation of tobacco control.

Chapter 7, "What We Know: Managing the Knowledge Content," focuses on the role of managing systems knowledge content, including research findings on knowledge management issues for health care environments, the results of a knowledge management review project to evaluate existing research dissemination efforts at the National Cancer Institute, recommendations for a general knowledge infrastructure for tobacco control efforts, and a systems-oriented conceptual modeling project used to develop the taxonomy for a tobacco control knowledge base.

The monograph closes in chapter 8, "Synthesis and Conclusions," by examining the critical issue of integrating component systems thinking disciplines within a broader framework of systems thinking in tobacco control. The chapter explores synergies across the areas studied in this project, existing trends toward systems approaches, and common methodological elements, together with consensus guidelines summarized in the "Major Conclusions" section of this chapter.

Two appendices describe the project's history and its formative decisions, as well as a potential framework for implementing systems thinking approaches in the real world of tobacco control.

Summary

To work efficiently and effectively in today's tobacco control environment, the tobacco control community must explore the systems methodologies that drive the competitiveness of the private sector. Such methodologies have strong potential for successful translation of science into practice and the achievement of desired outcomes. The goal of the first two years of the ISIS project was to take a critical first step toward bringing this potential to fruition.

The ISIS project represents a significant step in investigating approaches for systems thinking to improve outcomes of tobacco control efforts. It also serves as the framework for a new, rigorous approach to other public health issues. The findings and lessons learned in the first two years of this project were synthesized by its core members as a set of consensus guidelines for the future exploration and implementation of systems thinking approaches in tobacco control. The following "Major Conclusions" section and chapter 8 summarize these guidelines, which emphasize systems thinking as an ecological process rather than a cluster of methodologies.

The benefits of an integrated systems approach to tobacco control can go far beyond dollars and cents, to the estimated 1,200 people per day in the United States who die prematurely from smoking-related causes, according to the Centers for Disease Control and Prevention.[2] The vision is that by integrating technologies that address systems organizing, system dynamics, system networks, and systems knowledge in a framework of systems thinking, tobacco control organizations will be able to work more effectively and collaboratively and use evidence-based best practices more effectively in the field. More important, this effort leverages current systems research to create a bold new approach to integrating science and practice to achieve desired health outcomes.

Major Conclusions

1. Tobacco control is at a crossroads because tobacco use is increasingly recognized as a complex adaptive system involving biological, behavioral, and environmental influences.

2. Systems thinking has the potential to transform tobacco control research, practice, and policy by improving collaboration and by providing a more dynamic and adaptive evidence base for practice and a deeper knowledge about the impact of tobacco prevention and control activities.

3. Systems organizing encourages the transformation to a systems culture by addressing the core issues: vision and paradigm, barriers, leadership, and the need for an ongoing learning environment for systems thinking. Such an environment encompasses a wide variety of structured group processes, many of which may involve quantitative frameworks. Systems organizing implies a synthesis of the classic linear management processes of planning, organizing, leading, and controlling with a more adaptive environment expressed

around concepts of vision, structure, action, and learning.

4. System dynamics encompasses qualitative and mathematical simulation approaches to model dynamic relationships that evolve over time, and can simulate behavior including possible unintended consequences and long-term effects. Efforts to develop and apply systems methods and processes involve theory and research development, mixed-methods systems thinking, and participatory assessment of systems needs. At a practical level, the infrastructure for system dynamics is addressed by fostering an ecological perspective on implementation, as well as a systems approach to evaluation.

5. System networks of tobacco control stakeholders form a foundation for a systems environment in tobacco control, replacing "silos" with linkages of people and resources that transcend geography and discipline. This process involves building and maintaining stakeholder relationships by creating networks of stakeholders for systems thinking, studying the dynamics and effects of these networks, linking disciplines of stakeholders in tobacco control, and preparing for the impact of demographic change.

6. Systems knowledge management and translation form a key component of systems approaches for tobacco control, examining purpose, people, process, and products within a broader knowledge infrastructure. This involves building system and knowledge capacity by expanding public health data, integrating information silos, fostering the skills and culture to affect processes and outcomes, and creating networks for knowledge translation.

7. Integration and synthesis of systems approaches are key to a systems thinking environment for tobacco

control, moving toward a more adaptive system that changes public health outcomes. Approaches such as systems organizing, system dynamics modeling, network methods, and knowledge management contain synergies in areas ranging from participatory stakeholder networks to simulation and knowledge environments. Achievement of this goal involves creating a vision, developing capacity, building planning models, and establishing meaningful and adaptive evaluation measurements.

8. Capacity building for systems thinking touches on the resources needed for bringing a systems thinking environment to fruition in tobacco control. These include fundamental infrastructure issues such as creating networks and linking them with systems knowledge in other fields, as well as specific action items such as creating systems curricula for academia and national professional associations, and holding conferences for systems thinking in public health.

Chapter Conclusions

Chapter 2. Tobacco Control at a Crossroads

1. The prevalence of smoking among adults has been reduced by approximately one-half since 1950. However, tobacco use remains the nation's leading cause of premature preventable death. The success of efforts to reduce the prevalence of adult smoking to the Healthy People 2010 goals of 15% or less remains elusive.

2. Increasingly, tobacco use is seen as a population-level health problem that involves forces from the tobacco industry, current tobacco users and nonusers, and the environment.

3. Tobacco control efforts have evolved from a focus on individual interventions

toward population-level interventions, as the nature of tobacco use has become better understood. These efforts have evolved into a complex system involving multiple stakeholders and environmental factors, ranging from social attitudes toward smoking to the countervailing efforts of the tobacco industry.

4. Some research findings suggest that systems approaches are critical to further substantive gains in tobacco control. The success of early tobacco control efforts at the population level gives impetus to further exploration of this hypothesis.

Chapter 3. Systems Thinking: Potential to Transform Tobacco Control

1. The key challenges in tobacco control and public health today are fundamentally systems problems, involving multiple forces and stakeholders. Systems thinking is an innovative approach to address these challenges and improve health outcomes.

2. Numerous frameworks exist for systems thinking, a concept that encompasses a broad synthesis of systems approaches. These approaches provide a theoretical basis for applying specific systems methods, such as system dynamics modeling, structured conceptualization, and network analysis.

3. The Initiative on the Study and Implementation of Systems encompasses four key areas of systems thinking, and their integration: how people organize (managing and organizing as a system); how people understand dynamic complexity (system dynamics modeling); who people are (network analysis); and what people know (knowledge management and knowledge transfer).

4. Examination of systems approaches has the potential to address key questions and problems faced by the various stakeholder groups involved in tobacco control.

5. Potential benefits of systems thinking in tobacco control include improving collaboration among stakeholders; harnessing resources toward evidence-based practice; eliminating duplication of effort; and gaining deeper knowledge about the impact of tobacco control activities.

Chapter 4. How to Organize: Systems Organizing

1. Systems organizing implies a move away from the classical linear management processes of planning, organizing, leading, and controlling toward a more adaptive, participatory environment expressed here around the concepts of vision, structure, action, and learning:

- Vision encompasses a move from an environment of leading and managing to one of facilitating and empowering.

- Structure encompasses a move from organizing to self-organizing.

- Action encompasses a move from delegation to participation.

- Learning encompasses a move from discrete evaluation to continuous evaluation.

2. Two concept-mapping projects explored key areas of organizing as a system. One project, examining issues in accelerating the adoption of cancer control research into practice, yielded clusters of action items in areas of research, practice, policy, and partnerships. The other project examined components of strong local and state tobacco control programs and provided the framework for a logic model of process and outcome ranging from near-term to long-term objectives.

Chapter 5. How to Anticipate Change in Tobacco Control Systems

1. Tobacco control consists of dynamic relationships over time and requires

approaches, such as system dynamics modeling, that can address such dynamics.

2. Understanding of tobacco control and public health issues has evolved from simple cause-and-effect studies and logic models to more complex, ecological problems that involve feedback and evolving behavior.

3. System dynamics uses mathematical simulation approaches based on stocks, flows, and feedback loops, which can model system structures and simulate future system behavior, including possible unintended consequences and long-term effects.

4. Demonstration projects, such as the system dynamics simulation of tobacco prevalence and consumption developed for the Initiative on the Study and Implementation of Systems, show the potential to model and simulate future tobacco issues to design more effective interventions.

5. Opportunities are likely to surface for integrating system dynamics modeling and other systems thinking approaches at epistemological and methodological levels. Systems approaches can and should integrate within a larger systems thinking environment encompassing components such as systems organizing, networks, and knowledge management.

Chapter 6. Understanding and Managing Stakeholder Networks

1. Solving complex future issues in tobacco control will require replacing silos of information and activity with greater linkage of tobacco stakeholders through networks.

2. Networks of tobacco control stakeholders form a foundation of the systems environment envisioned for the future of tobacco control. Many components of a systems approach are built around the presumption of stakeholder networks

that span multiple levels of tobacco control activity and transcend geography and discipline. These components include building organizational capacity; participatory approaches to planning, implementation, and evaluation; optimization of resources and effort; and dissemination of knowledge and best practices.

3. Network analysis holds the potential for facilitating understanding and strategic management of linkages between stakeholder groups.

4. Numerous theories of network behavior currently coexist, and core concepts that describe networks now have broad acceptance, particularly those related to network attributes and behavior.

5. Network applications in public health are at an early stage. However, they have shown promise in recent studies, particularly in areas where disparate organizations have a common goal. Recent tobacco control applications of networks include the North American Quitline Consortium and Global Tobacco Research Network.

6. Network attributes potentially serve as a measure of the health of tobacco control efforts, as evidenced by a case study correlating network centrality with the strength of political and financial support for tobacco control.

7. In the future, tobacco control programs could consist of multiple networks with specific functional objectives, linked in turn as part of a "network of stakeholders."

Chapter 7. What We Know: Managing the Knowledge Content

1. Effective knowledge management is based on a social context revolving around knowledge production, use, and refinement, as well as an ecological context based on audience, motivations, and mechanisms.

2. A formal strategy for knowledge management is essential to the creation of a consistent knowledge environment. One framework defines knowledge capabilities in terms of purpose, people, process, and products, together with a knowledge management and translation infrastructure defined in terms of its underlying organization, technology, information, and finance infrastructures.

3. A review of resources for tobacco control knowledge at the National Cancer Institute confirmed the existence of extensive resources for tobacco control, combined with growth areas for the future, such as integration, visibility among stakeholders, and knowledge gaps.

4. A concept-mapping project that engaged stakeholders to examine specific information needed for tobacco prevention, control, or research yielded clusters of knowledge categories that helped form the taxonomy for a planned knowledge base for tobacco control.

References

1. U.S. Department of Health and Human Services. 2000. *Reducing tobacco use: A report of the Surgeon General*. Atlanta: U.S. Department of Health and Human Services, Centers for Disease Control and Prevention, National Center for Chronic Disease Prevention and Health Promotion, Office on Smoking and Health.

2. Centers for Disease Control and Prevention. 2002. Annual smoking-attributable mortality, years of potential life lost, and economic costs: United States, 1995–1999. *Morbidity and Mortality Weekly Report* 51 (14): 300–303.

3. U.S. Department of Health and Human Services. 2004. *The health consequences of smoking: A report of the Surgeon General*. Atlanta: U.S. Department of Health and Human Services, Centers for Disease Control and Prevention, National Center for Chronic Disease Prevention and Health Promotion, Office on Smoking and Health.

4. Centers for Disease Control and Prevention. 2004. Cigarette smoking among adults—United States, 2002. *Morbidity and Mortality Weekly Report* 53 (20): 427–31.

5. Best, A., R. Tenkasi, W. Trochim, F. Lau, B. Holmes, T. Huerta, G. Moor, S. Leischow, and P. Clark. 2006. Systemic transformational change in tobacco control: An overview of the Initiative for the Study and Implementation of Systems (ISIS). In *Innovations in health care: A reality check,* ed. A. L. Casebeer, A. Harrison, and A. L. Mark, 189–205. New York: Palgrave Macmillan.

Tobacco Control at a Crossroads

This chapter outlines key issues defining the state of tobacco control at the beginning of the twenty-first century and introduces the systems approaches under study in the Initiative on the Study and Implementation of Systems (ISIS) to improve public health outcomes related to tobacco use. The problem of tobacco use is discussed within a framework of the interaction of product, person, the tobacco industry, and the environment in which all exist. The chapter also discusses population-level efforts as early systems models for tobacco control, as well as some of the issues that frame the use of systems methods. The chapter concludes that the interaction of complex factors points to the need for a strategic systems approach to support future reductions in the prevalence of tobacco use.

For thy sake, tobacco, I would do anything but die.

—Charles Lamb (1775–1834)

Introduction

The need for systems approaches in tobacco control is largely framed by trends in the evolution of tobacco control and public health over the last few decades. These trends, and their role as a backdrop to the systems approaches addressed by ISIS, are examined here. Subsequent chapters present the argument for these systems approaches and explore them in more detail in a public health context. This chapter discusses (1) how the scientific view of tobacco use evolved from a model focused on individual behavior to a broader model that considers the full complexity of the problem and (2) how that evolution leads to a global systems orientation toward eradication of tobacco use.

Tobacco use is the most important preventable cause of disability and death in the United States[1] and is a risk factor for four of the five leading causes of death (heart disease, cancer, chronic obstructive lung disease, and stroke).[2] Analysis of the number of tobacco-related deaths from all causes during the 1997–2001 period shows that cigarette smoking was responsible for approximately 438,000 deaths each year in the United States.[3] Cigarettes and other tobacco products are highly engineered to create and maintain dependence. Many of the compounds in cigarette smoke are toxic, mutagenic, or carcinogenic.[2] Use of these products has long-term public health and economic consequences. Successful prevention of tobacco use and its associated morbidity and mortality is a national priority; it can also illustrate best practices and approaches to addressing other major public health problems.

Tobacco control research and practice have led to significant public health accomplishments in the past half-century. The prevalence of smoking among U.S. men decreased from nearly 60% in the 1950s to 24% in 2005.[4] During the same period, smoking prevalence among U.S. women decreased from approximately 30% to 18%.[4] Because tobacco use is the most important modifiable risk factor for chronic disease and early mortality, this represents a major victory for public health.

However, tobacco control is now at a critical juncture. Previous successes may be in jeopardy because of systematic barriers to tobacco control efforts. An ever-vigilant and highly profitable tobacco industry has become more sophisticated in its approach to marketing tobacco products and developing new marketing schemes and products that outstrip the responsiveness of tobacco control research and practice. Moreover, in some cases, research funds are being shifted to other health priorities, such as obesity.[5]

Healthy People 2010 provides the United States with a comprehensive, nationwide health promotion and disease prevention agenda. Among the many objectives to be achieved by 2010 are to reduce the adult smoking prevalence to 12% and to reduce high school student smoking prevalence to 16%.[6] However, it does not appear that the nation will meet these goals. More than 45 million U.S. adults are current cigarette smokers,[4] and each day, approximately 4,000 young people between the ages of 12 and 17 years initiate cigarette smoking.[7] Worldwide prevalence of smoking is increasing and, if current trends continue, tobacco use will become the leading global cause of death within 30 years.[8]

Tobacco manufacturers spent more than $15 billion in 2003 to advertise and promote tobacco products.[9] However, combined public and private resources for tobacco control amount to only a small fraction of this figure, and tobacco control initiatives are often fragmented. Additionally, because funds from tobacco taxes and other related sources often help sustain vital governmental infrastructure, the incentives to reduce or eliminate tobacco use and tobacco-related harm may not be as strong as they should be, despite tobacco's enormous negative impact on society.[10] The slow progress in tobacco control is likely due to many complex and overlapping factors that must be better understood if more effective action is to be taken.

Societal and environmental factors have continuously changed both tobacco use and the tobacco control environment. The resource-rich tobacco industry has paid close attention to the myriad intersecting threats to its business, with the aim of maintaining or increasing sales and undermining industry critics. The continued existence of the industry depends heavily on its ability to counter antitobacco efforts. The companies continue to invest billions of dollars in advertising and promotion, including payments to retailers.[11] They have advocated for state laws that preempt the ability of local communities to enact evidence-based tobacco control measures.[12,13] Tobacco use permeates the popular media, competing with the growing efforts of antitobacco advocates to decrease the acceptability of tobacco use.[14–16]

The battle against tobacco use has resulted in substantial victories. Today, more than one-half of all adults who have ever smoked have quit.[17] However, to increase the proportion of former smokers, more efficacious behavioral and pharmacological therapies must be developed and community and policy interventions need to be improved. In both clinical and community environments, translating research efficacy into real-world effectiveness is essential. For example, the efficacy of nicotine replacement therapy has been shown in numerous studies; however, these medications are often not used in the real world as they were in clinical trials.[18–20] As a result, changing nicotine replacement therapies from prescription to over-the-counter status does not seem to have had the predicted population effect.[21] Research is needed to better understand and address this issue.

To more effectively counter the tobacco industry's efforts, the tobacco control community must become better organized. Tobacco control resources must be used more judiciously and include approaches that have the greatest strategic effect in a system that optimizes the outcomes of all efforts. This goal of being more effective in practice is inexorably linked to construction of a more integrated system of scientific discovery, development, and delivery.

Need for a New Approach

Most twentieth century research has been driven by reductionism, the process of attempting to understand a problem by first deciphering its components.[22] The result has been an attempt to grasp the whole of tobacco use and tobacco control by understanding the parts, including the biological basis of nicotine addiction, the structure and function of cigarettes, the advertising and marketing of tobacco products, the economics of tobacco use, and the effectiveness of different tobacco control programs. Much has been learned about these dissociated aspects of tobacco use and tobacco control. However, few strides have been made in understanding the whole or in reducing tobacco use through systemwide change. Barabási puts it well: "Riding reductionism, we run into the hard wall of complexity."[22(p6)] A new paradigm must be adopted to address the complexities and ultimately improve the health of the public. Because of the complex problems involved, systems thinking is needed in tobacco control efforts.

Tobacco Use as a Complex System

To illustrate that population-level tobacco use and control involve a complex system, it is helpful to think in terms of the

Key Terms and Definitions

System: A set of elements interrelated among themselves and within the environment

Systems approaches: Theories that use systems methods in an organized framework to address systems (e.g., chaos theory or complexity theory)

Systems methods: Specialized techniques or procedures for researching and understanding systems (e.g., system dynamics modeling, structured conceptualization, or network analysis)

Systems thinking: Use of systems approaches to view the world

system of tobacco products: the industry that produces, distributes, and promotes the use of its products, and the people or populations who start, maintain, and stop using tobacco, or are harmed by exposure to secondhand smoke. In addition, the system includes the environment that helps to promote or prevent tobacco use and forces related to public policy, family and community norms, culture, and history.

Product

Tobacco products are diverse and include conventional cigarettes, pipes, cigars, smokeless tobacco, bidis, kreteks, and others.

Some of the complexity of the product is illustrated by conventional cigarettes. A commercial cigarette is not simply a column of tobacco wrapped in paper to which a filter is attached. The modern commercial cigarette is a highly engineered nicotine-delivery device. It is specifically designed for the rapid delivery of nicotine to the brain, allowing nicotine to enter a smoker's bloodstream via gas or particle deposition in the respiratory tract and mucous membranes. This rapidity of nicotine delivery results in immediate reinforcement

of smoking behavior and enables the smoker to exert exquisite control over his or her nicotine intake, from one puff to the next.[23] Smokers may self-dose with nicotine several hundred times a day. For example, a one-pack-per-day smoker likely inhales smoke 70,000–100,000 times per year.[23] Experienced smokers are expert at dose titration, with much of the process occurring with little conscious control.

Commercial cigarettes are engineered to allow significant flexibility in the delivery of nicotine and other components of smoke that reinforce smoking behavior. As smokers became more aware of the health consequences of smoking, tobacco manufacturers responded with changes to the cigarette's design that purported to reduce the delivery of toxins to the user. With the advent of filters, including ventilated filters, and porous cigarette papers, the average machine-measured, sales-adjusted yields of tar fell from 21.6 mg in 1968 to 12.0 mg in 1998,[24] while those for nicotine fell from 1.35 mg to 0.88 mg per cigarette.

These dramatic reductions might have been expected to yield significant public health benefits, but there is no convincing evidence that they have resulted in important health benefits to either smokers or the whole population.[25] The high degree of elasticity of delivery afforded by modern cigarettes has allowed smokers to compensate for the decreased machine-smoked yields of nicotine. Smokers use multiple compensatory mechanisms for increasing nicotine delivery, including increasing the number and volume of puffs and blocking filter ventilation holes.[26–31] Data indicate that cigarettes with low or medium quantities of nicotine are smoked much more intensely than is indicated by the test data from machine smoking analyses.

Moreover, use of the Federal Trade Commission method of measuring yields from machine-generated smoke leads to overestimations of the degree of exposure reduction afforded by low-yield cigarettes.[27,32] Most studies that compare smoking behavior in people who smoke cigarettes with different yields of nicotine reveal at least partial compensation for lower levels of nicotine by smoking behavior. This finding suggests that cigarettes with lower yields are smoked more intensely than are those with higher yields.[23]

Additionally, cigarettes may be manufactured to increase the potential for addiction by making more of the nicotine in smoke available for rapid transfer to the brain. The "free-base" (unprotonated) form of nicotine is volatile and is more rapidly and efficiently absorbed through the lungs and mucous membranes than is the "non-free-base"(monoprotonated) form of nicotine.[33–35] It has been postulated that rapid absorption increases the speed of nicotine delivery to the brain, increasing the potential for addiction.[36,37] The free-base form of nicotine has been likened to the free-base form of cocaine ("crack" cocaine)—both are rapidly absorbed, resulting in an explosive effect on the nervous system.[38]

The sensory and hedonistic qualities of cigarettes, including immediate perceptions of impact and satisfaction,[39,40] contribute to their high liability for abuse. The addictive consequences of swift delivery of nicotine to the brain became apparent when the subjective responses of smokers were examined. For example, a 1974 Liggett report demonstrates that a cigarette with a high proportion of free-base nicotine has "…more free nicotine in its smoke, and consequently, a higher nicotine impact."[39(Bates no. 2073832754)] Similarly, a 1976 R.J. Reynolds document describes free-base nicotine as "more rapidly absorbed by the body and more quickly gives a 'kick' to the smoker."[41(Bates no. 502420399)] Another document notes that nicotine in its free-base form is more readily absorbed through the body tissue.[42] Hence it is the free nicotine that is associated with impact; that

is, the higher the level of free nicotine, the higher the impact.[43]

It is apparent that the reinforcing and rewarding effects of cigarettes are such that the smoker is likely to become addicted and have great difficulty in stopping smoking. Personal characteristics also can make a person particularly susceptible to starting to smoke and having difficulty in stopping smoking.

Person

Nearly all people in the United States are exposed to advertising and promotion of tobacco products and to others smoking around them. However, not everyone initiates cigarette smoking or uses other tobacco products. Some people can stop smoking easily, while others may experience great difficulty.

Early research focused on the biobehavioral aspects of smoking initiation and cessation. For example, a person's level of educational attainment is an important predictor of smoking status. In 2004, smoking levels were higher among adults with a general equivalency diploma (43.2%) or 9–11 years of education (32.6%) than among adults with an undergraduate degree (women: 9.6%; men: 11.9%) or a graduate degree (women: 7.4%; men: 6.9%).[4] Additionally, cigarette smoking is more common among adults with incomes below the poverty level (29.9%) than among those with incomes at or above the poverty level (20.6%).[4]

The prevalence of smoking among adults has declined considerably in recent decades. However, cigarette smoking among adolescents rose in the late 1980s through the mid-1990s, before decreasing.[44] Among children and adolescents, associations have been reported between starting to smoke and factors related to the spheres of family, peers, personality, and environment. For example, higher smoking prevalence has been reported among adolescents who show symptoms of depression, have poor academic performance, or are prone to rebelliousness.[45] Smoking among family members and friends, and exposure to tobacco advertising and promotion, are associated with higher levels of childhood cigarette smoking.[45-49] Parental support and negative parental attitudes toward youth smoking are protective factors.[50-52] Traits such as impulsivity are associated with both starting to smoke and relapsing after attempting to stop smoking, suggesting that nicotine may be disproportionately rewarding for some people.[53]

The proportion of young adults (18–24 years old) who started to smoke cigarettes and who transitioned to regular smoking increased during the late 1990s.[54-57] In 2005, the prevalence of smoking among young adults was 24.4%, statistically equal to the rate of adults aged 25–44 years (24.1%),[4] the age group that traditionally had the highest prevalence. It is unlikely that the increase in smoking among college-age young adults is solely the result of adolescents aging into the group. Rather, specific targeting by advertising and promotion of tobacco companies has probably contributed to the increase.[55]

Emerging evidence suggests a genetic basis for some aspects of smoking behaviors in some individuals, which may explain part of the variation in smoking patterns among individuals. Behaviors in which genetics have been implicated include initiation of cigarette smoking, onset of addiction, and success in stopping smoking. Heritability has been implicated in starting to smoke, for men more than women, and for persistence in smoking.[58] Monozygotic twins have been shown to have a greater concordance for failure to stop smoking than have dizygotic twins.[59] One study of twins reported that genetic factors may account for 50% of the variance in risk for starting to smoke and 70% of the variance for continuing to smoke.[60] A review[61] of published studies

relates *DRD2 Taq1A, CYP2A6, DAT VNTR,* and *5HTT LPR* genetic polymorphisms (different forms of genes) to smoking patterns. The data were insufficient for performance of a meta-analysis. However, the authors conclude that the contribution of specific known genes to smoking behavior is probably modest.

Cigarette manufacturers place their product in the person's environment and promote its use. Particular activities of the tobacco industry are especially potent in countering public health efforts to eradicate tobacco use. These counterefforts underscore the need for a systems approach to tobacco control.

Tobacco Industry

Prior to the invention and patenting of the cigarette rolling machine in 1880, cigarettes were not the most popular tobacco product. The "cigarette market was small…. Cigarettes were expensive and hand rolled by the cigarette girls. Most manufacturers didn't see a use for that many cigarettes."[62] The advent of the cigarette rolling machine, which could produce 120,000 cigarettes in 10 hours, "led not only to the widespread use of cigarettes as America's favored form of tobacco, but to the modern era of mass-market advertising and promotion."[62] The success of mass marketing was also enhanced by the availability of bright (Virginia or flue-cured) tobacco, which produced smoke that was more easily inhaled than that of other tobaccos in previous use. In 2003, despite a ban on advertising on radio, television, and billboards,[63] the U.S. cigarette manufacturers together spent more than $15 billion—more than $41 million each day—to advertise and promote cigarettes.[9]

Tobacco companies maintain a sophisticated distribution system that results in the widespread availability of cigarettes. It is virtually impossible for consumers to avoid protobacco messages while going about their day-to-day activities. While communities often limit the number of outlets for the sale of alcohol by restricting the number of retail licenses or the density of stores, tobacco outlets are not similarly restricted. Most retail stores that sell necessities such as milk and bread also sell cigarettes. More than 80% of all cigarette advertising and promotional dollars are spent in ways that affect the retail environment. Ninety-seven percent of retail tobacco outlets contain at least one advertisement or promotional item, aside from the tobacco product itself. The average number of such items per store rose from 13 in 2001 to 17 in 2002 (P. I. Clark, pers. comm., October 21, 2005). No other consumer product is as heavily promoted in retail stores,[11,64] and the Master Settlement Agreement did not include provisions for restricting retail advertising.

In the earliest years of cigarette manufacturing, the tobacco companies had only to manufacture and distribute their products and convince people to buy and use them. However, by the early 1950s, reports about the association between smoking and adverse health outcomes began to appear in the scientific literature.[65,66] On January 11, 1964, Surgeon General of the Public Health Service Luther Terry released the report of the Surgeon General's Advisory Committee on Smoking and Health. The first Surgeon General's report, based on more than 7,000 articles from the biomedical literature, concluded that cigarette smoking causes lung cancer and stated that "cigarette smoking is a health hazard of sufficient importance in the U.S. to warrant appropriate remedial action."[67(p33)] The report was released to the public on a Saturday to avoid a strong reaction from Wall Street.[68]

Within weeks of the public release of the first Surgeon General's report, the tobacco companies fought back. George Weissman, then president of Philip Morris, reacted to the report by sending a confidential memorandum to Joseph Cullman III, then

Philip Morris's chair and chief executive officer, which referred to the report as a "propaganda blast" and provided ideas about how the tobacco industry could counteract it. In this memorandum, Mr. Weissman noted that he had originally supported a mild federal labeling act to thwart the efforts of the individual states, saying, "If possible, the state legislatures could be held off on the basis that this is a federal matter and the federal can be the subject of many hearings." He suggested working clandestinely to ridicule the findings of the Surgeon General's report, saying, "While it should not be done in the industry's name, someone ought to be contacting all the cartoonists, television gag writers, satirical reviews, etc...." He continued, "...However, at some point, reflecting the same seriousness with which we met the report, we must in the near future provide some answers which will give smokers a psychological crutch and a self-rationale to continue smoking...."[69(Bates no. 1005038559–8561)]

Since that time, the tobacco companies have countered every major public health initiative with varying degrees of success. An extensive body of peer-reviewed literature describes the diverse strategies and tactics the tobacco industry has used to undermine public health.[70–78] The industry has long been concerned that large-scale, comprehensive tobacco control programs would reduce smoking and thus reduce profits.[79] An important example of a program that the industry perceived as a threat was the American Stop Smoking Intervention Study for Cancer Prevention (ASSIST), a 17-state initiative that sought to reduce tobacco use by changing the sociopolitical environment through policy and media advocacy and through the development of state infrastructures to deliver tobacco control.[80–82] Given the scope of ASSIST, it is not surprising that the program caught the attention of the tobacco industry.[73,79] While local, state, and federal governments expended resources to reduce smoking rates and promote tobacco control, the tobacco industry expended significant resources to promote sales of their products, influence governmental bodies, and undermine programs such as ASSIST.[73,79]

The tobacco industry has relied heavily on lobbying and campaign contributions to oppose antitobacco legislative initiatives.[83–86] Some tobacco company efforts have made use of front groups or third-party allies to advance their goals.[87] For example, tobacco companies have used financial analysts from the investment banking industry, as though from an independent source, to promote the tobacco industry's public policy agenda.[74]

Early on, the tobacco industry realized that policies to reduce exposure to secondhand smoke were a serious threat to profits. For example, Philip Morris estimated that smoke-free workplaces would increase smoking cessation rates and reduce cigarette consumption by 11%–15% and that widespread restrictions on smoking in the workplace would severely affect the industry.[72] In response to the threat, the industry paid scientists and academicians to present research countering the evidence against the health hazards of exposure to secondhand smoke.[88–91] The tobacco

industry developed a network of experts on ventilation who represented themselves as independent consultants. However, these consultants promoted strategies of the tobacco industry under close, but generally undisclosed, industry supervision.[72] The ventilation consultants were used to steer public concerns about indoor air quality away from secondhand smoke, arguing that it was an insignificant component of a much larger problem of poor indoor air quality and inadequate ventilation. The consultants carried this message to businesses, particularly the hospitality business, and to regulatory and legislative groups.[72]

Over time, the tobacco companies developed strategies to counter or co-opt public health initiatives and maintain company profits. For many years, the major U.S. cigarette companies were able to coordinate their efforts through the Tobacco Institute, a trade association formed in 1958 to promote the tobacco industry's positions, primarily through public relations and lobbying activities. For many decades, the Tobacco Institute was a major force in the effort to counter antitobacco initiatives.[92] The Tobacco Institute was required to dissolve in 1998, pursuant to litigation brought by the state Attorneys General.

Tobacco and Public Officials: A Complex Relationship

While the tobacco industry is seen by tobacco control professionals as a "vector" for disease, its relationship with the public sector can be considerably more complex. The financial aftermath of the 1998 Master Settlement Agreement (MSA) is a case in point. As a result of a class action lawsuit in Illinois, Philip Morris was required to place billions of dollars in escrow while the case was appealed.[a] The company argued that such a bond could result in bankruptcy, jeopardizing funds the states were to receive under the MSA. In response, 37 state and territorial Attorneys General submitted a friend-of-the-court (amicus curiae) brief, requesting that Philip Morris be allowed to decrease the amount of bond required by the court. The court granted this request. It appears that, on occasion, dependence on MSA funds has provided an incentive for states to take positions that support the continued financial health of the tobacco industry.

[a]Altria Group. 2003. Illinois court reduces $12 billion bond: Philip Morris USA set to begin appeal; To make MSA payment to states. Press release. New York: Altria Group. http://www.altria.com/media/03_06_04_12_04_pricerpr.asp.

Image and the Tobacco Industry: A Systems Response

Market leader Philip Morris has demonstrated the tobacco industry's ability to change in response to pressure. In the early 1990s, Philip Morris faced pressure from the public health community and groups promoting the rights of nonsmokers. The company's own polling data showed that Philip Morris was viewed far less favorably by the public than other companies, including Exxon following the Exxon Valdez oil spill. In response, Philip Morris decided to revamp its corporate image by developing an image-enhancement campaign, "Philip Morris in the 21st Century," which included changing the company name to Altria, to distance itself from the negative image of a tobacco company.

Philip Morris and the other major U.S. tobacco companies have continued to use image-enhancement programs, including those focused on youth smoking prevention, and Web-based quit smoking assistance. Research to date demonstrates that these programs are either ineffective or actually harmful.[a] However, they may serve to help relieve some of the public pressure on the tobacco industry.[b]

The early years of the twenty-first century have been marked by decreased funding for tobacco control programs, including the near eradication of highly successful programs in Massachusetts and Florida. The transformation made by the tobacco companies provides evidence that tobacco control initiatives have been successful and that tobacco control strategies need to be sufficiently nimble to continue to apply pressure on the industry, especially in light of its recent efforts to reposition itself in the public eye. An integrated system of tobacco control will provide the needed agility.

[a]Henriksen, L., A. L. Dauphinee, Y. Wang, and S. P. Fortmann. 2006. Industry sponsored anti-smoking ads and adolescent reactance: Test of a boomerang effect. *Tobacco Control* 15 (1): 13–18.

[b]Hirschhorn, N. 2005. Corporate social responsibility and the tobacco industry: Hope or hype? *Tobacco Control* 13 (4): 447–53.

Sources. Smith, E. A., and R. E. Malone. 2003. Altria means tobacco: Philip Morris's identity crisis. *American Journal of Public Health* 93 (4): 553–56. Warner, K. E., and D. M. Burns. 2003. Hardening and the hard-core smoker: Concepts, evidence, and implications. *Nicotine & Tobacco Research* 5 (1): 37–48.

The tobacco industry continues to influence attitudes and behaviors toward smoking, particularly in areas in which it retains an economic influence. This influence occurs both at the micro level, through retailers, restaurant owners, and others, and at the macro level, where tobacco interests form a significant part of regional economies. At the micro level, tobacco interests often form coalitions with economic partners. For example, the industry may partner with hospitality industry allies to challenge a comprehensive clean indoor air law.[93,94] At the macro level, studies have shown that tobacco-producing states have substantially lower tobacco taxes,[95] fewer laws restricting smoking,[96] and less overall control of tobacco use[97] than do other states.

Economic factors such as these remain a challenge to address.

The product, the person, and the tobacco producer operate in an environment of national-, state-, and community-level factors. The significant influence of the environment on tobacco use is evident from the wide variation in smoking prevalence across the states. In 2005, the median prevalence of cigarette smoking among U.S. adults was 20.9%; however, the prevalence ranged from 11.5% in Utah to 28.7% in Kentucky.[98] Outside the 50 states and the District of Columbia, the median prevalence of cigarette smoking among adults was 13.6%, ranging from 10% in the U.S. Virgin Islands to 34% in Guam.[99]

Environmental factors such as clean indoor air laws and regulations, economic dependence on tobacco (e.g., tobacco-growing regions), and levels of taxation on tobacco products may contribute to this variation.

The interrelationship of environmental factors, combined with the broader relationship of product, person, and producer of tobacco products, provides a focus on understanding and managing behaviors associated with tobacco use as an integrated system. This approach is not entirely new, as is illustrated by the history of the evolution of systems thinking in tobacco control.

Population-Level Tobacco Control Efforts: Beginnings of an Integrated System

Tobacco use was once seen primarily as a problem of individual behavior, to be addressed at the individual level through interventions such as health education and assistance for smoking cessation. Today, experts recognize that population-level factors related to tobacco use function as a system. Moreover, population- and policy-level changes have a measurable influence on health outcomes. Indeed, this premise was reflected in the very first National Cancer Institute (NCI) Smoking and Tobacco Control Monograph, *Strategies to Control Tobacco Use in the United States: A Blueprint for Public Health Action in the 1990's.*[81] That seminal monograph delineated the framework for a "systems approach" by characterizing tobacco control as a complex interplay of priority populations, channels for reaching priority populations, and individual and community interventions.

Beyond the direct impact of these types of population-level interventions, the resulting changes in social attitudes toward smoking also affect overall tobacco use. For example, although clean indoor air laws are primarily aimed at protecting nonsmokers, they also help decrease smoking prevalence and consumption, which in turn, changes the social environment toward smoking.[1–8,100–102] Clean indoor air laws may also have helped to change attitudes toward secondhand smoke, including helping to decrease the social acceptability of smoking in homes and cars. Voluntary bans on smoking in the home are associated with longer and more frequent attempts by adults to stop smoking, lower rates of relapse to smoking in adults,[103,104] and lower rates of smoking among youth and young adults.[105]

Some tobacco control efforts focus on the biopsychosocial determinants of tobacco use. Interventions are targeted to the individual, such as use of medications to quit smoking. At the same time, some tobacco control interventions, such as banning smoking in bars and restaurants or increasing tobacco taxes, target policy and environmental influences on tobacco use. In the complex tobacco control environment, individual and policy approaches interact and influence each other in ways that need to be better understood. At the same time, tobacco companies continue to attempt to undermine individual and policy interventions. For example, major media campaigns encourage smokers who want information on quitting to visit the Philip Morris Web site.[106] Such campaigns may permit Philip Morris, a leading promoter of cigarette smoking, to gain credibility with the public. Philip Morris has also recently expressed support for legislation that would give the U.S. Food and Drug Administration authority to regulate tobacco products, despite having opposed this in the past. These and other efforts by the tobacco industry result in perturbations in the complex tobacco control system and will require new thinking, analysis, and action.

The growing realization that tobacco use is a systems problem has led to an increasing number of population-level tobacco control efforts, which serve as a precursor to the kinds of systems methods under study in ISIS. Three earlier efforts in Europe and the United States illustrate the evolution of thinking in tobacco control: the North Karelia Project, the Community Intervention Trial for Smoking Cessation (COMMIT), and ASSIST.

North Karelia Project

Tobacco use is mediated by social forces. Therefore, concerted efforts to change tobacco-related social and environmental influences may reduce tobacco use. An early intervention program attempted to approach tobacco use as a problem amenable to social change rather than individual change. The North Karelia (Finland) Project began in 1972 in response to unusually high rates of cardiovascular disease in Finland.[100] Three risk factors were identified for targeted community interventions: hypertension, hypercholesterolemia, and cigarette smoking. Health care personnel were trained to give advice on quitting smoking, to give dietary advice, and to conduct blood pressure and cholesterol measurements. A variety of activities were implemented to increase public awareness and to reduce risk factors of cardiovascular disease. These included, for example:

- Organization of cholesterol-lowering competitions between villages

- Working with food manufacturers and supermarkets to facilitate dietary changes, including development of low-fat dairy and meat products and the reduction of salt in a number of food items

- Workplace weight loss and smoking cessation programs, and the introduction of more vegetables in workplace cafeterias

- Broadcasts of nationwide television series in which people would volunteer to make healthy changes in their lifestyles with expert help

- A project that encouraged people to grow berries

Many factors contributed to the observed drop in smoking prevalence among men, including "buy in" from the media that resulted in extensive media coverage, educating health care providers to give advice on smoking cessation, group sessions for help with smoking cessation, using lay leaders to educate the public, prohibiting smoking in most indoor public places, eliminating tobacco advertising, and dedicating a portion of tobacco taxes for tobacco control programs. As a result of the program, smoking among men dropped by one-third. Although smoking increased among women, the prevalence was low. Fewer than one in six women smoked cigarettes.[101] The success of the project may be attributed to several factors, including

- Institution of a massive knowledge management process that integrated systems ranging from health care records to researchers

- Comprehensive efforts aimed at schools, workplaces, homes, and communities using a variety of channels and interventions

- Use of network-centric approaches to link networks within the province

The project was extremely influential and paved the way for several other community-based systems efforts. In the 1980s, three studies of community health education were conducted in the United States: the Stanford Five-City Project, the Minnesota Heart Health Program, and the Pawtucket Heart Health Program.[102,107] The effects of these interventions were modest and failed to reach statistical significance in many cases, perhaps because of positive changes in the environments of the control communities.[102,107]

COMMIT

In 1982, NCI's Division of Cancer Prevention and Control launched the Smoking, Tobacco, and Cancer Program. Recognizing that the link between tobacco use and cancer death had been persuasively demonstrated, this research effort was aimed at identifying, developing, and evaluating effective means of reducing tobacco use. Intervention trials were conducted to examine school-based prevention programs, self-help and minimal intervention strategies, advice delivered by physicians and dentists, mass-media approaches, and community-based programs. Interventions focused on youth, racial and ethnic minorities, women, users of smokeless tobacco, and heavy smokers. These interventions were later delivered through NCI's COMMIT, a randomized community trial to determine whether a community-level, multichannel effort could increase rates of smoking cessation.[108,109]

The intervention phase of COMMIT was conducted from 1988 to 1992. Trial activities were implemented through five major channels: community mobilization—an overarching effort to organize the community around tobacco control; health care providers; worksites and organizations; program services; and public education.[110] One community in each of 11 matched community pairs was randomly assigned to the intervention, and the other community in the pair served as a comparison community. Following the intervention, 10,019 heavy smokers and 10,328 light-to-moderate smokers were surveyed by telephone. There were no differences found between intervention and comparison communities among heavy smokers (more than 25 cigarettes per day). However, at the project's end, 30.6% of light-to-moderate smokers (less than 25 cigarettes

per day) in the intervention communities quit smoking, as compared with only 27.5% in the comparison communities.[110] COMMIT's impact on light-to-moderate smokers, although modest, had a significant public health impact. Additionally, the trial provided valuable lessons about how to mobilize communities to support environmental change. As in previous community trials, COMMIT's limited effectiveness was thought to result, at least in part, from secular trends in comparison communities.[109]

ASSIST

In 1991, NCI launched ASSIST to prevent or reduce cigarette prevalence and consumption, primarily through state policy-based approaches to alter the social environment.[81] The principal focus of ASSIST was to alter the environmental and social influences affecting cigarette smoking through development of skills in media advocacy; promotion of local and state clean indoor air laws; reduction of youth access to tobacco products; limitation of tobacco advertising, especially that targeting children, women, and members of minority groups; increases in tobacco taxes; and increases in demand for smoking cessation services.[111]

The COMMIT strategy, which ASSIST extended across entire states, recognized that powerful social forces affect tobacco use, and that the community must be mobilized to make smoking socially unacceptable. In community mobilization, networks of public and private organizations and special interest groups pool and coordinate resources—personnel, time, money, goods, and services—to support a broad range of tobacco control activities. Through ASSIST, state- and community-based coalitions for tobacco control were formed. These coalitions comprised community organizations capable of coordinating and delivering effective interventions.

NCI joined the American Cancer Society (ACS) and 17 state health departments in planning and managing ASSIST. ACS had long been involved in local smoking prevention and control activities and had a strong network of volunteers to mobilize communities and expand the delivery of tobacco use prevention and control interventions. Health departments—with their commitment to public health, experience in working in a culture of institutional partnerships, access to priority populations of smokers, and guaranteed continuing presence—competed to receive ASSIST contracts.

ASSIST was oriented toward developing, implementing, and evaluating multiple interventions, using a variety of channels to reach multiple populations. ASSIST used a three-dimensional cube (figure 2.1) as a model to define its scope.[111] This cube represents the domains of focus for states participating in ASSIST and provides a graphic reminder that the components (interventions, channels, and priority populations) are interrelated and represent critical constituents in a comprehensive approach to tobacco control.

By developing a matrix approach to the complex tobacco control enterprise, it was possible to create and improve on a framework for state tobacco control efforts. The ASSIST evaluation and modeling led to development of a revised model (figure 2.2) that retains the perspective that multiple variables interplay in a complex way, but includes factors not considered in the ASSIST cube (e.g., tobacco industry efforts to impede tobacco control). The evaluation effort was developed to enable both (1) a comparison of tobacco control in ASSIST and non-ASSIST states and (2) a modeling

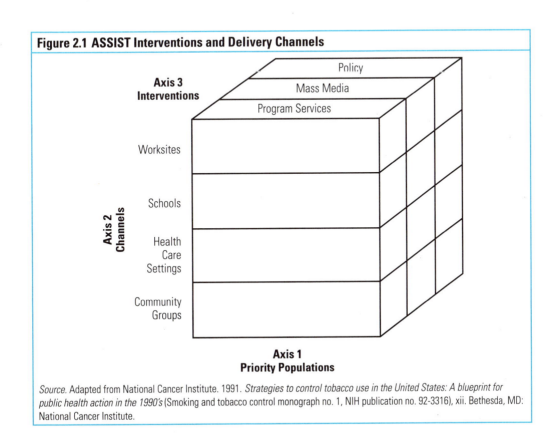

Figure 2.1 ASSIST Interventions and Delivery Channels

Axis 3
Interventions

Policy
Mass Media
Program Services

Worksites

Axis 2
Channels

Schools

Health Care Settings

Community Groups

Axis 1
Priority Populations

Source. Adapted from National Cancer Institute. 1991. *Strategies to control tobacco use in the United States: A blueprint for public health action in the 1990's* (Smoking and tobacco control monograph no. 1, NIH publication no. 92-3316), xii. Bethesda, MD: National Cancer Institute.

of the complex relationships among tobacco control program components to begin exploring their relative impacts.

ASSIST and similar intervention programs have been important to tobacco control efforts for several reasons. States that participated in ASSIST experienced a greater decrease in smoking prevalence than states that did not.[112] At a time of devolution from federal to state funding of tobacco control efforts, participating states demonstrated the ability to mobilize tobacco control resources. They also showed that investment in building state tobacco control capacity and in promoting tobacco control policy change was an effective strategy for reducing tobacco use.[112]

Before NCI and ACS instituted ASSIST, few state health departments had tobacco control programs of significance. In 1994, the Centers for Disease Control and

Prevention (CDC) funded the remaining non-ASSIST states (excepting California, which had Proposition 99 funding) and the District of Columbia to implement tobacco control programs through a program titled Initiatives to Mobilize for the Prevention and Control of Tobacco Use. The emphasis of these initiatives was to develop comprehensive state tobacco prevention and control programs involving participation of diverse community groups, coalitions, and community leaders. In 1999, CDC created the National Tobacco Control Program to provide funding to the state and territorial tobacco control programs.

In 1993, the Robert Wood Johnson Foundation founded the SmokeLess States Program, designating the American Medical Association to serve as the National Program Office. The goals of the program were to concentrate efforts in three general areas: (1) increased public awareness of the

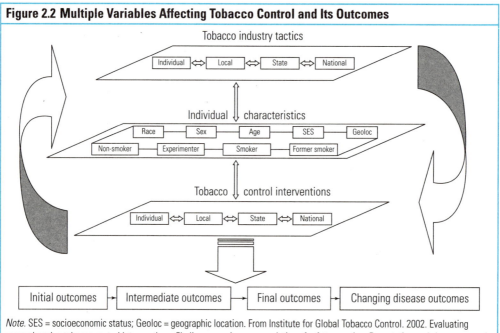

Figure 2.2 Multiple Variables Affecting Tobacco Control and Its Outcomes

Tobacco industry tactics

Individual ⟺ Local ⟺ State ⟺ National

Individual ↕ characteristics

Race — Sex — Age — SES — Geoloc
Non-smoker — Experimenter — Smoker — Former smoker

Tobacco ↕ control interventions

Individual ⟺ Local ⟺ State ⟺ National

Initial outcomes → Intermediate outcomes → Final outcomes → Changing disease outcomes

Note. SES = socioeconomic status; Geoloc = geographic location. From Institute for Global Tobacco Control. 2002. Evaluating comprehensive tobacco control interventions: Challenges and recommendations for future action. Report of a workshop convened by the Institute for Global Tobacco Control, Johns Hopkins Bloomberg School of Public Health. *Tobacco Control* 11 (2): 140–45. Figure 1. Framework for evaluating comprehensive tobacco control programmes, 141. Reproduced with permission from the BMJ Publishing Group.

dangers of tobacco use, (2) public education on effective tobacco control policies (e.g., increasing excise taxes, promoting clean indoor air), and (3) enhancement of local smoking prevention and treatment programs. The program initially funded statewide coalitions in 19 states; two years later, additional funding raised the number of coalitions to 30.[113]

Programs such as those described here highlight a growing focus on population-level tobacco control interventions that seek to create environmental change. They provide evidence that systems approaches make a difference in tobacco control efforts and tobacco use. These approaches represent an important evolutionary step, but alone they are not sufficient. There is a growing realization that relationships evolve among the individual and his or her environment, the tobacco product, and the industry that produces and promotes that product. It is increasingly important to approach tobacco control research and practice from a systems perspective, understanding the complex interactions among these components.

Current Tobacco Control Research and Practice: Systems Problems

The tobacco control problems that remain are systems problems—complex, interdependent issues that lie within the fundamental nature of today's tobacco control environment. Applying what is known about tobacco use as a system and what has been learned from earlier tobacco control efforts helped the ISIS team identify the following problems:

- Numerous disparate communities of interest and duplication of effort

- Ineffective integration of research and practice

- Competition from a well-financed and organized tobacco industry that has well-integrated dissemination and networking efforts

- In some cases, lack of evidence for effectiveness of specific tobacco control efforts on key outcomes such as smoking cessation, morbidity, and mortality

- Diffuse tobacco control efforts reflecting a lack of strategic, multipartner planning and execution

The ISIS team concluded that these substantial and often overlapping challenges must be overcome to bring tobacco control resources and efforts into an integrated system. Identifying problems provides direction for tobacco control efforts.

Moving tobacco control forward will require the recognition that the landscape today is different from that of 10 years ago. The tobacco industry has responded to tobacco control efforts with a new level of sophistication. As in many fields, good science frequently sits in scientific journals and reports, unused by many who could benefit from it. The tobacco control community is likely responsible for "tipping" the national consciousness in favor of reduced acceptance of tobacco use. However, the community has not adequately addressed long-term strategies and is, on occasion, at odds with itself over issues such as harm reduction.

To proceed to the next level and to more effectively translate scientific discoveries into practice, the ISIS team concluded that it is necessary to move beyond familiar approaches and toward systems methods that address fundamental issues of complexity, interdependency, knowledge management, and engagement of organizations as a system. Because the current challenges in tobacco control are related to the complexities and dynamics of the systems in which tobacco control is embedded, the solutions must lie in addressing those systems.

Lessons from ISIS

Unlocking the promise of systems approaches requires a participatory, collaborative environment among the stakeholders. In turn, this requires a fresh approach to management, leadership, and interactions within and among organizations. ISIS explored how organizations can function as systems through facilitation, empowerment, self-organization, participation, and continuous evaluation. The aim of ISIS was to apply methods of systems thinking to practices in tobacco control. Chapters 4 and 7 discuss systems thinking in the framework of a systems approach to organization and management and creation of a "combined toolbox" for the development of outcome-oriented implementation strategies for tobacco control.

ISIS is based on the idea that the growth of systems methods in areas such as epidemiology,[114] organizational behavior,[115] and national defense[116] are applicable to tobacco control. Here, the argument is made for applying integrated methods for strategic systems thinking in response to critical needs in tobacco control and as a proof of concept for applying these approaches to similar challenges in other key areas of public health. Six key facets of the ISIS perspective also are discussed here: (1) using a transdisciplinary approach; (2) transcending or integrating diverse cultures and missions; (3) accelerating transfer from discovery, to development, to delivery; (4) setting evidence-based priorities; (5) creating a federation of systems, also called "networks of stakeholders" in this monograph; and (6) setting long-term goals.

Using a Transdisciplinary Approach

Researchers, practitioners, policy makers, and other stakeholders approach tobacco control from the perspective of their own disciplines, which include law, economics, epidemiology, the behavioral sciences, neurobiology, toxicology, chemistry, addiction medicine, and public health. Members of these disciplines speak different languages, use different research and intervention tools and models, and read and contribute to different literature bases. To most researchers and practitioners, the composite whole of tobacco control and related literature is inaccessible and use of the full scientific basis for practice is unlikely.

Understanding the complex problems of tobacco use and tobacco control requires true transdisciplinary collaboration in both research and practice and between research and practice. However, creating the mind-set and functionality of a transdisciplinary approach is difficult, because it represents a worldview requiring increased teamwork across a wide array of fields and disciplines. This approach may also be more time consuming, at least initially, because it depends on the development and maintenance of relationships and infrastructures among diverse partners.

Disciplines serve a critical function by ensuring depth of knowledge in a particular field, partly through the exchange of information within discipline-specific social networks. They have also allowed relatively rapid gains in knowledge. However, disciplines may also become "stovepiped," in that the knowledge from one discipline gives rise to unique terminology that tends to isolate it from others. The lack of linkage among disciplines has created the effect of "silos dotting the landscape." These silos are effective in holding their contents but inefficient at allowing carryover from one silo to another.

Tobacco Control: A Multitude of Stakeholder Organizations

Organizations that focus on tobacco control vary greatly. For tobacco control efforts to succeed, it may be necessary to develop a strategic and collaborative vision and action. Major government research agencies such as the National Cancer Institute and the National Institute on Drug Abuse have different but overlapping areas of focus. The same holds true for more public health and practice-oriented government agencies, such as the Centers for Disease Control and Prevention and the Substance Abuse and Mental Health Services Administration. Furthermore, within the agencies that address public health research and practice, still more areas of focus overlap. When organizations such as the Robert Wood Johnson Foundation, the American Legacy Foundation, the Campaign for Tobacco-Free Kids, state health departments, and corporate leaders such as the Chief Executive Officer Roundtable on Cancer are also considered, the challenge of and opportunity for optimizing the missions of these many potential partners into a functional network oriented to achieving the greatest public good in the most efficient way are expanded. Fortunately, in diversity there is strength. Diversity allows for breadth of thinking and action. One key challenge is to harness and focus within that diversity to achieve the ultimate goal.

It is encouraging that efforts to link disciplines—to increase transdisciplinary and multidisciplinary thinking and action—are now recognized as valuable. For example, in 1999, NCI, the National Institute on Drug Abuse, and the Robert Wood Johnson Foundation provided funding for the Transdisciplinary Tobacco Use Research Centers. This paradigm shift has now been expanded beyond tobacco control; NCI also has funded several transdisciplinary centers to investigate obesity and energy balance.[117] Additionally, the National Institutes of Health (NIH) has recently created the "Roadmap Initiative," a transdisciplinary and transinstitutional initiative to identify major opportunities and gaps in biomedical research that no single NIH institute could tackle alone.[118] The gradual increase in linkage among disciplines could lead to more rapid knowledge discoveries, which could facilitate delivery of interventions.

Transcending or Integrating Diverse Cultures and Missions

Among the barriers to the creation of an integrated system is the reality that many partners and potential partners have different missions, practices, and cultures. In many cases, priorities overlap or are complementary, but little effort goes into exploring the areas of overlap and complementarity. On the other hand, planned redundancy may have value to ensure that a particular need is fully addressed and that decreased funding to one organization will not jeopardize survival of a critical infrastructure.

Accelerating Transfer from Discovery, to Development, to Delivery

Another major challenge in tobacco control, as in other domains of public health and medical care, is the less than optimal progression from scientific discovery to the development, delivery, and widespread use of interventions. One analysis indicated that 17 years can pass between the time of a discovery and its use in clinical practice.[119] This finding indicates a pipeline that is cumbersome and not oriented toward optimizing the flow and use of new knowledge. In this information age, it is time to optimize the progression from discovery to delivery. For example, in 2003, NCI provided $19 million for research on the treatment of tobacco addiction (C. Backinger, pers. comm.,

> **Moving from Clinical Trials to Real Life**
>
> The problem of effective dissemination and implementation often extends to clinical interventions as well. For example, once the U.S. Food and Drug Administration approved medications to help smokers stop smoking, these drugs were marketed rapidly to health care providers and the public, even though how they would be used in the "real world" was not well understood. The lack of a surveillance system to assess the effectiveness of medications being used to treat tobacco addiction has resulted in some confusion. Many in the scientific and public health communities cite numbers derived not from studies conducted in real-world settings but rather from highly controlled clinical trials. The development of surveillance systems to collect and analyze data on the progression of knowledge as a science-to-practice value chain could ensure that (1) those involved in each stage of discovery, development, and delivery are informed about what has been learned from each stage; and (2) delivery is not an end point but rather a rich environment for discovery through applied science. The process of progression from discovery, to development, to delivery is more interactive than linear.

October 18, 2005). However, insufficient infrastructure exists to ensure that the knowledge gained through this research will be shared systematically with other investigators. Furthermore, not enough effort has been made to develop a network of scientists studying the treatment of tobacco addiction, so that these investigators can rapidly share knowledge of methods and research outcomes.

Despite the existence of Web-based social networks that allow the rapid exchange of information and rapid publication via scientific e-journals, the scientific community has largely held to the practices of the past. In addition, once new knowledge is developed about interventions for clinics and communities, little effort is made to link scientists and community interventionists to determine the most effective strategies for disseminating and implementing the interventions. There are examples of timely, successful transition from discovery to delivery of interventions for tobacco control and development of networked collaboration between scientists and public health practitioners—for example, the proliferation of toll-free telephone quitlines to provide smoking cessation assistance. Unfortunately, these examples demonstrate the potential rather than common experience.

Setting Evidence-Based Priorities

Despite evidence that it is cost effective, disease prevention is not the primary paradigm of the U.S. health care system. The system's orientation toward diagnosis and treatment of disease, which is fundamental to the training of health care providers, continues because a different paradigm has not gained prominence. The United States spends billions of dollars to care for patients with health conditions caused by tobacco use but does not consistently support preventing these conditions. A greater focus on prevention may be viewed as a zero-sum gain, because it may require decreased spending on diagnosis and treatment in the short term, absent new investments. Changing the status quo is not easy, even in the face of mounting evidence that prevention is a good long-term investment.

Creating a Federation of Systems: Can Tobacco Control Learn a Lesson from the Department of Defense?

In the U.S. military, command and control issues are widely discussed and developed. Krygiel[116] defines an environment in which there is no direct command and control (i.e., no top-down hierarchy) as a federation of systems. For example, the U.S. military operated collaboratively within the command and control structure of the North Atlantic Treaty Organization during the Bosnian War; no single controlling organization existed.[116] To function optimally, the military forces had to work together to compromise and develop a coordinated and collaborative mission based on common goals and objectives. This orientation is similar to what exists in tobacco control.

Perhaps the best comparison in tobacco control was the process of developing and implementing the World Health Organization's Framework Convention for Tobacco Control (FCTC). As a result of leadership and collaboration by the World Health Organization, many organizations around the world developed a common goal and worked together to achieve that goal.[120] The FCTC is an important example of what can be accomplished by developing synchronous networks of organizations or a federation of systems that direct their efforts toward a common outcome. This collaborative effort is also an excellent example of using the fruits of scientific discovery to develop effective policies that can benefit humanity.

Setting Long-Term Goals

Little organized consideration of the long-term goals of the tobacco control movement has occurred. Stakeholder goals may vary widely from reducing the prevalence of smoking to the lowest possible level, to dismantling tobacco companies as they now exist.[121] The long-term goals envisioned by the tobacco companies must also be considered. For example, a strategic analysis by Philip Morris considered the complex interacting influences in the business system, changes in knowledge, network-enabled direct marketing, and a shift in the corporate paradigm toward development as a pharmaceutical company.[69]

Unfortunately, the tobacco control community has not implemented efforts to model the many complex components that support and impede tobacco control efforts, so as to develop a more strategic vision of the future. Such an effort would not be simple, in part because different groups may identify and pursue different long-term strategies. However, exploring these strategies and the structures and functions needed to achieve them has the potential to inform the tobacco control community and supportive policy makers about what can and cannot be achieved. Working backward from various long-term goals would make it possible to better understand which structures and functions are needed to achieve them. The scenarios would likely represent new, highly nonlinear models with complex and dynamic components, requiring large quantities of data over time. By exploring both data-driven and theoretical (or simulation) models, the scientific and public health communities also could encourage the development of data sources that can be used to develop data-driven models, which have the potential to predict outcomes of known interventions.

Summary

Moving tobacco control forward requires the recognition that the landscape today is fundamentally different from that of even 10 years ago. Many significant advances have occurred in tobacco control, but the tobacco industry has responded to these successes with a new level of sophistication. ISIS identified several critical needs and priorities for addressing tobacco and other public health threats in the future:

- Using a transdisciplinary approach
- Transcending or integrating diverse cultures and missions

- Accelerating transfer from discovery, to development, to delivery

- Setting evidence-based priorities

- Creating a federation of systems (or networks of stakeholders)

- Setting long-term goals

Thus, the tobacco control community needs to set long-term goals that take into account changing tobacco industry tactics. Progress toward improving the translation of discoveries into practice will require moving beyond familiar approaches and toward systems methods that address fundamental issues of complexity, interdependency, knowledge management, and engagement of organizations as a system. Current challenges are related to the complexities and dynamics of the systems in which tobacco control is embedded. Therefore, the solutions must lie in addressing those systems.

ISIS was a pilot effort to better understand the complexities of addressing tobacco use as a major public health threat. However, it also reflects a continuation of the vision delineated in the very first NCI tobacco control monograph to better understand those complexities. Just as the ideas put forth in the first monograph led to new thinking and action on tobacco control, it is believed that the implementation and integration of systems approaches have the potential to further advance tobacco control and improve the public's health.

Conclusions

1. The prevalence of tobacco use and levels of cigarette consumption among adults have dropped considerably since 1950. However, tobacco use remains the nation's leading cause of premature preventable death. The success of efforts to reduce the prevalence of adult smoking to the *Healthy People 2010* goal of 12% or less remains elusive.

2. Increasingly, tobacco use is seen as a population-level health problem that involves forces from the tobacco industry, current tobacco users and nonusers, and the environment.

3. Tobacco control efforts have evolved from a focus on individual interventions toward population-level interventions, as the nature of tobacco use has become better understood. These efforts have evolved into a complex system involving multiple stakeholders and environmental factors, ranging from social attitudes toward smoking to the countervailing efforts of the tobacco industry.

4. Some research findings suggest that systems approaches are critical to further substantive gains in tobacco control. The success of early tobacco control efforts at the population level gives impetus to further exploration of this hypothesis.

References

1. U.S. Department of Health and Human Services. 2000. *Reducing tobacco use: A report of the Surgeon General*. Atlanta: U.S. Department of Health and Human Services, Centers for Disease Control and Prevention, National Center for Chronic Disease Prevention and Health Promotion, Office on Smoking and Health.

2. U.S. Department of Health and Human Services. 2004. *The health consequences of smoking: A report of the Surgeon General*. Atlanta: U.S. Department of Health and Human Services, Centers for Disease Control and Prevention, National Center for Chronic Disease Prevention and Health Promotion, Office on Smoking and Health.

3. Centers for Disease Control and Prevention. 2005. Annual smoking-attributable mortality, years of potential life lost, and productivity losses—United States, 1997–2001. *Morbidity and Mortality Weekly Report* 54 (25): 625–28.

4. Centers for Disease Control and Prevention. 2006. Tobacco use among adults—United States, 2005. *Morbidity and Mortality Weekly Report* 55 (42): 1145–48.

5. Yach, D., M. McKee, A. D. Lopez, and T. Novotny. 2005. Improving diet and physical activity: 12 lessons from controlling tobacco smoking. *British Medical Journal* 330 (7496): 898–900.

6. U.S. Department of Health and Human Services. 2000. *Healthy People 2010: Understanding and improving health.* 2nd ed. Washington, DC: U.S. Department of Health and Human Services.

7. Substance Abuse and Mental Health Services Administration. 2006. *Results from the 2005 National Survey on Drug Use and Health: National findings* (DHHS publication no. SMA 06-4194). NSDUH Series H-30. Rockville, MD: U.S. Department of Health and Human Services, Substance Abuse and Mental Health Services Administration, Office of Applied Studies. http://www.samhsa.gov or http://www.oas.samhsa.gov.

8. World Health Organization. 2007. Why is tobacco a public health priority? http://www.who.int/tobacco/health_priority/en/index.html.

9. Federal Trade Commission. 2005. Federal Trade Commission cigarette report for 2003. http://www.ftc.gov/reports/cigarette05/050809cigrpt.pdf.

10. Will, G. F. 2006. The states' tobacco addiction. *Washington Post,* January 1.

11. Feighery, E. C., K. M. Ribisl, P. I. Clark, and H. H. Haladjian. 2003. How tobacco companies ensure prime placement of their advertising and products in stores: Interviews with retailers about tobacco company incentive programmes. *Tobacco Control* 12 (2): 184–88.

12. Gorovitz, E., J. Mosher, and M. Pertschuk. 1998. Preemption or prevention? Lessons from efforts to control firearms, alcohol, and tobacco. *Journal of Public Health Policy* 19 (1): 36–50.

13. Siegel, M., J. Carol, J. Jordan, R. Hobart, S. Schoenmarklin, F. DuMelle, and P. Fisher. 1997. Preemption in tobacco control. Review of an emerging public health problem. *JAMA: The Journal of the American Medical Association* 278 (10): 858–63.

14. Glantz, S. A., K. W. Kacirk, and C. McCulloch. 2004. Back to the future: Smoking in movies in 2002 compared with 1950 levels. *American Journal of Public Health* 94 (2): 261–63.

15. Sargent, J. D., M. L. Beach, M. A. Dalton, L. T. Ernstoff, J. J. Gibson, J. J. Tickle, and T. F. Heatherton. 2004. Effect of parental R-rated movie restriction on adolescent smoking initiation: A prospective study. *Pediatrics* 114 (1): 149–56.

16. Glantz, S. A. 2004. Effect of viewing smoking in movies on adolescent smoking initiation: A cohort study. *Journal of Pediatrics* 144 (1): 137–38.

17. Centers for Disease Control and Prevention. 2004. *Percentage of adult ever smokers who are former smokers (prevalence of cessation), overall and by sex, race, Hispanic origin, age, and education. National Health Interview Surveys, selected years—United States, 1965–2000.* Atlanta: U.S. Department of Health and Human Services, Centers for Disease Control and Prevention, National Center for Chronic Disease Prevention and Health Promotion, Office on Smoking and Health, Tobacco Information and Prevention Source. http://www.cdc.gov/tobacco/research_data/adults_prev/adstat4.htm.

18. Pierce, J. P., and E. A. Gilpin. 2002. Impact of over-the-counter sales on effectiveness of pharmaceutical aids for smoking cessation. *JAMA: The Journal of the American Medical Association* 288 (10): 1260–64.

19. Leischow, S. J., J. Ranger-Moore, M. L. Muramoto, and E. Matthews. 2004. Effectiveness of the nicotine inhaler for smoking cessation in an OTC setting. *American Journal of Health Behavior* 28 (4): 291–301.

20. Leischow, S. J., M. L. Muramoto, G. N. Cook, E. P. Merikle, S. M. Castellini, and P. S. Otte. 1999. OTC nicotine patch: Effectiveness alone and with brief physician intervention. *American Journal of Health Behavior* 23 (1): 61–69.

21. Lawrence, W. F., S. S. Smith, T. B. Baker, and M. C. Fiore. 1998. Does over-the-counter nicotine replacement therapy improve smokers' life expectancy? *Tobacco Control* 7 (4): 364–68.

22. Barabási, A.-L. 2002. *Linked: The new science of networks.* New York: Perseus Books.

23. Clark, P. I., and M. V. Djordjevic. 2003. *The role of smoking topography in assessing human smoking and its utility*

for informing machine-smoking protocols. Report to the World Health Organization. Geneva: World Health Organization.

24. Federal Trade Commission. 2003. Federal Trade Commission cigarette report for 2001. http://www.ftc.gov/os/2003/06/2001cigreport.pdf.

25. Thun, M. J., and D. M. Burns. 2001. Health impact of "reduced yield" cigarettes: A critical assessment of the epidemiological evidence. *Tobacco Control* 10 Suppl. 1: i4–i11.

26. Bridges, R. B., J. G. Combs, J. W. Humble, J. A. Turbek, S. R. Rehm, and N. J. Haley. 1990. Puffing topography as a determinant of smoke exposure. *Pharmacology, Biochemistry, and Behavior* 37 (1): 29–39.

27. Djordjevic, M. V., J. Fan, S. Ferguson, and D. Hoffmann. 1995. Self-regulation of smoking intensity: Smoke yields of the low-nicotine, low-"tar" cigarettes. *Carcinogenesis* 16 (9): 2015–21.

28. Kozlowski, L. T., W. S. Rickert, M. A. Pope, J. C. Robinson, and R. C. Frecker. 1982. Estimating the yield to smokers of tar, nicotine, and carbon monoxide from the "lowest yield" ventilated filter-cigarettes. *British Journal of Addiction* 77 (2): 159–65.

29. Kozlowski, L. T. 1981. Tar and nicotine delivery of cigarettes: What a difference a puff makes. *JAMA: The Journal of the American Medical Association* 245 (2): 158–59.

30. Kozlowski, L. T., R. C. Frecker, V. Khouw, and M. A. Pope. 1980. The misuse of "less-hazardous" cigarettes and its detection: Hole-blocking of ventilated filters. *American Journal of Public Health* 70 (11): 1202–3.

31. Djordjevic, M. V., R. Moser, A. A. Melikian, J. Szeliga, S. Chen, J. E. Muscat, J. P. Richie Jr., and S. D. Stellman. 2002. Puffing characteristics and dosages of mainstream smoke components among black and white smokers of regular and mentholated cigarettes. Slides presented at the first Conference on Menthol Cigarettes, Atlanta.

32. Djordjevic, M. V., S. D. Stellman, and E. Zang. 2000. Doses of nicotine and lung carcinogens delivered to cigarette smokers. *Journal of the National Cancer Institute* 92 (2): 106–11.

33. Pankow, J. F. 2001. A consideration of the role of gas/particle partitioning in the deposition of nicotine and other tobacco smoke compounds in the respiratory tract.

Chemical Research in Toxicology 14 (11): 1465–81.

34. Armitage, A. K., and D. M. Turner. 1970. Absorption of nicotine in cigarette and cigar smoke through the oral mucosa. *Nature* 226 (252): 1231–32.

35. Bergstrom, M., A. Nordberg, E. Lunell, G. Antoni, and B. Langstrom. 1995. Regional deposition of inhaled 11C-nicotine vapor in the human airway as visualized by positron emission tomography. *Clinical Pharmacology and Therapeutics* 57 (3): 309–17.

36. Pankow, J. F., A. D. Tavakoli, W. Luo, and L. M. Isabelle. 2003. Percent free base nicotine in the tobacco smoke particulate matter of selected commercial and reference cigarettes. *Chemical Research in Toxicology* 16 (8): 1014–18.

37. Watson, C. H., J. S. Trommel, and D. L. Ashley. 2004. Solid-phase microextraction-based approach to determine free-base nicotine in trapped mainstream cigarette smoke total particulate matter. *Journal of Agricultural and Food Chemistry* 52 (24): 7240–45.

38. Henningfield, J. E., and R. M. Keenan. 1993. Nicotine delivery kinetics and abuse liability. *Journal of Consulting and Clinical Psychology* 61 (5): 743–50.

39. Newsome, J. R. Progress during 730000 on Project TE 5001: Development of a cigarette with an inceased smoke pH. 29 Jan 1974. Philip Morris. Bates No. 2073832754/2755. http://legacy.library.ucsf.edu/tid/zfr85c00.

40. Rose, J. E., F. M. Behm, E. C. Westman, and M. Johnson. 2000. Dissociating nicotine and nonnicotine components of cigarette smoking. *Pharmacology, Biochemistry, and Behavior* 67 (1): 71–81.

41. McKenzie, J. L. Product characterization definitions and implications. Letter. 21 Sep 1976. R.J. Reynolds. Bates No. 502420398/0400. http://legacy.library.ucsf.edu/tid/lya19d00.

42. Creighton, D. E., and T. D. Hirji. 1988. The significance of pH in tobacco and tobacco smoke. http://tobaccodocuments.org/product_design/3223.html.

43. State of Minnesota. 1998. Direct examination—Dr. Channing Robertson. http://www.tobacco.org/resources/documents/980205minnesota.html.

44. Centers for Disease Control and Prevention. 2004. Cigarette use among high school

students—United States, 1991–2003. *Morbidity and Mortality Weekly Report* 53 (23): 499–502.

45. Conrad, K. M., B. R. Flay, and D. Hill. 1992. Why children start smoking cigarettes: Predictors of onset. *British Journal of Addiction* 87 (12): 1711–24.

46. Flay, B. R., F. B. Hu, O. Siddiqui, L. E. Day, D. Hedeker, J. Petraitis, J. Richardson, and S. Sussman. 1994. Differential influence of parental smoking and friends' smoking on adolescent initiation and escalation of smoking. *Journal of Health and Social Behavior* 35 (3): 248–65.

47. Flay, B. R., J. Petraitis, and F. B. Hu. 1999. Psychosocial risk and protective factors for adolescent tobacco use. *Nicotine & Tobacco Research* 1 Suppl. 1: S59–S65.

48. Flay, B. R., F. B. Hu, and J. Richardson. 1998. Psychosocial predictors of different stages of cigarette smoking among high school students. *Preventive Medicine* 27 (5 pt. 3): A9–A18.

49. Chassin, L., C. C. Presson, M. Todd, J. S. Rose, and S. J. Sherman. 1998. Maternal socialization of adolescent smoking: The intergenerational transmission of parenting and smoking. *Developmental Psychology* 34 (6): 1189–1201.

50. Jackson, C., and L. Henriksen. 1997. Do as I say: Parent smoking, antismoking socialization, and smoking onset among children. *Addictive Behaviors* 22 (1): 107–14.

51. Jackson, C., D. J. Bee-Gates, and L. Henriksen. 1994. Authoritative parenting, child competencies, and initiation of cigarette smoking. *Health Education Quarterly* 21 (1): 103–16.

52. Jackson, C., L. Henriksen, and V. A. Foshee. 1998. The Authoritative Parenting Index: Predicting health risk behaviors among children and adolescents. *Health Education and Behavior* 25 (3): 319–37.

53. Doran, N., B. Spring, D. McChargue, M. Pergadia, and M. Richmond. 2004. Impulsivity and smoking relapse. *Nicotine & Tobacco Research* 6 (4): 641–47.

54. Jamner, L. D., C. K. Whalen, S. E. Loughlin, R. Mermelstein, J. Audrain-McGovern, S. Krishnan-Sarin, J. K. Worden, and F. M. Leslie. 2003. Tobacco use across the formative years: A road map to developmental vulnerabilities. *Nicotine & Tobacco Research* 5 Suppl. 1: S71–S87.

55. Lantz, P. M. 2003. Smoking on the rise among young adults: Implications for research and policy. *Tobacco Control* 12 Suppl. 1: i60–i70.

56. Rigotti, N. A., J. E. Lee, and H. Wechsler. 2000. US college students' use of tobacco products: Results of a national survey. *JAMA: The Journal of the American Medical Association* 284 (6): 699–705.

57. Wechsler, H., N. A. Rigotti, J. Gledhill-Hoyt, and H. Lee. 1998. Increased levels of cigarette use among college students: A cause for national concern. *JAMA: The Journal of the American Medical Association* 280 (19): 1673–78.

58. Heath, A. C., and N. G. Martin. 1993. Genetic models for the natural history of smoking: Evidence for a genetic influence on smoking persistence. *Addictive Behaviors* 18 (1): 19–34.

59. Carmelli, D., G. E. Swan, D. Robinette, and R. Fabsitz. 1992. Genetic influence on smoking—A study of male twins. *New England Journal of Medicine* 327 (12): 829–33.

60. True, W. R., A. C. Heath, J. F. Scherrer, B. Waterman, J. Goldberg, N. Lin, S. A. Eisen, M. J. Lyons, and M. T. Tsuang. 1997. Genetic and environmental contributions to smoking. *Addiction* 92 (10): 1277–87.

61. Munafo, M. R., T. G. Clark, E. C. Johnstone, M. F. G. Murphy, and R. T. Walton. 2004. The genetic basis for smoking behavior: A systematic review and meta-analysis. *Nicotine & Tobacco Research* 6 (4): 583–98.

62. Borio, G. 2005. The tobacco timeline. http://www.tobacco.org/History/Tobacco_History.html.

63. National Association of Attorneys General. 1998. Master Settlement Agreement and amendments. Washington, DC: National Association of Attorneys General. http://www.naag.org/backpages/naag/tobacco/msa.

64. Feighery, E. C., K. M. Ribisl, N. C. Schleicher, and P. I. Clark. 2004. Retailer participation in cigarette company incentive programs is related to increased levels of cigarette advertising and cheaper cigarette prices in stores. *Preventive Medicine* 38 (6): 876–84.

65. Doll, R., and A. B. Hill. 1950. Smoking and carcinoma of the lung: Preliminary report. *British Medical Journal* 2 (4682): 739–48.

66. Wynder, E. L., and E. A. Graham. 1950. Tobacco smoking as a possible etiologic

factor in bronchiogenic carcinoma: A study of 684 proved cases. *JAMA: The Journal of the American Medical Association* 143 (4): 329–36.

67. U.S. Department of Health, Education, and Welfare. 1964. *Smoking and health: Report of the Advisory Committee to the Surgeon General of the Public Health Service* (PHS publication no. 1103). Washington, DC: U.S. Department of Health, Education, and Welfare, Public Health Service, Center for Disease Control.

68. Parascandola, J. 1997. The Surgeons General and smoking. *Public Health Reports* 112 (5): 440–2.

69. Weissman, G. Surgeon General's report. 29 Jan 1964. Philip Morris. Bates No. 1005038559/8561. http://legacy.library.ucsf.edu/tid/ctv74e00.

70. Bialous, S. A., and S. A. Glantz. 2002. ASHRAE Standard 62: Tobacco industry's influence over national ventilation standards. *Tobacco Control* 11 (4): 315–28.

71. Dearlove, J. V., S. A. Bialous, and S. A. Glantz. 2002. Tobacco industry manipulation of the hospitality industry to maintain smoking in public places. *Tobacco Control* 11 (2): 94–104.

72. Drope, J., S. A. Bialous, and S. A. Glantz. 2004. Tobacco industry efforts to present ventilation as an alternative to smoke-free environments in North America. *Tobacco Control* 13 Suppl. 1: i41–i47.

73. Trochim, W. M., F. A. Stillman, P. I. Clark, and C. L. Schmitt. 2003. Development of a model of the tobacco industry's interference with tobacco control programmes. *Tobacco Control* 12 (2): 140–47.

74. Alamar, B. C., and S. A. Glantz. 2004. The tobacco industry's use of Wall Street analysts in shaping policy. *Tobacco Control* 13 (3): 223–27.

75. Ibrahim, J. K., and S. A. Glantz. 2006. Tobacco industry litigation strategies to oppose tobacco control media campaigns. *Tobacco Control* 15 (1): 50–58.

76. Lopipero, P., and L. A. Bero. 2006. Tobacco interests or the public interest: 20 years of industry strategies to undermine airline smoking restrictions. *Tobacco Control* 15 (4): 323–32.

77. Landman, A. 2000. Push or be punished: Tobacco industry documents reveal aggression against businesses that discourage tobacco use. *Tobacco Control* 9 (3): 339–46.

78. Francis, J. A., A. K. Shea, and J. M. Samet. 2006. Challenging the epidemiologic evidence on passive smoking: Tactics of tobacco industry expert witnesses. *Tobacco Control* 15 Suppl. 4: iv68–iv76.

79. White, J., and L. A. Bero. 2004. Public health under attack: The American Stop Smoking Intervention Study (ASSIST) and the tobacco industry. *American Journal of Public Health* 94 (2): 240–50.

80. Stillman, F., A. Hartman, B. Graubard, E. Gilpin, D. Chavis, J. Garcia, L. M. Wun, W. Lynn, and M. Manley. 1999. The American Stop Smoking Intervention Study: Conceptual framework and evaluation design. *Evaluation Review* 23 (3): 259–80.

81. National Cancer Institute. 1991. *Strategies to control tobacco use in the United States: A blueprint for public health action in the 1990's* (Smoking and tobacco control monograph no. 1, NIH publication no. 92-3316). Bethesda, MD: National Cancer Institute. http://cancercontrol.cancer.gov/tcrb/monographs/1/index.html.

82. Manley, M., W. Lynn, R. P. Epps, D. Grande, T. Glynn, and D. Shopland. 1997. The American Stop Smoking Intervention Study for Cancer Prevention: An overview. *Tobacco Control* 6 Suppl. 2: S5–S11.

83. Givel, M. S., and S. A. Glantz. 2001. Tobacco lobby political influence on US state legislatures in the 1990s. *Tobacco Control* 10 (2): 124–34.

84. Glantz, S. A., and M. E. Begay. 1994. Tobacco industry campaign contributions are affecting tobacco control policymaking in California. *JAMA: The Journal of the American Medical Association* 272 (15): 1176–82.

85. Moore, S., S. M. Wolfe, D. Lindes, and C. E. Douglas. 1994. Epidemiology of failed tobacco control legislation. *JAMA: The Journal of the American Medical Association* 272 (15): 1171–75.

86. Monardi, F., and S. A. Glantz. 1998. Are tobacco industry campaign contributions influencing state legislative behavior? *American Journal of Public Health* 88 (6): 918–23.

87. Dearlove, J. V., and S. A. Glantz. 2002. Boards of health as venues for clean indoor air policy making. *American Journal of Public Health* 92 (2): 257–65.

88. Muggli, M. E., J. L. Forster, R. D. Hurt, and J. L. Repace. 2001. The smoke you don't see: Uncovering tobacco industry scientific

strategies aimed against environmental tobacco smoke policies. *American Journal of Public Health* 91 (9): 1419–23.

89. Barnoya, J., and S. Glantz. 2002. Tobacco industry success in preventing regulation of secondhand smoke in Latin America: The "Latin Project." *Tobacco Control* 11 (4): 305–14.

90. Ong, E. K., and S. A. Glantz. 2001. Constructing "sound science" and "good epidemiology": Tobacco, lawyers, and public relations firms. *American Journal of Public Health* 91 (11): 1749–57.

91. Muggli, M. E., R. D. Hurt, and D. D. Blanke. 2003. Science for hire: A tobacco industry strategy to influence public opinion on secondhand smoke. *Nicotine & Tobacco Research* 5 (3): 303–14.

92. Morley, C. P., K. M. Cummings, A. Hyland, G. A. Giovino, and J. K. Horan. 2002. Tobacco Institute lobbying at the state and local levels of government in the 1990s. *Tobacco Control* 11 Suppl. 1: I102–I109.

93. Samuels, B., and S. A. Glantz. 1991. The politics of local tobacco control. *JAMA: The Journal of the American Medical Association* 266 (15): 2110–17.

94. Traynor, M. P., M. E. Begay, and S. A. Glantz. 1993. New tobacco industry strategy to prevent local tobacco control. *JAMA: The Journal of the American Medical Association* 270 (4): 479–86.

95. National Cancer Institute. 2006. *Evaluating ASSIST: A blueprint for understanding state-level tobacco control* (Tobacco control monograph no. 17, NIH publication no. 06-6058). Bethesda, MD: National Cancer Institute. http://cancercontrol.cancer.gov/tcrb/monographs/17/index.html.

96. Chaloupka, F. J., and H. Saffer. 1992. Clean indoor air laws and the demand for cigarettes. *Contemporary Policy Issues* 10 (2): 72–83.

97. Chriqui, J. F., M. Frosh, R. C. Brownson, D. M. Shelton, R. C. Sciandra, R. Hobart, P. H. Fisher, R. El Arculli, and M. H. Alciati. 2002. Application of a rating system to state clean indoor air laws (USA). *Tobacco Control* 11 (1): 26–34.

98. Centers for Disease Control and Prevention. 2006. State-specific prevalence of current cigarette smoking among adults and secondhand smoke rules and policies in homes and workplaces—United States, 2005. *Morbidity and Mortality Weekly Report* 55 (42): 1148–51.

99. Centers for Disease Control and Prevention. 2002. Annual smoking-attributable mortality, years of potential life lost, and economic costs: United States, 1995–1999. *Morbidity and Mortality Weekly Report* 51 (14): 300–303.

100. Guest, I. 1978. Preventing heart disease through community action: The North Karelia Project. *Developmental Dialogue* 1: 51–58.

101. Korhonen, T., A. Uutela, H. J. Korhonen, and P. Puska. 1998. Impact of mass media and interpersonal health communication on smoking cessation attempts: A study in North Karelia, 1989–1996. *Journal of Health Communication* 3 (2): 105–18.

102. Fortmann, S. P. , and A. N. Varady. 2000. Effects of a community-wide health education program on cardiovascular disease morbidity and mortality: The Stanford Five-City Project. *American Journal of Epidemiology* 152 (4): 316–23.

103. Farkas, A. J., E. A. Gilpin, J. M. Distefan, and J. P. Pierce. 1999. The effects of household and workplace smoking restrictions on quitting behaviours. *Tobacco Control* 8 (3): 261–65.

104. Gilpin, E. A., M. M. White, A. J. Farkas, and J. P. Pierce. 1999. Home smoking restrictions: Which smokers have them and how they are associated with smoking behavior. *Nicotine & Tobacco Research* 1 (2): 153–62.

105. Clark, P. I., M. W. Schooley, B. Pierce, J. Schulman, A. M. Hartman, and C. L. Schmitt. 2006. Impact of home smoking rules on smoking patterns among adolescents and young adults. *Preventing Chronic Disease* 3 (2): A41.

106. Philip Morris USA. 2007. Our initiatives and programs: QuitAssist. http://www.philipmorrisusa.com/en/our_initiatives/quit_assist.asp.

107. Winkleby, M. A., H. A. Feldman, and D. M. Murray. 1997. Joint analysis of three U.S. community intervention trials for reduction of cardiovascular disease risk. *Journal of Clinical Epidemiology* 50 (6): 645–58.

108. American Journal of Public Health. 1995. Community Intervention Trial for Smoking Cessation (COMMIT): 1. Cohort results from a four-year community intervention. *American Journal of Public Health* 85 (2): 183–92.

109. Bauman, K. E., C. M. Suchindran, and D. M. Murray. 1999. The paucity of effects

in community trials: Is secular trend the culprit? *Preventive Medicine* 28 (4): 426–29.

110. National Cancer Institute. 1995. *Community-based interventions for smokers: The COMMIT field experience* (Smoking and tobacco control monograph no. 6, NIH publication no. 95-4028). Bethesda, MD: National Cancer Institute. http://cancercontrol.cancer.gov/tcrb/monographs/6/index.html.

111. National Cancer Institute. 2005. *ASSIST: Shaping the future of tobacco prevention and control* (Tobacco control monograph no. 16, NIH publication no. 05-5645). Bethesda, MD: National Cancer Institute. http://cancercontrol.cancer.gov/tcrb/monographs/16/index.html.

112. Stillman, F. A., A. M. Hartman, B. I. Graubard, E. A. Gilpin, D. M. Murray, and J. T. Gibson. 2003. Evaluation of the American Stop Smoking Intervention Study (ASSIST): A report of outcomes. *Journal of the National Cancer Institute* 95 (22): 1681–91.

113. Gerlach, K. K., and M. A. Larkin. 2005. The SmokeLess States Program: To improve health and health care. http://www.rwjf.org/files/publications/books/2005/chapter_02.pdf.

114. Centers for Disease Control and Prevention. 2005. Syndemics overview: When is it appropriate or inappropriate to use a syndemic orientation? Atlanta: U.S. Department of Health and Human Services, Centers for Disease Control and Prevention, National Center for Chronic Disease Prevention and Health Promotion, Syndemics Prevention Network. http://www.cdc.gov/syndemics/overview-uses.htm.

115. Senge, P. M. 1990. *The fifth discipline: The art and practice of the learning organization.* New York: Currency Doubleday.

116. Krygiel, A. J. 1999. *Behind the wizard's curtain: An integration environment for a system of systems.* Washington, DC: Institute for National Strategic Studies.

117. National Institutes of Health. 2006. Clinical Nutrition Research Unit Core Centers. RFA announcement. http://grants.nih.gov/grants/guide/rfa-files/RFA-DK-06-013.html.

118. National Institutes of Health. 2006. Exploratory Centers for Interdisciplinary Research. Bethesda, MD: U.S. Department of Health and Human Services, National Institutes of Health, Office of Portfolio Analysis and Strategic Initiatives. http://nihroadmap.nih.gov/interdisciplinary/exploratorycenters.

119. Institute of Medicine. 2004. *The chasm in quality: Select indicators from recent reports.* Washington, DC: Institute of Medicine. http://www.iom.edu/?id=14991.

120. World Health Organization. 2003. World Health Assembly Resolution 56.1. Geneva: World Health Organization. http://www.who.int/tobacco/framework/final_text/en.

121. Callard, C., D. Thompson, and N. Collishaw. 2005. Transforming the tobacco market: Why the supply of cigarettes should be transferred from for-profit corporations to non-profit enterprises with a public health mandate. *Tobacco Control* 14 (4): 278–83.

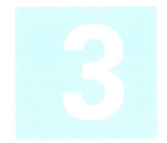

Systems Thinking: Potential to Transform Tobacco Control

The preceding chapter explored contemporary challenges faced by proponents of tobacco control, particularly with respect to improving public health outcomes. This chapter presents a view of systems thinking as an endeavor that encompasses a broad and rich historical tradition of systems fields that could help address the increasingly complex challenges that tobacco control faces. The chapter addresses the application of systems approaches to tobacco control by examining

- *Current systems thinking approaches, including theories and issues encompassed by or closely allied to systems thinking*

- *Four promising systems approaches under study in the Initiative on the Study and Implementation of Systems (ISIS) project, which are explored in detail in subsequent chapters within the broader context of an integrated systems environment*

- *Key questions of tobacco control practitioners, researchers, and policy makers that are addressed by systems thinking*

The goals of this chapter are to describe several frameworks for understanding what is meant by systems thinking, present a brief overview of the vast terrain of systems concepts, suggest an integrated view of the idea of systems thinking that is emerging in part from the work conducted in this project, and outline some of the implications of systems thinking for three key stakeholder groups in tobacco control—practitioners, policy makers, and researchers.

First come hints, then fragments of systems, then defective systems, then complete and harmonious systems. [And] thus, the great progress goes on.

—Thomas Babington Macaulay (1800–59)

Introduction

This chapter begins to frame the process of applying systems thinking to key issues in tobacco control as a prelude to more detailed examinations of individual systems approaches and their synthesis in subsequent chapters. The first section offers a brief overview of the idea of systems thinking and the many systems concepts that help inform it. The next section suggests the contours of an integrated framework for systems thinking. It does so by introducing the four systems approaches that were the specific focus of the ISIS project (systems organization, system dynamics, network analysis, and knowledge management and transfer). The central role of participatory approaches to human systems is described, and suggestions are offered about how these might be integrated within a new field of study. The chapter concludes with specific questions these systems approaches might help answer for several groups of tobacco control stakeholders: practitioners, researchers, and policy makers.

Public health issues such as tobacco control are not simple, linear cause-and-effect problems. They are systems bound together by a network of factors that influence and react with each other, much like a living organism. The prevalence of tobacco use and tobacco product consumption has decreased substantially in the United States in the past few decades in response to interventions such as consumer education, telephone quitlines for smoking cessation, advertising restrictions, increased taxation, clean indoor air restrictions, and health warnings. Nevertheless, tobacco use remains responsible for hundreds of thousands of preventable deaths each year. Moving past the current plateau in tobacco control outcomes requires dealing with a complex interplay of evolving actors and factors that must be addressed as a system. The purpose

of ISIS has been to explore the potential of key systems approaches that address challenges in tobacco control, including

- Disparate communities of interest and frequent duplication of effort

- Limited integration of research and practice, so that the best science frequently sits unread and unimplemented

- A paucity of organized dissemination and collaboration methods

- Competition from a well-financed and well-organized tobacco industry that has integrated dissemination and networking efforts

- The need for more experience in evaluating (1) the interconnected dynamics of the tobacco control system and efforts of the tobacco industry and (2) the effects of these dynamics on key outcomes such as tobacco cessation and morbidity and mortality due to tobacco use

Successful program development in any field requires both effective strategy and powerful implementation—sometimes characterized as "doing the right thing right." The ultimate primary goal of these systems approaches in tobacco control is to improve performance. Documentation of improvement requires direct measures of outputs and outcomes, such as (1) decreases in smoking prevalence; (2) greater efficiency in terms of the number of smokers served by direct contact programs (e.g., clinics, Web sites, and hotlines) per dollar invested and over time; and (3) higher proportions of programs and policies meeting standards for "evidence-based" interventions. The promise of systems approaches, backed by a growing body of evidence, is increased facilitation of progress toward such desired outcomes.

Systems approaches may help cast new light on issues that affect program delivery in the real world: staff turnover, the glut of information and directives, isolation, multiple demands on programs, and multiple roles for managers. The world does not stand still as proponents of tobacco control attempt to manage this environment. A well-funded tobacco industry has the resources to anticipate and thwart novel initiatives. Even well-intentioned, beneficial efforts can have unintended negative-feedback effects. Therefore, flexible strategies based on widely accepted philosophy and best practices are essential. However, these strategies also must enable response to emerging science and systemic feedback.

At the broadest level, a fresh, trans-disciplinary approach to thinking about intervention systems is likely needed, one that integrates a balanced and comprehensive blend of program and policy tools. Program, policy, budgetary, and legislative issues all arise from the identification and implementation of strategies for best practice, which are themselves often in flux. Moreover, the underlying philosophy of public health continues to evolve. As stated in an overview of the syndemics initiative of the Centers for Disease Control and Prevention,[1] "The medical model of disease specialization, once praised for its utility and versatility, is proving inadequate for confronting. . . contemporary public health challenges." The statement echoes a growing move toward researching public health problems as both multidimensional population-level issues and individual issues. Unless these crosscutting factors are viewed from a systems perspective, it is likely that progress on any initiative can become mired in the many interacting and competing forces. Developing capacity for integrated strategies to tackle the complexity of these issues is a major focus of ISIS.

Already, developments in tobacco control and in public health in general are starting to move in this direction. As outlined in chapter 2, tobacco control strategy has mirrored the shift in emphasis from individual behavior change to population-level and policy-level change. There is a concomitant shift from controlled studies of individuals to population-level efforts involving logic models, networks, and collaborations among multiple stakeholders—all historical precursors to the systems approaches described here. The ISIS project springs from a clear trend that these approaches—and more important, their synthesis—hold a potential key to solving more complex issues in the prevalence of tobacco use and tobacco product consumption and, in turn, making further substantive positive changes in public health.

Systems and Systems Thinking

The *Merriam-Webster Dictionary* offers 12 distinct definitions of "system."[2] The principal definition is "a regularly interacting or interdependent group of items forming a unified whole."[2] In the field of systems theory, system is defined as "a set of elements standing in interrelation among themselves and with the environment."[3(p159)] Hidden within these simple definitions is considerable complexity, a history of ideas spanning centuries, and the basis of a new scientific and philosophical paradigm.

In this monograph, *systems methods* are considered specialized techniques or procedures for researching and understanding systems (e.g., system dynamics modeling, structured conceptualization, or network analysis). *Systems approaches* are broader theories or traditions that use systems methods within an organizing framework to address systems (e.g., general systems theory, chaos theory, and complexity theory). *Systems thinking* is the use of systems approaches and the general logic that underlies them to view the world.

The modern idea of systems theory is credited to the biologist Ludwig von Bertalanffy, who wrote *General System Theory: Foundations, Development, Applications*[4] in 1968. However, thinking about systems has a much longer history. The relationship between part and whole that serves as a foundation for systems-based approaches[5–7] is as old as European philosophy.[3] Aristotle's hypothesis that formal nature (e.g., the whole form) is of greater importance than material nature—more commonly known today as the principle that "the whole is more than the sum of its parts"—still is an accurate description of one of the central premises of systems theory.[8] In the 15th century, Nicholas of Cusa linked medieval mysticism with the origins of modern science through the idea of *coincidentia oppositorum*—the "fight" between part and whole.[3]

Systems thinking spans 2,600 years to the time of Lao Tzu and the first formal description of a complex system in the yin and yang of the Tao. Systems thinking was not "born yesterday."[3] However, its modern incarnation has risen simultaneously from several fields, including quantum physics, biology, ecology, cybernetics, psychology, and sociology.[3,6] It can be found in the physical, natural, and social sciences and is common in business[9–11] and education.[9,12–18] Depending on how wide one casts the net, systems thinking approaches span centuries, hundreds of fields, and thousands of scholars.[19] A family tree of systemic thought[20] includes in its "genealogy" ancient and contemporary scholars in a wide range of fields[19] and illustrates the variety of traditions in systems thinking.

The reader who is new to systems thinking may be daunted by the complexity and volume of literature. However, these variations and distinct traditions of systems

thinking have some common themes. These themes include the notions of holism, integration, interconnectedness, organization, perspective taking, nonlinearity, and constructivism. Biological, ecological, and organismic metaphors are widely used to describe these themes.[4,6,7,21–29]

Common misconceptions are (1) that systems thinking rejects traditional scientific views[3,4,6,28–30] that emphasize linear, reductionist, mechanistic, and atomistic thinking; and (2) that systems thinking is framed by mechanical metaphors.[31] These are not correct. Although systems thinking does emphasize holistic thinking,[3,4,6,28–30] it complements traditional reductionist science rather than rejecting it. Von Bertalanffy wrote that it "is apparent that [systems epistemology] is profoundly different from the epistemology of logical positivism or empiricism even though it shares their scientific attitude."[4(pxxii)]

Another misconception is that systems thinking superficially emphasizes holistic thinking and lacks the rigor of traditional science. To the contrary, systems thinking uses differential equations and other more complex mathematics to describe system dynamics,[3,32,33] formalized qualitative systems methods,[34] and well-reasoned systems metaphors,[3,24,28,30,35,36] along with specific applications in virtually every field.[6,10,11,37]

The roots of systems theory[4,19] have grown into what is sometimes described as the "new sciences": general systems theory;[4] complexity science;[33,38–41] chaos theory and nonlinear dynamics;[42,43] cybernetics;[44,45] control theory, information theory, and computational simulation;[46] relational mathematics, game theory, decision theory, and system dynamics;[11,32] and ecology and set, graph, and network theory.[47–50] Systems thinking is used to better understand system behaviors and to identify systems principles such as feedback loops, stocks and flows, open versus closed systems, decentralized versus hierarchical systems, self-organization,[33,40] autopoiesis,[35,51] nonlinear systems,[43] complex adaptive systems (CAS),[33,38,40,41,45,52] boundary conditions, scaling and power laws, silo effects, small-world phenomena,[47,48] emergence,[53] cellular automata,[45] and fractal self-similarity.[54]

Many examples of systems thinking contribute to an understanding of the world. From the systems thinking of chaos theory, one can learn that minuscule changes in initial conditions can lead to dramatic emergent effects and that resistant systems can be directed to change. From complexity science, one can see that complexity emerges from simple rules acting locally on independent variables. That is, biological and social systems often do not have hierarchical controls that coordinate their behavior but are instead self-organizing. From system dynamics one can learn that, as systems thinker Senge puts it, "cause and effect are not closely related in time and space"[9(p63)] and that feedback can lead to unintended and unforeseen outcomes. Understanding of control systems has been expanded from an "input-blackbox-output" paradigm[3] to one that includes inputs, outputs, feedback, processes, flows, and control. These are just a few examples of systems thinking concepts from a broad range of disciplines.

Frameworks for Systems Thinking

There is no single and correct method of systems thinking. Borrowing an idea from Collins and Porras,[55] systems thinking rejects the "tyranny of either/or" and embraces the "genius of and/both." Systems thinking is a worldview that balances part and whole and focuses on complex interrelationships and patterns from multiple perspectives.[28,37] An inherently transdisciplinary approach that blends many perspectives, it has been characterized as

an Odyssean thinking style that combines Apollonian and Dionysian perspectives.[56,57] Systems thinking is an epistemological stance transcending reductionist, critical realist, and constructivist perspectives. As an applied science, it bridges theory and practice. It is a conceptual revolution that has led to an emerging understanding of the complexities of the systems that make up the world. Systems thinking provides new tools to address practical, complex problems in much the same way mechanical thinking enabled previous generations to build agricultural or industrial structures.

A number of scholars have developed frameworks for systems thinking—sets of principles, rules, skills, or ideas that they claim underlie systems thinking. Each framework has advantages and disadvantages and was developed in the context of a particular purpose. Each was created from a different perspective or systems tradition. The summaries of some of the frameworks presented here are not meant to be exhaustive or definitive. However, each one gives a glimpse of systems thinking, and collectively they help to convey the essence of systems thinking.

Some scholars see system dynamics as a branch of systems theory. Others see systems theory as a branch of system dynamics. Scholars of system dynamics often use the term "systems thinking" to refer to system *dynamics* thinking,[9,58–64] dropping the word "dynamics" as a descriptor. For example, "systems thinking" is defined by one source as follows:

Systems thinking is an approach for studying and managing complex feedback systems, such as one finds in business and other social systems. In fact, it has been used to address practically every sort of feedback system. System dynamics is more or less the same as systems thinking, but [it] emphasizes the usage of computer-simulation tools. System dynamics is based on systems thinking, but [it] takes the additional steps of constructing and testing a computer-simulation model.[65]

Richmond offers an example of a framework for system dynamics thinking in his book *The "Thinking" in Systems Thinking: Seven Essential Skills.*[59] He compares seven skills of systems thinking that are derived from system dynamics with skills of traditional styles of thinking (table 3.1).[59] Richmond's framework illustrates some of the key notions of systems (dynamics), including the ideas of causal linkages and feedback loops. Chapter 5 in this monograph explores system dynamics in greater depth.

System dynamics is a type of systems thinking that has gained popularity in business settings such as organizational learning. In *The Fifth Discipline: The Art and Practice of the Learning Organization,*[9]

Senge lays out five disciplines for building a "learning organization." According to Senge, learning organizations are adaptive and generative and are necessary for survival and competition. His five disciplines[66] are as follows:

1. **Systems thinking:** The integrative [fifth] discipline that fuses the other four into a coherent body of theory and practice

2. **Personal mastery:** Approaching life and work "as an artist would approach a work of art"

3. **Mental models:** Deeply ingrained assumptions or mental images "that influence how we understand the world and how we take action"

4. **Shared vision:** With genuine vision "people excel and learn, not because they are told to, but because they want to"

Table 3.1 Richmond's Seven Skills of Systems Thinking

Traditional skill	Systems thinking skill
Static thinking Focusing on particular events	**Dynamic thinking** Framing a problem in terms of a pattern of behavior over time
System-as-effect thinking Viewing behavior generated by a system as driven by external forces	**System-as-cause thinking** Placing responsibility for a behavior on internal actors who manage the policies and plumbing of the system
Tree-by-tree thinking Believing that really knowing something means focusing on the details	**Forest thinking** Believing that to know something requires understanding the context of relationships
Factors thinking Listing factors that influence or are correlated with some result	**Operational thinking** Concentrating on causality and understanding how a behavior is generated
Straight-line thinking Viewing causality as running in one direction, with each cause independent from other causes	**Closed-loop thinking** Viewing causality as an ongoing process, not a one-time event, with effect feeding back to influence the causes and the causes affecting each other
Measurement thinking Searching for perfectly measured data	**Quantitative thinking** Accepting that one can always quantify, even though one cannot always measure
Proving-truth thinking Seeking to prove models to be true by validating them with historical data	**Scientific thinking** Recognizing that all models are working hypotheses with limited applicability

Note. From Richmond, B. 2000. *The "thinking" in systems thinking: Seven essential skills.* Toolbox Reprint series. Waltham, MA: Pegasus Communications. Used with permission.

5. **Team learning:** Engagement of team members in true dialogue, with assumptions suspended

Senge[9] outlines 11 laws of the fifth discipline, which he derives from lessons in fields as diverse as chaos theory, complexity theory, organizational theory, management theory, and system dynamics:

1. Today's problems come from yesterday's solutions.

2. The harder you push, the harder the system pushes back.

3. Behavior grows better before it grows worse.

4. The easy way out usually leads back in.

5. The cure can be worse than the disease.

6. Faster is slower.

7. Cause and effect are not closely related in time and space.

8. Small changes can produce big results, but the areas of highest leverage often are the least obvious.

9. You can have your cake and eat it too, but not all at once.

10. Dividing an elephant in half does not produce two small elephants.

11. There is no blame.

Similarly, Gelb sees systems thinking as the glue that binds his seven principles of effective thinking. Gelb proposes that effective thinking in today's world can be framed by seven principles[67,68] he claims are characteristic of Leonardo da Vinci's genius:

1. An insatiable quest for knowledge and continuous improvement

2. Learning from experience

3. Sharpening the senses

4. Managing ambiguity and change

5. Whole-brain thinking

6. Body–mind fitness

7. Systems thinking

Gelb believes[68] that da Vinci's principles will help people to cultivate creativity every day, balance analysis with imagination, sustain continuous learning, embrace ambiguity and uncertainty, nurture creativity and innovation in the workplace, and apply systems thinking to problem solving.

Capra, a physicist and systems thinker, proposed ecological thinking, a systems thinking model he defines as "core concepts in ecology that describe the patterns and processes by which nature sustains life."[6(p231)] Table 3.2 illustrates his six principles of ecology. Like system dynamics thinking, ecological thinking emphasizes cyclic thinking, processes over time, and feedback. However, it also gives more salience to networks, being nested, and development.

Checkland developed soft systems methodology in the 1960s. In the classic form of these methods,[69,70] a researcher or an observer experiencing a problem makes as few presumptions about the nature of the problem as possible. A "rich picture" then is developed by attempting to capture in detail the logic, relationships, value judgments, and feel (tone) of the problem situation. Essential features of the system (root definition) are then characterized. The mnemonic device CATWOE is used in this step: customers, who are beneficiaries of the system; actors, who transform inputs to outputs; transformation of input to output; weltanshauung (relevant worldviews); owners, who have veto power over the system; and environmental constraints. CATWOE is used to construct the root definition, which takes the following form: "A system that does P (what) by Q (how) to contribute to achieving R (why)." Then a "cultural analysis" is undertaken to explore the roles, norms, values, and politics

Table 3.2 Capra's Six Principles of Ecology

Networks	At all scales of nature, we find living systems nesting within other living systems— networks within networks. Their boundaries are not boundaries of separation but boundaries of identity. All living systems communicate with one another and share resources across their boundaries.
Cycles	All living organisms must feed on continual flows of matter and energy from their environment to stay alive, and all living organisms continually produce waste. However, an ecosystem generates no net waste, one species' waste being another species' food. Thus, matter cycles continually through the web of life.
Solar Energy	Solar energy, transformed into chemical energy by the photosynthesis of green plants, drives the ecological cycles.
Partnership	The exchanges of energy and resources in an ecosystem are sustained by pervasive cooperation. Life did not take over the planet by combat but by cooperation, partnership, and networking.
Diversity	Ecosystems achieve stability and resilience through the richness and complexity of their ecological webs. The greater their biodiversity, the more resilient they will be.
Dynamic Balance	An ecosystem is a flexible, ever-fluctuating network. Its flexibility is a consequence of multiple feedback loops that keep the system in a state of dynamic balance. No single variable is maximized; all variables fluctuate around their optimal values.

Note. From Capra, F. 2002. *The hidden connections: Integrating the biological, cognitive, and social dimensions of life into a science of sustainability,* 231. New York: Doubleday.

relevant to the root definition. A systems model is developed by using only the elements of the root definition and cultural analysis in a way that flows logically from the two elements. The focus of this step is to limit the number of possible components to the six or fewer CATWOE elements, while demonstrating all the properties of the system. Thus, the focus is to balance the simplicity of few components with the complexity of system properties. Different root definitions and CATWOE elements are used to construct several models illustrating how multiple perspectives relate to the problem. Finally, these models are discussed, compared, and contrasted by using the problem situation and insight from this process to identify ways to improve the problem situation.

In his book *Hidden Order: How Adaptation Builds Complexity,*[71] Holland details a framework for studying CAS, proposing seven basics.[71(p10)] "We *aggregate* similar things into categories (and) then treat them as equivalent."[71(p10)] Aggregations are reusable and recombinable and, once formed, can act as agents or meta-agents. "*Tagging* facilitates the formation of aggregates."[71(p12)] Holland gives the example of a banner or flag that "is used to rally members of an army or people of similar political persuasion."[71(p13)] He explains that CAS use tagging to "manipulate symmetries" and to "ignore certain details while directing our attention to others."[71(p12)] Another property of CAS is *nonlinearities,* which "almost always make the behavior of the aggregate more complicated than would be predicted by summing or averaging."[71(p23)] A property Holland calls *flows* includes two types of effects: multiplier and recycling. The property of flows explains how resources move and change as they proceed through the system. In describing the property of *diversity,* Holland writes, "it should be evident then that we will not find CAS settling to a few highly adapted types that exploit all opportunities. Perpetual novelty is the hallmark of CAS."[71(p31)] Anticipation is a critical capability for CAS. CAS anticipate or make predictions by using *internal models.* For example, "insectivorous birds anticipate the bitter taste of butterflies with a particular orange and black wing pattern."[71(p31)] One paradox CAS must solve is how to use internal models based on repetition in constantly changing and novel situations. How can CAS use an internal model based on a repeating pattern if each situation is slightly different or totally novel? Holland proposes that *building blocks* are used and reused, allowing CAS to decompose novel situations into parts, as a child's building blocks are used to create novel structures.

Systems Concepts

Important systems concepts are relevant to different types of systems and constitute a unique lexicon of systems thinking. Here, several major systems concepts that inform systems thinking are introduced. Rather than being comprehensive, the intent is to present notable systems concepts within this rich historical tradition. Each concept

may represent an entire specialized field of study, networks of scholars and researchers, scientific journals, conferences, and societies.

CAS self-organize, adapt, and evolve over time. In a CAS, semiautonomous agents interact on the basis of simple local rules. The term "complex adaptive system" often is used interchangeably with the term "complexity theory," which proposes that higher level complexity emerges from lower level simplicity. In an example highlighted in this chapter (see sidebar, this page), the boids, sporting fans, fish, or birds are *adaptive agents* because they adapt to their environments. The environment of an adaptive agent includes other adaptive agents.

Interaction between adaptive agents or systems often is called *feedback*, which refers to the mutual causality of the relationship (e.g., positive/exciting or negative/dampening). In a similar vein, the term *cellular automata*, originally developed

---

Simple Rules and Superorganisms

In 1986, Reynolds made a computer model of coordinated animal motion such as bird flocks and fish schools, calling the simulated flocking creatures "boids."[a] The basic flocking model consisted of three simple "steering behaviors":

- Separation: Steer to avoid crowding local "flockmates."
- Alignment: Steer toward the average heading of local flockmates.
- Cohesion: Steer to move toward the average position of local flockmates.

Each boid reacts "only to flockmates within a small neighborhood," so the boids are interacting only with neighbors. Flockmates that lie outside the individual boid's neighborhood are ignored.

Reynolds's computational experiment models the complex flocking behavior of boids, fish, and birds by using simple local rules acting on independent variables. The result is emergent complexity—a collection of individual organisms that act like a single superorganism.

An even simpler example of the complex behavior of superorganisms that is based on simple rules can be found at national sporting events. The stadium wave, in which fans simulate an undulating elliptical blanket around the stadium, is based on a single, simple, local rule: if your left neighbor stands up, then stand up. The initial starting condition for this complex phenomenon is a single line of standing people.

Note. Adapted from Cabrera, D. 2002. Patterns of knowledge: Knowledge as a complex, evolutionary system; An educational imperative. In *Creating learning communities,* ed. R. Miller. Brandon, VT: Solomon Press.

[a]Reynolds, C. 2006. Boids: Background and update. http://www.red3d.com/cwr/boids.

by von Neumann[72] in the computing arena, also refers to the idea of modeling biological or artificial self-reproduction by using simple interacting "cells" that follow simple, local rules.[72] Computational cellular automata models are popular and useful because they explicate many of the essential patterns found in more complex, self-organizing, real-world systems. *Self-organization* occurs in CAS as spontaneous patterns or features of a system that emerge at macro levels resulting from the collective interactions of microscale independent agents and local rules. These features are often called *dissipative structures,* because they persist as stable structures for longer durations, even though, internally, there is a continuous and dynamic flow of matter or energy. The concept of *emergence* is related because it refers to the existence of properties at a higher level (e.g., the level of the whole) that cannot be found at a lower level (e.g., the level of the parts).

The concept of *autopoiesis* (literally, self-production), which refers to self-producing systems, also is related. Two Chilean biologists, Maturana and Varela,[51] developed the concept of autopoiesis. Autopoiesis is similar to Kauffman's autocatalytic theory of sets in which the origin of life occurs when a collection of molecules catalyze each other. Kauffman writes, "Whenever a collection of chemicals contains enough different kinds of molecules, a metabolism will crystallize from the broth."[33(p43),40]

Nonlinear systems are systems in which the whole does not equal the sum of its parts or, more technically, systems that can be represented by a curvilinear pattern, rather than a linear pattern. Nonlinear systems are capable of self-organization and chaos. There are many implications of chaos. Chief among them is the understanding that small changes in initial conditions can result in large, systemwide effects (sensitivity to initial conditions). The popularized story of Lorenz's butterfly—an insect that by flapping its wings causes a chain of events leading to a hurricane on the other side of the world—often is used as an anecdote for understanding chaos theory.

Both linear and nonlinear systems are attracted to a subset of their phase space called an *attractor.* Attractors are modes or phases of system behavior. Attractors (e.g., fixed-point, periodic, or strange) determine the behavior of a system within a particular space. A marble tossed into a salad bowl will, over time, settle into an attractor at the bottom of the bowl (the basin of attraction). A chaotic (strange) attractor is fractal. *Fractals* are geometric patterns, a set of points, or structures that are self-similar across different levels of scale. Fractals, discovered by Mandelbrot, have become popular in science and art; many fractal patterns are strikingly beautiful. When a system exhibits fractal geometry, the parts appear to be similar to the whole, even though they belong to different scales. The branching pattern of trees is fractal, as are the coastline of England and the branching alveoli of the lung.[54] All systems evolve in some way. *Evolution* can be defined in Darwinian terms as natural selection and the descent of species, or in more general terms, as behavior over time.

Finally, *network theory* is a general theory used throughout physics, biology, and the social sciences that explores the behaviors, structure, and function of an interacting set of items (e.g., objects, people, concepts, or points).[47,48,50,54,73,74] Networks are made up of *vertices* (a set of items) and *edges* (connections among the items). Vertices and edges are called sites and bonds in physics, nodes and links in computer science, and actors and bonds in sociology.[50] Chapter 6, "Understanding and Managing Stakeholder Networks," in this monograph, presents network approaches to systems thinking.

Systems thinking can be simple and complex, theoretical and practical, scientifically rigorous and philosophically grounded. In the context of tobacco control, it is important to consider the types of systems questions that people with different roles in tobacco control need to address. Chapters 4 through 7 address in depth four broad systems approaches—systems organizing and management, system dynamics modeling, network analysis, and knowledge management—and their implications for tobacco control.

Systems Thinking: Toward an Integrated View

As understanding of systems thinking, systems approaches, and systems methods increases, it becomes apparent that there is a need to integrate the diverse and myriad traditions into a more coherent whole. The ISIS project is an initial and somewhat limited foray into such an endeavor. Nevertheless, one can begin to sketch some of the central components of a more integrated view of systems for tobacco control and public health, based on the work done to date. In addition to consideration of the construct of systems thinking, an integrated approach to systems thinking would include the following components (and likely much more):

- **Case studies of systems approaches.** This would include studies of the variety of systems approaches and the methods that are associated with them. The ISIS project has begun studies in four systems approaches: systems organizing, system dynamics, network analysis, and knowledge management.

- **Participatory methods for systems thinking.** In human systems like tobacco control and public health, better participatory methods for modeling systems and for thinking from a systems perspective need to be developed.

- **Evolution of systems studies.** As more studies of systems approaches and methods are developed, the evolution of a "field" of systems studies that integrates across diverse traditions will be encouraged.

Case Studies of Systems Approaches

An integrated approach to systems thinking should involve trial-and-error experimenting with a variety of potentially promising systems approaches and methods to learn how they work and what their potential advantages and costs are in real-world contexts. A central purpose of ISIS has been to identify several promising approaches and apply them to help "navigate" current problems in tobacco control.

The four core systems approaches examined by ISIS are outlined in table 3.3 along with brief descriptions of the goals of each approach and the case studies conducted in the ISIS project. Many of these approaches are newly developing. Other approaches, such as system dynamics, have been available for years but have rarely been applied in this area. Because the application of systems thinking to tobacco control is in its early stages, the excitement and the promise of this undertaking are just beginning to be realized.

These approaches all serve as parts of a broad, systems-based view of the world that can be applied specifically to tobacco control and more generally to public health. More important, these approaches reflect more general trends of using systems approaches to understand and manage increasingly complex phenomena in all walks of life, ranging from organizational behavior[9] to national defense.[75] These four approaches were chosen because of their promise in key areas of tobacco control. They are not the only systems approaches, nor are they necessarily the best. They are part of a much

Table 3.3 Core Areas Examined by ISIS and Goals

Core area	Long-term goals	ISIS case studies
How we organize: Systems organizing	Participatory, stakeholder-based approaches to systems organizing	Concept-mapping studies of local strength of tobacco control factors and of designing for research dissemination
How we understand dynamic complexity: System dynamics modeling	• Development of systems models for tobacco control factors and processes for analyzing and evaluating them • Telling the tobacco control "story" in qualitative as well as quantitative terms, so it can reach a wider audience	• Causal model for tobacco cessation based on data in clinical and community guides • Quantitative simulation of intervention impacts in different age groups
Who we are: Network analysis	Network-based structures for future collaborative tobacco control efforts	• Examination of network issues in the Global Tobacco Research Network • Case study of network analysis in ongoing multistate tobacco control evaluation project
What we know: Knowledge management and knowledge transfer	Infrastructure for knowledge management and transfer in tobacco control efforts, incorporating both explicit and tacit knowledge	Review of current dissemination efforts (e.g., NCI's Cancer Control PLANET initiative)[a] and analysis of knowledge management needs

Note. ISIS = Initiative on the Study and Implementation of Systems; NCI = National Cancer Institute; PLANET = Plan, Link, Act, Network with Evidence-based Tools.

[a]Cancer Control PLANET is an NCI-funded portal providing on-line access to research results, partner organizations, and evidence-based programs and products for cancer control, available at http://cancercontrolplanet.cancer.gov.

larger diverse mosaic of potential systems approaches hinted at in the review earlier in this chapter.

The methods described here as part of the ISIS project have the potential to deliver incremental improvements in tobacco control and public health outcomes. However, each method also complements the others. Together, these methods provide a fundamentally new way to address the complex root causes of current tobacco use. Frameworks that enable integration of a number of systems-based approaches also would be useful.

An integrated approach to systems thinking will likely result in the evolution of one or more fields of study that enable researchers and practitioners to learn about the construct of systems thinking, and the history and variety of approaches and methods, and to begin to develop crosscutting and cross-disciplinary perspectives on systems thinking. Such fields already are emerging. For example, frameworks such as Integration and Implementation Sciences[76] (described in table 3.4 and in the sidebar in Appendix B, p. 272) propose a core theoretical base from which systems methodologies may be developed and applied to specific areas. They provide a potential transdisciplinary base for studying system-level problems faced in tobacco control efforts and may help fill important gaps in methodologies between complementary disciplines. For example, chaos and complexity theory often takes an exploratory approach to the behavior of a system based on simulations of interactions of individual agents who follow simple rules, whereas traditional system dynamics seeks to identify relationships and optimize

Figure 3.1 Combining ISIS Approaches for Applications

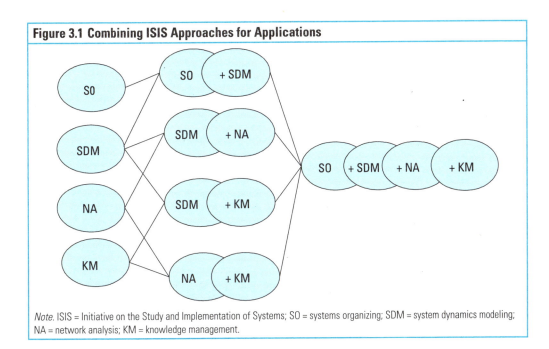

Note. ISIS = Initiative on the Study and Implementation of Systems; SO = systems organizing; SDM = system dynamics modeling; NA = network analysis; KM = knowledge management.

Table 3.4 Framework of Integration and Implementation Sciences

Integration and Implementation Sciences framework	ISIS case studies
Systems thinking and complexity science	System dynamics simulation
Participatory methods	System dynamics simulation; concept-mapping projects with multiple stakeholders
Knowledge management, exchange, and implementation	Network analysis Knowledge management and knowledge transfer

outcomes.[77] An integrated systems study field can enhance understanding of the advantages of these different approaches and suggest how new hybrid approaches might be formed by combining or integrating features of each. For example, figure 3.1 illustrates how the four systems approaches studies in the ISIS project can potentially be coupled in various pairings and even integrated as a set. The framework of Integration and Implementation Sciences (table 3.4) serves as one example of using an integrative approach to link these disciplines to address core problems in public health (e.g., the paradox of society's inability to implement known cost-effective solutions to the 10 leading causes of preventable death worldwide, as identified by the World Health

Organization).[78] The ISIS project sought to apply key components from this framework to existing problems in tobacco control, as a proof of concept for how they can integrate to form a new approach to complex public health issues.

ISIS is only a first step in applying systems approaches to tobacco control. An aim of this monograph is to show the potential value of these approaches individually and in combination and to point to broader frameworks for further development of these approaches. In this sense, ISIS attempts both to encourage and model how an emergent field of systems studies might approach its task. It is not clear at this point whether such a field eventually will be a formal academic discipline, a transdisciplinary specialization, or some other form. But however the field evolves, the idea of systems studies is one whose time has come.

Participatory Methods for Systems Thinking

An integrated approach to systems thinking needs to include the recognition that participatory methods are integral to human systems approaches. All four of the systems approaches studied in the ISIS project integrate participatory methods into how they address systems. An integrated approach would have the study and evolution of participatory methods as a major focus.

Brown and colleagues[79] outline a framework for stakeholder inclusion that views participatory methods as forms of structured engagement among researchers, community representatives, business groups, and policy makers to accomplish the collective solution of problems as a system. They recognize the importance of individuals, societies, and cultures as aspects of complexity.

Participatory methods encompass a wide range of engagements, including action research, Delphi methods, consensus building, and numerous intuitive unnamed methods.[80] These methods involve two or more parties and a range of disciplines and sectors, can be short- or long-term, can challenge elites or be controlled by them, and can vary in the degree to which they empower marginalized groups. Participatory methods enable practitioners and researchers to learn together about problems of mutual interest in a way that provides reciprocal benefits. They can combine perspectives to build new concepts, insights, and/or practical innovations that they could not produce alone.

The four key elements in contemporary thinking about participatory methods

are (1) paradigms, goals, and interests; (2) relationships and organization; (3) methods and technologies; and (4) contextual forces and institutions. Engagement between researchers and practitioners must take into account different social, political, and ethical paradigms; different engagement goals and interests; and different expectations about accountability. Furthermore, the relationships and organization must be able to accommodate power differences; build trust; and develop effective control, ownership, division of work, and decision-making processes. The methods and technologies used within this framework can be divided into four types:

1. **Participatory, focused, puzzle-solving methods** are appropriate when answers to well-defined problems are needed. Such methods make efficient use of the comparative advantages of each party and do not require expensive ongoing relationships.

2. **Exploration of issues and agenda setting** are appropriate when multiple views are needed for understanding complex, ill-structured problems. These methods allow many voices to be involved in identifying issue patterns and implications and set the stage for wide participation in problem solving.

3. **Participatory intervention and assessment methods** document, analyze, and improve the quality of interventions and best practices. They focus on existing programs and activities and are particularly useful for identifying the costs and benefits of possible solutions.

4. **Participatory methods for long-term development** of domains involve ongoing co-inquiry to build perspectives, theory, and practice in new domains. These methods are particularly useful in providing in-depth analysis of poorly understood problems over the longer term. They can produce new paradigms for understanding intractable problems

and lead to fundamental changes in theory and/or practice.

Contextual forces and institutions are the final element of the framework. They take into account the broad range of factors such as political, social, and economic forces on global, national, and local levels that are at play at the time of engagement. This element also allows for the impact of the auspices under which the participatory methods are conducted and of the institutional bases of the researchers and practitioners.

Participatory methods are central to bringing stakeholders into the consideration of complex problems. Ideally, their use enables those affected to have a say in the management of uncertainties and of the inability to find perfect solutions. However, strategies for guiding researchers on which methods to use still are being created, and experience with key issues (such as how to build trust) is limited. This scenario underscores the need for continuous evolution of closer links between systems thinking and participatory methods. Chapter 4 of this monograph considers participatory methods in greater detail and describes their critical role in systems organization and management.

Application of Systems Thinking in Tobacco Control

Systems thinking approaches are by their very nature context dependent. Public health issues such as tobacco control provide an ideal laboratory for their implementation. The next section describes several frameworks for understanding systems thinking and presents a brief overview of the vast terrain of systems concepts, suggests an integrated view of the idea of systems thinking that is emerging in part from the

work conducted in this project, and outlines some of the implications of systems thinking for three key stakeholder groups in tobacco control—practitioners, policy makers, and researchers.

Case Studies of Systems Approaches

On a practical level, stakeholders certainly will question how systems thinking and systems approaches apply to real-life situations they regularly encounter. Each of the approaches, either in part or in combination, provides promising methods for tackling the sometimes disparate problems faced by various stakeholder groups. The next three subsections present some of the "real-world" questions several groups of tobacco control stakeholders might pose about their most pressing issues. Here, three stakeholder groups that are especially important for early implementation of systems thinking and approaches in tobacco control are considered:

1. **Practitioners:** Stakeholders and managers of "agencies" that deliver state or local programs for prevention and cessation of tobacco use.

2. **Researchers:** Scientists and analysts who develop the evidence base for effective tobacco control, such as heads of research institutes or those working at the interface of tobacco control programs and research.

3. **Policy makers:** Politicians and national agency executives who make decisions about policy and strategy.

ISIS and the Practitioner

Practitioners often represent the front line in delivering tobacco control interventions to individuals and populations. The following questions suggest practitioner issues that could be addressed via systems approaches.

- **How can I cope with competition from other organizations for scarce resources?** Funding is almost always a concern for practitioners. The changing political climate and the previous successes of tobacco control efforts make it difficult for practitioners to argue effectively for resources that often are scarce. Practitioners frequently are faced with competition from similar organizations and must find a balance between effectively stating a need for funding and presenting their organization and previous accomplishments positively.

- **How do I communicate the positive outcomes my organization has achieved while arguing for continued/ additional funding?** When applying for a continuation of funds, practitioner organizations face a dilemma. The program must appear to be effective, yet justify the need for continued work. This is a common issue in which practitioners and policy makers interface. It is particularly salient in the evidence-based environment of tobacco control efforts.

- **How can I maintain trust with my clients when changes in funding levels alter the services I am able to provide?** Practitioners committed to tobacco control and to their clientele may find it difficult to reduce or restrict services they view as necessary. Frequently, little notice is given when changes occur. Practitioners must be prepared to communicate "bad news" to smokers and other clients who rely on their services and who may feel unimportant, frustrated, and angry. Decisions about the changing nature of services often are made outside the organization, and practitioners may feel as though they are voiceless in the policy arena.

- **How can I spend more time in the field and less time with administrative details?** The effects of top-down decision making also are evident in the amount of bureaucratic paperwork that requires increasingly more of the practitioner's time. In an attempt to ensure that money is being spent only on high-quality, effective programs, policy makers frequently require increased reporting from funded agencies. These requirements often take valuable time away from the "real work" that needs to be accomplished. Moreover, it may seem as though more time is spent reporting on what is being done than on doing anything to help smokers. This situation is especially frustrating when funding levels are reduced or when increased reporting responsibilities accompany reductions in funding.

- **Where can I find succinct, clear, and practical information on best practices?** Because of the limited time practitioners often have to accomplish their goals, keeping abreast of the latest research discoveries and finding information relevant to the practitioner's organization can be particularly difficult. Research journals are designed for researchers rather than practitioners and often are not organized for simple access to knowledge.

ISIS and the Researcher

Researchers play a key role in developing the evidence base and underlying science behind tobacco control efforts. The following questions present researcher issues that could be addressed via systems approaches.

- **How do we keep our research from sitting unread in journals?** Academic institutions place a high value on publications in peer-reviewed journals and frequently discount writing that is geared toward practitioners. Taking the time to write for a more general audience is not highly valued, and researchers often are pressed for time. Research discoveries are shared with other researchers from similar fields in journals or at conferences, but the ideas are rarely put into practice.

- **Why don't more people use the science that we develop?** Researchers often work in isolated groups and do not have access to practitioners and others who might put their work into practice. Although dissemination often is a goal, the existing pathways of dissemination are not highly effective. Moreover, as described here, practitioners frequently have trouble finding time to keep abreast of research. At a deeper level, research may not connect with the immediate goals and priorities of practitioners.

- **Where can we connect with other researchers who have common or complementary interests but are in different departments or fields?** In addition to dealing with weak networks between researchers and practitioners, researchers often struggle to make connections with other researchers outside their primary disciplines. Although tobacco control is a transdisciplinary field that relies on knowledge from a wide variety of areas, it often is difficult to identify appropriate collaborators with different backgrounds.

At another level, even though funding agencies are increasingly interested in transdisciplinary collaborations, partnerships are difficult to form in an environment in which research silos are the predominant force. Collaborations traditionally have been formed by researchers who work in the same field, read the same journals, and attend the same conferences. The changing environment makes the development of extended, well-funded networks a challenge for ongoing research.

- **How can we streamline the process of approval and funding for our work?** Large funding bodies make it more difficult for individual researchers and laboratories to obtain funding, because their focus increasingly shifts toward funding large-scale projects involving multiple principal investigators. Such projects require (1) a great deal of logistical support, not only to conduct the project, but also to organize proposals and apply for funding; (2) a high level of understanding of the needs of the target population; and (3) the ability to adequately articulate practical implications of the research to the funding organizations.

ISIS and the Policy Maker

Policy makers not only provide leadership among tobacco control stakeholders groups, but also play a key role in the funding decisions and policy interventions that are increasingly becoming central to tobacco control efforts. The following questions focus on policy maker issues that could be addressed via systems approaches.

- **What priorities dictated past resource allocation, and what priorities does the future dictate?** Policy makers, as the primary source of funding for both research and tobacco control programs, have the unique role of bridging both research and practice. Financial implications are at the forefront of many decisions and are a critical concern for most policy makers.

- **How can we get more "bang for our buck" in research expenditures?** The changing tobacco control environment alters the amount of funding available and places limitations on how available funds can be spent. Lessons learned must be considered when decisions about future allocations are made, and the available money must be stretched to cover many pressing needs.

- **How can we synthesize all of the "silos" of information out there?** To accomplish more for less, research endeavors need to be more streamlined and collaboration across disciplines must increase. There is a constant struggle between the desire to fund short-term projects with immediate results versus longitudinal projects that explore long-term health outcomes.

- **How can we reduce or eliminate duplication of effort among stakeholder organizations?** Coordinating the sharing of resources and information also is a struggle for practitioners. Policy makers have the responsibility to ensure that efforts are not duplicated and that ineffective practices are not implemented.

- **How can we persuade more professionals to make use of evidence-based practices?** Holding organizations accountable and requiring reporting are the tools policy makers use to address these concerns. However, organizations frequently complain that they do not have the time or resources to conduct complex evaluations that will provide the necessary information. Without proper evaluations, policy makers cannot determine whether funds are wisely spent, whether organizations are achieving desired outcomes, or whether best practices are being used.

From Stakeholders to Synthesis

Questions such as those discussed previously highlight issues of concern to specific stakeholders in tobacco control. Systems approaches hold the potential to address these issues. However, they also speak to a much broader area, moving from an environment of "What's in it for me?" to one in which professionals have sufficient understanding of their own systems to ask, "What's in it for all of us?" With improved linkage, visibility, and participation—driven by approaches such as systems models, networks, and knowledge bases—stakeholders such as those discussed here have the potential to address broader questions:

- How can we engage the public generally and people at risk from smoking to build a consensus agenda for how best to reduce smoking prevalence and tobacco consumption?

- How can we link our efforts to work more efficiently?

- How can we learn from each other's knowledge to forge better solutions to the problems we address?

- How can we better integrate research and practice?

Within the answers to such questions are the keys to realizing the potential of systems approaches to make substantive change in tobacco control, while at the same time addressing individual stakeholder issues such as those outlined here. The lesson of many systems, whether they are successful organizations or natural ecosystems, is that fundamental interconnectedness is, unto itself, critical to achieving successful outcomes. A major aim in the ISIS project was to combine systems approaches that address specific needs by setting a much broader goal, namely, the linkage of these approaches and their communities of interest into a new tobacco control environment that holds a much greater benefit for all parties.

Summary

The current tobacco control environment consists of a broad mosaic of individuals and organizations with a common goal of reducing smoking prevalence and tobacco consumption and associated morbidity and mortality. The path to this goal still suffers from a gap in the linkage between current science and clinical and public health practice. The general premise offered here is that integrated systems thinking, approaches, and methods can help fill this gap. The application of systems thinking to tobacco control holds the promise of an integrated, dynamic process with several potential benefits, including the following:

- Development of clearer, collaborative relationships within the tobacco control community

- Improved alignment of resources and networks toward effective, evidence-based practices

- More efficient, nonduplicating use of resources

- Better understanding of the impact of tobacco control activities on public health outcomes

One goal of ISIS was to examine and explore the integration of four key approaches to systems thinking—systems organizing, system dynamics modeling, network analysis, and knowledge management. Such an effort, while potentially useful for many issues, may be especially apt for helping to create an integrated framework that will facilitate efficient and effective dissemination and implementation of evidence-based tobacco control practices. One hope is that efforts of ISIS will contribute to the foundation extant in the *Guide to Clinical Preventive Services*[81] and *Guide to Community Preventive Services*[82] and existing dissemination efforts to create a new, scientific, integrated systems approach to evidence-based public health practice. This would involve a shift in approach—one that seeks to transform a profession, not just to integrate methodologies. With this in mind, the role of ISIS could be framed with the following arguments:

- Tobacco control is at a crossroads, with many tasks accomplished, but difficult and complex challenges lie ahead.

- Approaches that are known to work are not being adopted in practice,[83] despite significant efforts. One hypothesis is that tobacco control efforts have not succeeded because the systems of research and the systems of practice do not intersect effectively.

- To reach the next level of outcomes, professionals in the system have to work more effectively and efficiently as a system. The most significant challenges today are systems challenges.

- Therefore, a goal of ISIS was to transform tobacco control by addressing systems issues to encourage more effective integration of research and practice and dramatically improve health outcomes.

Applying systems thinking to more effectively integrate the systems of research and practice is key to achieving more effective use of science in tobacco control initiatives and, more important, within public health as a whole. The chapters that follow outline in detail the specific systems approaches and methodologies studied in the ISIS project. Collectively, they point to a new and more comprehensive view of the field— as a systems problem that can be addressed by using systems approaches to achieve dramatic improvements in outcomes.

Conclusions

1. The key challenges in tobacco control and public health today are fundamentally systems problems, involving multiple forces and stakeholders. Systems thinking is an innovative approach to address these challenges and improve health outcomes.

2. Numerous frameworks exist for systems thinking, a concept that encompasses a

broad synthesis of systems approaches. These approaches provide a theoretical basis for applying specific systems methods, such as system dynamics modeling, structured conceptualization, and network analysis.

3. The Initiative on the Study and Implementation of Systems encompassed four key areas of systems thinking, and their integration: how people organize (managing and organizing as a system); how people understand dynamic complexity (system dynamics modeling); who people are (network analysis); and what people know (knowledge management and knowledge transfer).

4. Examination of systems approaches has the potential to address key questions and problems faced by the various stakeholder groups involved in tobacco control.

5. Potential benefits of systems thinking in tobacco control include improving collaboration among stakeholders; harnessing resources toward evidence-based practice; eliminating duplication of effort; and gaining deeper knowledge about the impact of tobacco control activities.

References

1. Centers for Disease Control and Prevention. 2005. Syndemics overview: When is it appropriate or inappropriate to use a syndemic orientation? Atlanta: U.S. Department of Health and Human Services, Centers for Disease Control and Prevention, National Center for Chronic Disease Prevention and Health Promotion, Syndemics Prevention Network. http://www.cdc.gov/syndemics/overview-uses.htm.

2. Merriam-Webster Online Dictionary. 2006. http://www.m-w.com/dictionary/system (object name system).

3. von Bertalanffy, L. 1975. *Perspectives on general system theory: Scientific-philosophical studies,* ed. E. Taschdjian. New York: Braziller.

4. von Bertalanffy, L. 1968. *General system theory: Foundations, development, applications.* New York: George Braziller.

5. Hoffman, W. C. 1998. The topology of wholes, parts and their perception-cognition. *Psycoloquy* 9 (3). http://psycprints.ecs.soton.ac.uk/archive/00000552.

6. Capra, F. 1994. From the parts to the whole: Systems thinking in ecology and education. Berkeley, CA: Center for Ecoliteracy.

7. Capra, F. 1995. *Characteristics of systems thinking.* Audiocassette. Big Sur, CA: Dolphin Tapes.

8. Aristotle. 1991. *The metaphysics.* New trans. by J. H. McMahon. Amherst, NY: Prometheus Books.

9. Senge, P. M. 1994. *The fifth discipline: The art and practice of the learning organization.* New York: Currency.

10. Gharajedaghi, J. 1999. *Systems thinking: Managing chaos and complexity; A platform for designing business architecture.* Burlington, MA: Elsevier/Butterworth-Heinemann.

11. Sterman, J. D. 2000. *Business dynamics: Systems thinking and modeling for a complex world.* New York: McGraw-Hill/Irwin.

12. Sweeney, L. B., and J. D. Sterman. 2000. Bathtub dynamics: Initial results of a systems thinking inventory. *System Dynamics Review* 16 (4): 249–86.

13. Zalewski, J., ed. 1996. *Real-time systems education.* Los Alamitos, CA: IEEE Computer Society Press.

14. Sanders, T. I., and J. A. McCabe. 2003. *The use of complexity science: A survey of federal departments and agencies, private foundations, universities, and independent education and research centers. A report to the U.S. Department of Education.* Washington, DC: Washington Center for Complexity and Public Policy.

15. Bar-Yam, M., K. Rhoades, L. B. Sweeney, J. Kaput, and Y. Bar-Yam. 2003. Complex systems perspectives on education and the education system. http://nesci.org/projects/edresearch/index.html.

16. McMaster, G. 2003. Complexity science and reforming education. Alberta: Univ. of Alberta, Department of Education. http://www.uofaweb.ualberta.ca/education/news.cfm?story=20726.

17. Davies, L. 2004. *Education and conflict: Complexity and chaos.* New York: RoutledgeFalmer.

18. Kaput, J., Y. Bar-Yam, M. Jacobson, E. Jakobsson, J. Lemke, and U. Wilensky. 2003. *Planning a national initiative on complex systems in K–16 education.* Cambridge, MA: New England Complex Systems Institute.

19. Schwarz, E. 2001. *Some streams of systemic thought.* Neuchâtel, Switzerland: International Institute for General Systems Studies. http://www.iigss.net/gPICT.jpg.

20. International Institute for General Systems Studies. 2005. Genealogy: A family tree of systemic thinking. http://www.iigss.net.

21. von Bertalanffy, L., and P. A. LaViolette. 1981. *A systems view of man.* Boulder, CO: Westview Press.

22. von Bertalanffy, L. 1933. *Modern theories of development: An introduction to theoretical biology.* Trans. J. H. Woodger. London: Oxford Univ. Press.

23. von Bertalanffy, L. 1968. *The organismic psychology and systems theory.* Heinz Werner lectures. Worcester, MA: Clark Univ. Press.

24. Capra, F., and B. D. Steindl-Rast. 1993. *New paradigm thinking.* Audiocassette. San Francisco: New Dimensions Foundation.

25. Capra, F. 1991. *MindWalk: A film for passionate thinkers.* Hollywood: Paramount.

26. Capra, F. 1997. *The web of life: A new scientific understanding of living systems.* New York: Anchor Books.

27. Laszlo, E. 1996. *The systems view of the world: A holistic vision for our time.* Cresskill, NJ: Hampton Press.

28. Cabrera, D. 2001. *Remedial genius: Thinking and learning using the patterns of knowledge.* Loveland, CO: Project N Press.

29. Capra, F. 1991. *The turning point: A transformative vision for an ecological age.* Audiocassette. Emeryville, CA: Enhanced Audio Systems.

30. Capra, F. 1998. Ecology, systems thinking and project-based learning. Talk presented at the sixth annual conference on project-based learning of the Autodesk Foundation, San Francisco.

31. Petrina, S. 1993. Under the corporate thumb: Troubles with our MATE (Modular Approach to Technology Education). *Journal of Technology Education* 1 (5).

http://scholar.lib.vt.edu/ejournals/JTE/v5n1/petrina.jte-v5n1.html.

32. Forrester, J. W. 1971. *World dynamics.* 2nd ed. Waltham, MA: Pegasus Communications.

33. Kauffman, S. A. 1995. *At home in the universe: The search for the laws of self-organization and complexity.* New York: Oxford Univ. Press.

34. Checkland, P. 1985. From optimizing to learning: A development of systems thinking for the 1990s. *Journal of the Operational Research Society* 36 (9): 757–67.

35. Maturana, H. R. 1992. *The tree of knowledge: The biological roots of human understanding.* Rev. ed. Ed. F. J. Varela and R. Paolucci. Boston: Shambala.

36. Bateson, G. 1972. *Steps to an ecology of mind.* New York: Ballantine Books. Repr. with foreword by M. C. Bateson. 2000. Chicago: Univ. of Chicago Press.

37. Cabrera, D. 2002. Patterns of knowledge: Knowledge as a complex, evolutionary system; An educational imperative. In *Creating learning communities,* ed. R. Miller. Brandon, VT: Solomon Press.

38. Gell-Mann, M. 2003. *The quark and the jaguar: Adventures in the simple and the complex.* New York: W. H. Freeman.

39. Pines, D., ed. 1988. *Emerging synthesis in science: Proceedings of the founding workshops of the Santa Fe Institute.* Vol. 1. Reading, MA: Addison-Wesley.

40. Kauffman, S. A. 1993. *The origins of order: Self-organization and selection in evolution.* New York: Oxford Univ. Press.

41. Gell-Mann, M. 1995–96. Let's call it plectics. *Complexity* 1 (5): 3.

42. Gleick, J. 1988. *Chaos: Making a new science.* Repr. ed. New York: Penguin.

43. Strogatz, S. H. 1994. *Nonlinear dynamics and chaos: With applications in physics, biology, chemistry, and engineering (studies in nonlinearity).* Reading, MA: Addison-Wesley.

44. Young, J. F. 1969. *Cybernetics.* London: Iliffe Books.

45. Wolfram, S. 2002. *A new kind of science.* Champaign, IL: Wolfram Media.

46. Kitano, H. 2002. Computational systems biology. *Nature* 420 (6912): 206–10.

47. Watts, D. J. 1999. *Small worlds: The dynamics of networks between order and randomness.* Princeton: Princeton Univ. Press.

48. Watts, D. J. 2003. *Six degrees: The science of a connected age.* New York: Norton.

49. Strogatz, S. H. 2003. *Sync: The emerging science of spontaneous order.* New York: Hyperion.

50. Newman, M. E. J. 2003. The structure and function of complex networks. *SIAM Review* 45 (2): 167–256.

51. Maturana, H. R., and F. J. Varela. 1980. *Autopoiesis and cognition: The realization of the living.* Vol. 42. Boston: D. Reidel.

52. Waldrop, M. M. 1992. *Complexity: The emerging science at the edge of order and chaos.* New York: Simon and Schuster.

53. Johnson, S. 2001. *Emergence: The connected lives of ants, brains, cities, and software.* New York: Simon and Schuster Adult Publishing Group.

54. Mandelbrot, B. B. 1982. *The fractal geometry of nature.* New York: W. H. Freeman.

55. Collins, J. C., and J. I. Porras. 1994. *Built to last: Successful habits of visionary companies.* New York: HarperBusiness.

56. Gell-Mann, M. 1987. The concept of the institute. In *Emerging syntheses in science: Proceedings of the founding workshops of the Santa Fe Institute,* 1–15. Reading, MA: Addison-Wesley.

57. Nietzsche, F. W. 1995. *The birth of tragedy.* New York: Dover Publications.

58. Forrester, J. W. 1961. *Industrial dynamics.* Waltham, MA: Pegasus Communications.

59. Richmond, B. 2000. *The "thinking" in systems thinking: Seven essential skills.* Toolbox Reprint series. Waltham, MA: Pegasus Communications.

60. Haines, S. G. 1999. *The manager's pocket guide to systems thinking and learning.* Amherst, MA: Human Resource Development Press.

61. Weinberg, G. M. 2001. *An introduction to general systems thinking.* Silver anniv. ed. New York: Dorset House.

62. Anderson, V., and L. Johnson. 1997. *Systems thinking basics: From concepts to causal loops.* Waltham, MA: Pegasus Communications.

63. Senge, P. M. 1994. *The fifth discipline fieldbook: Strategies and tools for building a learning organization.* New York: Currency.

64. Sherwood, D. 2002. *Seeing the forest for the trees: A manager's guide to applying systems thinking.* London: Nicholas Brealey.

65. Forrester, J. R. 2004. Systems dynamics—System thinking. http://www.valuebasedmanagement.net/methods_forrester_system_dynamics.html.

66. Senge, P. 2004. Five disciplines. http://www.valuebasedmanagement.net/methods_senge_five_disciplines.html.

67. Gelb, M. 1998. *How to think like Leonardo da Vinci: Seven steps to genius every day.* New York: Delacorte Press.

68. Gelb, M. 2004. *How to think like Leonardo da Vinci.* New York: Random House. http://www.michaelgelb.com.

69. Mathison, S. 2004. *Encyclopedia of evaluation.* Thousand Oaks, CA: Sage.

70. Checkland, P. 1981. *Systems thinking, systems practice.* Chichester, UK: John Wiley and Sons.

71. Holland, J. H. 1996. *Hidden order: How adaptation builds complexity.* Reading, MA: Addison-Wesley.

72. von Neumann, J. 1966. *The theory of self-reproducing automata.* Ed. A. W. Burks. Urbana: Univ. of Illinois Press.

73. Barabási, A. L., and E. Bonabeau. 2003. Scale-free networks. *Scientific American* 288 (5): 60–69.

74. Strogatz, S. H. 2001. Exploring complex networks. *Nature* 410 (March 8): 268–76.

75. Krygiel, A. J. 1999. *Behind the wizard's curtain: An integration environment for a system of systems.* Washington, DC: Institute for National Strategic Studies.

76. Bammer, G. 2005. Integration and implementation sciences: Building a new specialization. *Ecology and Society* 10 (2): 6. http://www.ecologyandsociety.org/vol10/iss2/art6.

77. Phelan, S. E. 1999. A note on the correspondence between complexity and systems theory. *Systems Practice and Action Research* 12 (3): 237–46.

78. World Health Organization. 2002. The world health report 2002: Reducing risks, promoting healthy life. http://www.who.int/whr/2002/en/.

79. Brown, L. D., G. Bammer, S. Batliwala, and F. Kunreuther. 2003. Framing practice-research engagement for democratizing knowledge. *Action Research* 1 (1): 81–102.

80. Moore, C. M. 1987. *Group techniques for idea building (applied social research methods).* Thousand Oaks, CA: Sage.

81. Agency for Healthcare Research and Quality. 2005. *Guide to clinical preventive services.* Rockville, MD: U.S. Department of Health and Human Services, Agency for Healthcare Research and Quality. http://www.ahrq.gov/clinic/cps3dix.htm.

82. Centers for Disease Control and Prevention. 2005. *Guide to community preventive services.* Atlanta: Department of Health and Human Services, Centers for Disease Control and Prevention, National Center for Health Marketing, Community Guide Branch. http://thecommunityguide.org.

83. Institute of Medicine. 2001. *Crossing the quality chasm: A new health system for the 21st century.* Washington, DC: National Academies Press.

How to Organize: Systems Organizing

Unlocking the promise of systems approaches in tobacco control requires a participatory, collaborative environment among stakeholders. This in turn requires a fresh approach to management, leadership, and interactions in and between organizations. This chapter describes an adaptive systems view of organizing that represents a well-documented evolution in management theory and serves as a cornerstone to implementation of systems methods and approaches.

The chapter reviews the evolving field of management theory and explores possible changes in traditional management theory with the addition of a systems perspective. It proposes a model for facilitating and organizing purposeful and adaptive organizations and describes associated "systems-friendly" methods that researchers and practitioners can use. The framework for the model includes four major interrelated dimensions:

- Vision: *From leading and managing to facilitating and empowering*

- Structure: *From organizing to self-organizing*

- Action: *From delegation to participation*

- Learning: *From discrete evaluation to continuous evaluation*

The chapter presents two real-world case studies that use concept mapping, a method for organizing participatory systems, to address two tobacco control issues: integration of research and practice and development of criteria for high-quality state and local initiatives to control tobacco use.

Science is organized knowledge. Wisdom is organized life.

—Attributed to Immanuel Kant (1724–1804)

Introduction

The springboard for this chapter is the premise that traditional approaches to management will not be sufficient to address the complex environment of systems in tobacco control specifically and public health generally in the twenty-first century. Traditional management theory is predicated on the notion of the corporation and focuses primarily on command and control using hierarchical structures and theories of directive leadership to accomplish planning, implementation, and control functions. These traditional approaches to management are evolving as the complex management challenges of today are addressed.

This chapter also focuses on *how to organize* tobacco control efforts from the viewpoint of systems thinking, and its central purpose is reconciliation of the tension between the idea of a *purposeful organization* and an *adaptive* one. Organizations generally are thought of as purposeful, with goals, vision, and planning toward specific means and ends. Purposeful organizations purportedly do what they were designed to do. However, they might be expected to have greater difficulty adapting to novel situations. In contrast, adaptive organizations are subject to the processes of evolution, with no prescribed purpose, no a priori design, and no rational designer. Both purposeful and adaptive organizations are systems, composed of parts brought into relationship as a whole. Purposeful organizations benefit from the command-and-control structures that bring about goal-seeking activities. Adaptive organisms benefit from the adaptivity that enables survival in unpredictable and changing environments.

This chapter suggests how systems thinking can be used to better understand both types of systems and to incorporate their features into tobacco control efforts. The term *organization* is used in this chapter in a broad "ecological" sense encompassing loose affiliations, traditional organizations, and more complex interorganizational structures, such as coalitions, networks, initiatives, collaborations, and partnerships comprising many distinct organizations.

In chapter 2, tobacco control is shown to be a complex and continually evolving collaboration of stakeholders and organizations that increasingly requires cooperation in networks to accomplish crosscutting tasks. Contemporary practice of public health in general increasingly depends on cross-organizational collaborations and networks to address complex problems. In this increasingly networked environment, member groups come to the table with mixed agendas, competing interests, and often, dramatically different resources and capabilities. Typically, no overarching command-and-control decision structure exists.

Collaborating organizations create their own governance mechanisms and negotiate differences as they evolve. Frequently, the system has a motivating purpose (e.g., desire for greater efficiency, need for better coordination, or intent to concentrate efforts). However, the organizations usually serve voluntarily or because of overt or covert inducements or incentives. In a rapidly changing environment, such systems are extremely fragile, and many do not survive for long. Members can and do leave, and the system changes and either adapts or dissolves when leadership of member organizations changes, strategic interests of key members become threatened, or the political and economic context is dramatically altered. Organization is really about how these complex systems are steered toward a purpose without sacrificing their profoundly powerful adaptive qualities.

Chapter 3 introduces the idea of systems thinking as a more effective approach to understanding and adapting to complexity. In this chapter, systems thinking is viewed as it applies to organizational and management theory. A model and methods for managing from a systems thinking perspective are outlined. A systems approach to management is essential for enabling collaborative networks in tobacco control to organize, learn, and adapt to a rapidly changing environment and to the competitive forces of the continuously subversive and creative tobacco industry.[1] These evolving approaches to management will be required to achieve more effective integration of research and practice, build a tobacco control system with sufficient agility to anticipate and counter strategies of the tobacco industry, efficiently use diminishing resources, and reach the next level of health outcomes in today's public health environment.

Traditional Management Theory

Concepts of management have evolved considerably over the past century. Management experts have arrived at broad agreement on the general contours of the evolution. In approximate chronological order, management theory has progressed through four general phases:[2,3] (1) classical or technical management, (2) humanistic or behavioral perspective, (3) management science or quantitative perspective, and (4) integrative or contemporary management approaches.

Classical or *technical management* originated during the industrial revolution of the late nineteenth and early twentieth centuries. This approach tends to use a mechanistic metaphor, viewing organizations as machines, leaders as engineers, and workers as mechanical parts. It emphasizes (1) the division of labor that divides work into a subseries of basic tasks

and (2) the use of production or assembly lines that incorporate efficient application of technology. Taylor[4] called these strategies "scientific management."

The *humanistic* or *behavioral perspective* arose in the late 1920s through the human relations movement, born of research at the Hawthorne facilities of the Western Electric Company and led by Elton Mayo. In these approaches, the organization is viewed through the behavioral and social sciences, with an emphasis on the concept that workers are people rather than simply parts of a machine. These perspectives include the human relations movement and origins of the fields of organizational development and organizational behavior. The focus generally is on human behaviors, motivation, and the socioemotional factors of organizational life.

The *management science* or *quantitative perspective* originated after World War II. Frequently confused with the classical or technical perspective, this viewpoint was distinctive for its reliance on quantitative modeling as a general approach to management issues. The approach includes the fields of management science, operations research, operations management, and information sciences.

Integrative or *contemporary management theories* tend to combine or integrate across traditional approaches, using each perspective as appropriate. For instance, the contingency perspective argues that the management approach in any organization or situation should be contingent on the circumstances. In this approach, managers adapt methods from classical, behavioral, or quantitative traditions as needed and required.

Most surveys of management theory include systems perspectives within contemporary management theories. This scenario suggests both their recent evolution and the degree to which management is adopting them. The history of management and organization theory supports the contention in this monograph that management theory is evolving to a form that incorporates systems thinking as a major emphasis.

The basic management process as presented in typical courses in management is multiphased. The assumptions are that the organization is the primary unit of management and that such organizations are hierarchical, use command-and-control procedures, and have leaders who initiate and implement planning and control of key processes. This process is described in multiple texts on contemporary management.[2,3] Four functions typically are associated with this traditional view of the management process: planning, organizing, leading, and controlling.

The *planning* function in management emphasizes actions that can achieve goals. Planning typically occurs in a specialized department (planners) and is implemented by the executive team and disseminated to the lower ranks. Planning involves a short-term (often 1 to 2 years or less) or a long-term (5-year) timeline tied to goals and more efficient processes. Planning is conceived as a linear process that proceeds from mission, goals, and objectives to actions and timelines.

The *organizing* function in management involves "…the assignment of tasks, the grouping of tasks into departments, and the assignment of authority and allocation of resources across the organization."[3(p7)] Organizing also includes allocation of resources and authority into hierarchical levels and often is associated with individuals or departments (organizers).

The *leading* function is rooted in the idea of a top-down organization motivated and driven by the passions, foresight, and charisma of its leader. Leadership is thought of as a function of the executive,

and the power to lead is ascribed through status roles, with decreasing power through each lower level. In this view, the leader is metaphorically a driver and the corporation is a well-engineered and well-oiled machine.

The *controlling* function is associated with monitoring activities and making corrections. Specialized individuals or departments (controllers) perform essential control functions. In addition, control frequently is derived from financial or legal structure.

The model of the four-phase management process also is consonant with a long tradition in planning and evaluation that construes the basic planning–evaluation cycle as consisting of three phases— planning, implementation, and evaluation.[5] In this model, the *planning* function is retained, the two functions of organizing and leading are integrated into the broader function of *implementing,* and the term *evaluation* is substituted for the related "controlling function."

The four functions of management theory are derived from a number of assumptions about how organizations work. The organization is viewed as a type of machine, driven and directed by one or more leaders, in which ideas, resource allocation, power, and information flows are pushed through the hierarchical levels. The metaphor of a machine is a derivative of the time and thinking in which the classical management theory was developed—the preindustrial and industrial ages. Power is allocated by positions of ascribed status in a hierarchical structure that is broad at the base and small and exclusive at the pinnacle. Organizations are controlled by controllers; strategy and execution could be planned by planners, managed by managers, and led by leaders; specialization yields efficiency; and little crossover of duties or roles exists. The four functions are related to common descriptors in table 4.1.

Table 4.1 Four Functions of Classical Management Theory and Descriptors

Management function	Descriptors
Planning	<ul><li>Leadership driven and vision of leader enforced</li><li>Motivation through charisma of leadership team</li></ul>
Organizing	<ul><li>Goal oriented, efficiency centered, hierarchical</li><li>Agenda set by planners</li><li>Exclusive planning process, few executives/planners, 1- to 5-year plans, and planning department</li><li>Structured</li><li>Starts with mission, goals, objectives, and timeline</li></ul>
Leading	<ul><li>Assignment of tasks and grouping of tasks into departments</li><li>Allocation of resources and authority</li><li>Hierarchical</li></ul>
Controlling	<ul><li>Activities monitored and corrections made</li><li>Departmental function</li><li>Hierarchical</li><li>Exercise of control at regular intervals</li></ul>

This management paradigm yielded results that were judged as positive by those who benefited. The Industrial Revolution owes its dominance to the classical management approach, but times are changing. The world's peoples and nations are increasingly more interconnected and interdependent as the result of globalization. Information flows rapidly in many directions. Organized arrangements are more complex. Traditional command-and-control structures are difficult to establish and maintain. Even the relationship between employee and employer has been reframed so that both intrinsic and extrinsic motivations and motivational strategies are different. Chapter 2 of this monograph presents the recent evolution of tobacco control and points to the need for new models that deal with systems issues. Systems thinking offers promising extensions to a classical management theory that is not adequate to handle these complexities.

Systems Organizing Model

Moving tobacco control toward a systems approach to management does not mean abandonment of the traditional functions of management. Some degree of planning, organizing, leading, and controlling, or alternatively, planning, implementation, and evaluation, will always be required in organizations. A new model is offered here that integrates the advantages of the traditional and the systems views of organizations and enables leaders or agents to deal flexibly with myriad organizational contexts. A continuum ranging from the traditional management model to a systems organizing model is envisioned. This model is based on four principles (**v**ision, **s**tructure, **a**ction, and **l**earning [VSAL]) that enable movement between these two hypothetical end points, as a bead moves on a string (figure 4.1). The VSAL model is adapted from Cabrera's "operating system"[6] and is offered here as an organizing framework for its utility and applicability in managing complex systems.

Using these four principles, organizational leaders may choose a balance of traditional approaches (such as leadership, management, delegation, organized structures, and discrete evaluations) and systems approaches (such as facilitation and empowerment, self-organizing structures, participatory action, and continuous

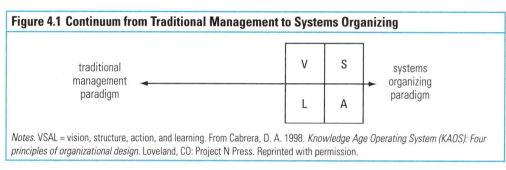

Figure 4.1 Continuum from Traditional Management to Systems Organizing

traditional management paradigm ←————————————→ systems organizing paradigm

V	S
L	A

Notes. VSAL = vision, structure, action, and learning. From Cabrera, D. A. 1998. *Knowledge Age Operating System (KAOS): Four principles of organizational design.* Loveland, CO: Project N Press. Reprinted with permission.

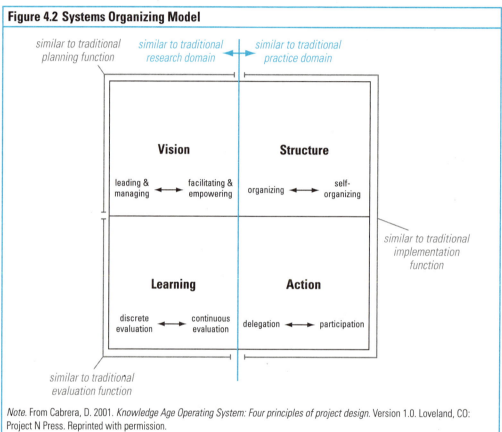

Figure 4.2 Systems Organizing Model

similar to traditional planning function   *similar to traditional research domain* ←→ *similar to traditional practice domain*

Vision

leading & managing ←→ facilitating & empowering

Structure

organizing ←→ self-organizing

similar to traditional implementation function

Learning

discrete evaluation ←→ continuous evaluation

Action

delegation ←→ participation

similar to traditional evaluation function

Note. From Cabrera, D. 2001. *Knowledge Age Operating System: Four principles of project design.* Version 1.0. Loveland, CO: Project N Press. Reprinted with permission.

evaluation), depending on the context and circumstances. This "systems organizing" model is compatible with both traditional and systems perspectives (figure 4.2). The continua within each principle illustrate how a leader has the freedom to move among positions on the four continua much as one tunes the equalizer on a stereo, matching the organizational situation to a particular style for each of the principles.

However, because of the uniqueness and complexity of the interorganizational structures of contemporary tobacco control initiatives, much of value will be found in the systems organizing end of the continuum. This is not to say that the systems approach eclipses the traditional approach. In many organizations, a top-down, leader-centered, command-and-control structure is ideal, and subsystems better suited to more traditional approaches may exist within the larger tobacco control network. However, as was illustrated in chapter 2, tobacco control efforts typically have many interorganizational parts, each with its own policies, culture, history, expertise, and methods. To manage such a system from a traditional approach is to neutralize the system's most potent advantages—diversity, adaptivity, self-organization, and creativity.

The systems organizing model shown in figure 4.2 has four principles: vision, structure, action, and learning. Each of these principles is associated with a different continuum. On the left side of each continuum is a descriptor of that principle from a traditional view. On the right side is a descriptor associated with a systems view as follows:

- Vision: From leading and managing to facilitating and empowering

- Structure: From organizing to self-organizing

- Action: From delegation to participation

- Learning: From discrete evaluation to continuous evaluation

The four principles can be thought of as similar to the traditional progression of planning, implementation, and evaluation. In figure 4.2, the planning, implementation, and evaluation functions are depicted by the outer lines that enclose the VSAL boxes. Therefore, vision is associated with the traditional planning function; learning, with the traditional evaluation function; and structure and action, with the traditional implementation function. These similarities help ease the transition from a traditional linear model to a continuous systems model, but they also may hinder an understanding of the integrated nature of systems organizing. The traditional model of planning, implementation, and evaluation

is a linear and discrete progression usually performed by "experts": planning comes first, then implementation, then evaluation. In the systems organizing model, planning, implementation, and evaluation can occur throughout the system, continuously over time; they are not the private domain of expert planners or evaluators.

Likewise, there are similarities between the systems organizing model and the traditional domains of research and practice. The center line in figure 4.2 distinguishes between the traditional research domain (vision and learning) and the traditional practice domain (structure and action). Because VSAL is an integrated model, these distinctions are relatively unimportant. However, it is relevant that there are areas in common between traditional functions and the newer systems organizing model. The traditional view assumes that (1) research is distinctly separate from practice, (2) research is the driver of practice, and (3) research and practice are the domains of specialized experts. In contrast, the systems organizing model makes no such distinctions. An organization is just as likely to benefit from evidence-based practice as from practice-based research. The boundaries between planning, implementation, and evaluation and between research and practice are blurred in the systems organizing model.

Both the traditional and systems models have four interrelated components. In the traditional management process, the four components are considered to be management *functions*. However, in the systems organizing model, they are more analogous to *principles*. It is tempting to assume that the planning, organizing, leading, and evaluating functions are analogous to the VSAL principles. Although these functions appear to be similar, they are subtly and importantly different. For example, consider the following descriptions of the four functions of traditional management (table 4.1):

- Planning: Select goals and ways to attain them

- Organizing: Assign responsibility for accomplishment of tasks

- Leading: Use influence to motivate

- Controlling: Monitor activities and make corrections

The perspective of each function is leader–follower centered. A *leader* selects goals, assigns responsibilities to followers, uses influence to motivate followers, and monitors activities and makes corrections. The traditional management functions are based on leadership and management, because the assumption is that leaders and managers can direct, delegate, motivate, and control their organizations. Thus, although traditional functions and systems principles appear to be similar, they are not similar. The systems principles are *agent–system* centered, rather than *leader–follower* centered. For example, the vision principle does not live in the private domain of people at the top of the organization. Any agent in the system can possess and be directed by a vision. Consider, for example, that many innovations in science and society do not "trickle down from the top." Instead, they "percolate up from the bottom." Another

key difference between the traditional and systems views is the role of "thinking" versus "doing," which is alternatively an alias for "ideal versus real" or "research versus practice." In the traditional paradigm, these functions are differentiated, whereas in the systems paradigm, they are integrated.

In general, contemporary tobacco control efforts are likely to be better served by systems perspectives toward the right side of these continua. The proposed location of tobacco control initiatives is depicted in figure 4.3. Likewise, most tobacco control efforts are better served by the right side of the specific continua associated with VSAL (figure 4.2).

Same but Different

Within a systems organizing context, the traditional roles of planning, organizing, leading, and controlling take on a different perspective:

- The traditional *planning* function is goal oriented, with an emphasis on actions that can achieve leader-defined goals. Reaching organizational goals is predicated on a paradigm centered on leaders and followers, in which the leader

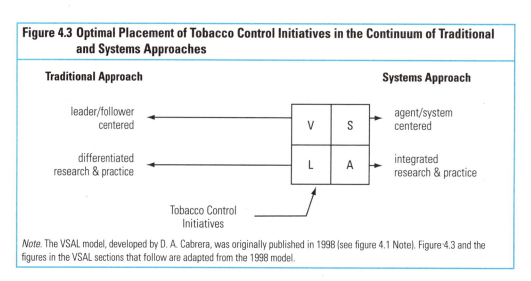

Figure 4.3 Optimal Placement of Tobacco Control Initiatives in the Continuum of Traditional and Systems Approaches

Note. The VSAL model, developed by D. A. Cabrera, was originally published in 1998 (see figure 4.1 Note). Figure 4.3 and the figures in the VSAL sections that follow are adapted from the 1998 model.

sets the goals and motivates, organizes, and controls followers. In the systems organizing perspective, leaders become more like facilitators. The focus is shifted to a principle of collaboratively developed vision, suggesting a more collective sense of purpose.

- The *organizing* function in traditional management involves "…the assignment of tasks, the grouping of tasks into departments, and the assignment of authority and allocation of resources across the organization."[3] In a systems organizing perspective, the emphasis is shifted to include both purposefully organized structure and provision for self-organizing structures.

- The traditional *leading* function, which is described as "using influence to motivate," has been transformed to an *agent-centered* principle. Individual agents of a system are not thought of as inert bodies waiting for a leader to delegate and motivate them to action. Instead, they are self-motivated individuals or organizations alternatively capable of motivating other agents and driven by internal goals and constraints. Agents are not merely active; they also are participatory.

- Finally, the *controlling* or *evaluation* function in the traditional model is transformed into agent and systemwide *learning*. Evaluation is not merely a discrete and linear process accomplished by impact assessments or by counting outcomes. Instead, evaluation is a continuous process of evaluative feedback that is critical to adaptation, creativity, innovation, and survival.

Other subtle differences exist between the two approaches. First, in the systems organizing model, these categories are not discrete, whereas in the traditional management model they are discrete. The principles of systems organizing are

themselves a system, so the four systems organizing principles are integrally interconnected.

Second, systems organizing principles have no set order, whereas there is an assumed phasing of the four traditional management functions. In a systems organizing model, participants may self-organize, learn together, and then realize they are working toward a common vision. In addition, agents may develop a common vision and then self-organize, adapt, and learn who needs to take what action to achieve the vision. The VSAL sections that follow describe a family of potentially useful methodological models that could be used to manage the four principles of systems organizing.

Third, the systems organizing model, like its traditional predecessor, also is related to the three phases of planning, implementation, and evaluation.[5] However, a systems perspective transforms the meaning of these three functions. Like the four principles, they are not discrete and/or sequential; they can be entered into in any sequence. Sometimes one implements and then learns; in other situations, one may evaluate and then implement. The three functions are continually interacting.

Finally, the systems organizing model explicitly incorporates the ideas of research and practice. In general, the traditional view of research is associated with planning and evaluation, whereas a traditional view of practice is associated with implementation. The dynamic relationship between research and practice in the systems organizing model suggests that systems thinking may help to address the integration of research and practice.

Many aspects of traditional management must be used to effectively manage systems. Consequently, the four principles (vision, structure, action, and learning) can be adapted to a more traditional approach by "moving the slider" to the left on any one of the continua. For example, it is common for a catalytic and influential leader to "have a vision" and then use a more traditional leadership style (e.g., ascribed power or influence) to promote that vision. However, at a critical point, the leader may realize that shifting to more participatory action will better accomplish the vision than will delegating actions to individuals. The four principles allow for this type of transition across each of their dimensions. Some of the differences highlighted here demonstrate the transformation that is occurring in management and that more aptly addresses the complexities of systems environments, especially in tobacco control settings.

It is tempting to describe the systems organizing approach as an "end of the chapter" tool for increasing the understanding of contemporary management. In almost every chapter of every current textbook on management, a future-looking section near the end of the chapter explores the latest thinking in management theory and is populated with phrases such as[3] "new workplace"; "learning organization"; "virtual organization approach"; and "increasing participation in decision making." Such wording gives a glimpse into the future of contemporary management theory. These sections reveal that management thinking is evolving to address a more complex, networked, and dynamic world. The suggestions in this chapter and in the model of systems organizing that is presented are not meant to be antithetical to contemporary management thinking. These suggested approaches seem to be right there, at the end of the chapters of nearly every modern textbook on management.

The following sections discuss each of the four principles and primary methods associated with them. Because all of the principles are interrelated, the methodologies are interrelated as well. Although methods are discussed in connection with specific principles, they should be viewed as crosscutting.

Vision: From Leadership and Management to Facilitation and Empowerment

A collective vision is one that is shared throughout the organization. It is not the exclusive purview of the "leaders" or hierarchy in an organization but is "held" in common by each of the agents in the network. The more agents in a network share the same vision and "see" the same possibilities, the more a system can be said to have a collective vision. The job of a leader is to facilitate the acquisition of a collective vision. Because each agent holds part of the collective vision, each is capable of influencing another agent's vision and, in turn, the whole system. In this way, collective vision takes on three important qualities that are different from the traditional vision.

First, collective vision is *distributed* throughout the network. Second, collective vision is a *dissipative* structure, that is, the structure remains stable despite changing flows through it. This characteristic makes collective visions more durable and timeless, because they are not radically changed by the natural recidivism of the network. Third, collective vision is *adaptive* and *dynamic*. Although the vision is a durable dissipative structure, it also is susceptible to the dynamics of the network and can adapt over time. The systems organizing leader will find that many traditional techniques of planning remain useful in facilitating collective vision. However, he or she should reframe these traditional planning techniques in light of the characteristics of these important changes to the traditional vision (e.g., distributed, dissipative, adaptive, and dynamic).

Vision is not always a *collaborative* process, but it should always be *collective.* Organizational leaders may need to establish a vision. However, one that is not broadly held to be important will have little support and thus lack the necessary support from individual agents. Also, it is not necessary to establish the vision before moving to the other systems organizing principles. A collective vision could be an emergent property of a complex system or the catalyst for a set of discrete agents to self-organize into a network. Some of the methods discussed later in this chapter are well suited for facilitating a collective vision. Systems leaders play a key role in facilitating processes that help agents link local and semiautonomous action (mission) to the collective vision.

The idea of "management," which has the same Greek root as "manipulate" and implies an action "at the hand of" a leader (L. *manus,* hand), is challenged by the evolving paradigm toward systems. The organizational leader does not manage per se but becomes a facilitator of organization (L. *facilis,* to make easier). A leader makes self-organization *easier* by removing constraints on the system, rather than adding them.

In the traditional management framework, planning usually is considered a top-down process with leadership from the highest levels of the organization. This traditional view has been challenged, especially in the area of strategic planning, where it became clear that the planning function often was in conflict with the development of strategy. Mintzberg argues that planning efforts often stifle commitment and innovation and confine the organization and its members.[7] He proposes a model in which planners are more facilitative and supportive, rather than structural and proscriptive. The past decade brought a transformation of the idea of planning along these lines that parallels the shift to systems thinking generally. Historically, planning in large organizations tended to be confined to a department or unit. The planners worked with top management in a tightly structured process that proceeded from the statement of mission and goals to objectives, actions, and delineation of timelines, responsibilities, and costs. Today, planning has evolved into a more collaborative and collective endeavor, in which planners are facilitators, rather than leaders. Moreover, the process itself has shifted from being a goal-oriented exercise to more of an adaptive one.

A broad range of methods and processes can be applied in systems planning to encourage development of a collective vision. Here the territory is briefly sketched, and more detailed descriptions of methodological choices are cited.[8] Many of these strategies fall within the broad rubric of collaborative *needs assessment.*[9] One of the oldest collaborative group methods used in planning is traditional *brainstorming.*[10] The *nominal groups* approach[11] is a structured participatory method in which people work individually to brainstorm and then share ideas. *Focus groups*[12] essentially are a type of group interview to generate ideas in response to a focus prompt or stimulus. The *Delphi technique*[13] began as a relatively delimited, iterative, structured group method of surveying participants and, through feedback of results, moving the group toward consensus. As they evolved, Delphi methods became so broadly defined as to be virtually indistinguishable from any structured collaborative methods for identifying and assessing planning options.

A broad range of planning methods are particularly relevant to the notion that "vision" has as a root the idea of a "visual" model. Visual models involve the construction and use of maps of ideas. Some, such as the *concept-mapping* methods of Novak[14] or Buzan and Buzan's[15] *mind maps,* are primarily tools for use by individuals, although collaborative use may be possible. Explicitly collaborative *concept mapping,*[16] sometimes referred to as structured conceptualization, is a participatory mixed-methods approach that integrates group process activities (brainstorming, unstructured pile sorting, and rating of brainstormed items) with multivariate statistical analyses (multidimensional scaling and hierarchical cluster analysis) to yield both statistical and graphic representations of a conceptual domain. This approach is designed around a well-informed, group-oriented, decision-making process that drives both planning and evaluation. In public health, it has been used to address statewide planning in Delaware[17] and Hawaii,[18] development of an evaluation framework for a center grant initiative of the National Cancer Institute (NCI),[19] and articulation of an expert model of the activities the tobacco industry uses to undercut public health efforts.[1] This concept-mapping method is illustrated in detail in the case study later in this chapter. Other map-based approaches to planning incorporate the idea of causation and consist of sequential paths of expected or predicted activities and outcomes:

- *Strategy maps*[20] pictorially link perspectives in an organization to encourage strategic alignment that leads to greater value.

- *Cognitive maps*[21] are among the earliest causal maps that were widely used.

- *Logic models*[22] are designed to link planning and evaluation by mapping the causal connections between program activities and outputs and outcomes.

- *System dynamics models*[23,24] are causal maps that can be integrated into the planning function. Chapter 5 considers these models in detail.

- *Outcome maps*[25] are ways of depicting the changes in behavior of an individual, group, or organization with which a program or intervention works.

An array of collaborative, participatory methods that have value in the planning function come from the field of organizational development and are used in large-scale efforts toward organizational change. Many are ideal for facilitating and empowering a collective vision. Such methods include the following:

- *Future-search conferences* are events, typically approximately three days in duration, designed to help an organization find an ideal future and aim for it.[26·]

- The *conference model*[27,28] is a comprehensive system designed for a top-to-bottom redesign of an organization. It involves factors such as a customer/supplier conference, vision conference, technical conference, and design conference, across separate two- or three-day events.

- The *large-scale interactive process*[29] is an intervention encompassing mix-and-match table groups of 8 to 10 people usually over approximately three days.

- *Real-time strategic change*[30] is an approach that grew out of Dannemiller and Jacobs's[29] work in large-group interventions and also is used to implement organization-wide change, as the beginning of a process that aims to change the way an organization works, rather than planning only one event.

- *Participative work redesign*[31] emphasizes a democratic approach to job design, in which the people who do the work determine how it should be done, in groups of 8 to 10. It often follows a search conference, and the vision for the future of the organization frequently is established before this event occurs.

- *Open-space meetings*[32–34] are minimally structured events where a group gathers, a blank page on the wall constitutes the agenda, and participants are encouraged to sponsor a discussion by writing the title of the session on one of the many flipcharts in the room.

- *Appreciative inquiry summit methodology*,[35] pioneered by Cooperrider and Whitney, cofounders of the Taos Institute (Chagrin Falls, Ohio), focuses attention on expanding an organization's capacity for positive change through inquiry into its positive core of strengths, gifts, and life-giving forces.

- The *search conference*[36] is a highly participative and democratic planning process developed to empower an organization to identify, design, and enact its most desired future, in which people create strategic goals and action plans that develop the organization or system.

The variety of methods available for participatory, collaborative planning and the establishment of a collective vision illustrate both the potential and the challenge for systems organizers. Many of the methods share common features (e.g., brainstorming and ranking). Moreover, systematic, empirical comparative evidence of relative strengths and weaknesses needs to be developed. Even so, explicit structured processes for participatory planning and for helping systems develop maps describing the collective vision of the group or organization are critical tools for systems organizers.

Structure: From Organizing to Self-Organizing

Despite the limitations of the traditional management paradigm, one of its strengths is its usefulness in leading an organization toward a predefined purpose. However, no organizational leader, no matter how skilled or charismatic, can single-handedly move a complex organization toward a desired goal. Organizations are complex and evolving "organisms" encompassing diverse stakeholder groups, political and cultural processes, and competing demands. Especially in the context of tobacco control efforts, in which loosely knit coalitions and collaboratives form with limited central control, the traditional approach alone is not sufficient. Therefore, the central task of a new management model is to reconcile the paradox between *purposeful organization* and *adaptive self-organization.* The real power of complex organizations is the ability to self-organize, adapt, and evolve. However, the self-organization and evolution must be directed toward a *purposeful* goal. These countervailing forces speak to fundamental issues of power and infrastructure in organizations, particularly as they move toward a systems environment.

When Darwin wrote his treatise on evolution by natural selection,[37] he began with examples of domestic breeding for selective traits in pigeons to provide an analog for what would prove to be a profoundly influential argument: a similar kind of selection that resulted from *natural* causes, rather than divine inspiration or intelligent design[38] (W. B. Provine, pers. comm., 2004). The phylogeny of organs like the human eye, organisms like the kangaroo, or superorganisms like a colony of ants, is the result of good genes combined with a modest amount of good fortune.[38,39]

Instead of developing traditional command-and-control systems, the systems manager facilitates (eases the formation of) systems that encourage self-organization. This end frequently is accomplished by reducing restraining forces, instead of adding directing forces. Systems organizing leaders must facilitate and empower *interaction* of all kinds. When adaptive agents are allowed to freely interact, self-organization typically results. Many of the structures, policies, and rules in a traditional organization are designed to direct, control, or otherwise inhibit interaction. Departmentalization and imposed specialization are driving forces for organization, but they restrain self-

Going with the Flow

Consider the following anecdote, which differentiates between purposeful organizing and adaptive self-organizing. In the world of river-raft guiding, novice guides can be distinguished from seasoned guides because novices work harder and expert guides work smarter. Novice guides rely on raw power and young muscles to maneuver the raft. A great deal of effort is expended fighting against the natural flow of the river. The seasoned guide surrenders the boat to the flow of the river and pays close attention to critical moments when a single stroke in the right place, at the right time, with the right amount of force can alter the course of the raft, transitioning the boat from one turbulent flow to another. The differences between the novice and expert guide are subtle but profound.

The parallels to management and organizations are obvious: the leader, manager, or agent of change floating on the turbulent flows of a complex organization cannot hope to move an organization toward a goal or objective. However, well-placed and well-timed actions, based on a thorough understanding of the system's complexities and behaviors, can lead to purposeful and adaptive change. In this anecdote, "going with the flow" does not mean simply letting the river take the boat wherever it takes it without a care for outcomes or path. Instead, going with the flow means understanding the effects of the larger systems at work and coordinating one's actions to use and leverage these systems toward purposeful ends.

organization. Self-organizing systems may cluster into subsystems that may adapt to fill specialized roles, but they do so organically.

Systems organizers understand that systems allowed to form naturally are better able to adapt and evolve. When agents self-organize, they often form novel bonds in the network that can help decrease the relative distances in the network, making the world smaller.[40] In turn, a "smaller" world can be navigated more quickly and may be better able to adapt to rapid changes in the environment. Because these novel, "long" bonds connect discrete clusters, they facilitate the flow of critical system components, such as information, resources, knowledge, learning, and power, from one part of the system to another.

The issue of structure in systems organizing is closely related to the issue of networks, because networks either constitute the structure or can be used to represent it. This finding is consonant with a literature on collaboration in networks[41] and the idea of "network organizations"[42] that addresses structural issues (types of networks) and how to perform facilitation effectively in networked contexts. Chapter 6 considers networks and network analysis as they relate to systems thinking. However, much of that discussion is relevant here.

The systems organizing leader recognizes similarities between efforts to encourage structures that enable self-organization and the traditional implementation functions. However, the paradigm shift to systems thinking requires a transformation of traditional thinking. The rules of the traditional manager become "recipes"[43] to the systems organizer. Where rules attempt to control, recipes suggest. Encouraging structures that allow self-organization is a complex and difficult process, but it need not be any more difficult than traditional approaches. The systems organizer must develop a keen sense of the behavior of complex adaptive systems and must be a catalyst for systems change at critical times, while "letting go" to self-organizing processes at other times.

The organizational environment that currently characterizes tobacco control can be viewed as a *loosely coupled system,* a term Weick[44] coined in studying educational organizations. Loosely coupled systems are distinguishable from the command-and-control environments normally found in the business sector. They are characterized by several factors.[44] They exist in situations in which several means can produce the same result. There is a lack of coordination or dampened coordination and an absence of regulations throughout the system. These systems consist of connected networks with very slow feedback times. The various subsystems evidence causal independence, and planned unresponsiveness exists in the system. Orton and Weick[45] summarize major advantages and disadvantages of loose coupling:

- *Persistence:* Stability and continued operation in the good sense; resistance to change and reduced responsiveness in the bad sense

- *Buffering:* Inclination to seal off and prevent the spread of problems, which also can manifest itself in the lack of communications that may have led to problems such as the Three Mile Island accident[46]

- *Adaptability:* Great tendency to experiment and find local solutions to problems

- *Satisfaction:* Fostering of efficacy and self-determination[44] and creation of an environment in which deviance and experimentation are protected;[47] loosely coupled systems can also contribute to loneliness,[48] reducing satisfaction levels

Orton and Weick reach several conclusions on the best management of loosely coupled systems.[45] They recommend subtle leadership that focuses on providing centralized direction and coordination while recognizing the value of increased discretion on the part of agents. The investigators suggest focusing attention on specific relationships in the system by use of strategies such as carefully selecting targets; managing/controlling resources; and initiating focused, forceful action as appropriate. Orton and Weick

advise an emphasis on shared values and tight cultural couplings to counteract loose couplings between policies and actions.[45] The study of loosely coupled systems suggests four insights about navigating collaborations in public health:

1. The focus should be on the *interfaces*—defining the inputs and end products required for each participating organization, rather than activities that occur within each.

2. The system should rely less on detailed instructions and more on encouraging mutually agreed upon operational milestones for each partner and facilitating economic incentives that are driven by fulfilling explicit operational milestones.

3. The systems organizer should anticipate that in the course of the system's evolution, it may be necessary to substitute new participants for others who have left or are not performing well.

4. Structuring the system's work so that it can be accomplished with minimal disruption to the system is essential.

Moreover, the systems organizer should encourage development of distinctive competencies by (1) providing opportunities for partners to become involved in activities that use their expertise and (2) reassigning activities that can be better performed by other partners.

While this chapter maintains that tobacco control is a loosely coupled system, this should not be taken to suggest that it cannot or should not organize. Many issues in tobacco control are best addressed through well-coordinated, orchestrated, organized efforts on the part of the system. For example, efforts to lobby state legislatures around specific tobacco control legislation being considered (e.g., cigarette taxes, clean indoor air laws) need to be planned and executed carefully to be effective. In a loosely coupled system, this often will require that multiple groups or organizations come together and self-organize to achieve such ends.

Power, Conflict, and Structure

The structure that is used in a system is directly related to the potential for power and conflict to arise. For example, issues surrounding the distribution of power among key stakeholders are a common theme whenever researchers and community members form a partnership. Historically in such cases, researchers control the resources and thus are the primary decision makers. Community-based participatory research, which is discussed later in this chapter, attempts to adjust the balance so that researchers and community members equally share power, funds, and responsibility.[49] This research has important insights for systems organizing in situations of power disparities. If participants do not address issues of power and develop relationships built on trust, they are unlikely to embrace the results of the research,[50–52] a factor that may contribute to the lack of research utilization in public health practice.

The literature on open systems and self-managed teams is particularly relevant to the issue of structure and its relationship to power and conflict in systems. Proponents of the open systems framework[53] argue that, in any environment, there is a set of factors so interrelated that a change in one may create changes in the others. As factors of a system interact, members of the organization receive feedback on whether they are accomplishing their goals.[53,54] This feedback is especially apt in a context of contemporary dynamic systems that require participants to monitor and adapt to external changes to survive.[55] Within this context, systems must themselves be able to adapt.

In traditional management, the idea of self-managing teams emerged as a solution to

help organizations manage the dynamics of a more complex environment.[54,55] The concept of self-management often is used interchangeably with terms such as self-controlling and self-regulating. The idea behind self-managing teams is that when the manager is removed from the interaction, the team is left to self-regulate and consequently becomes better able to adapt to the organization's changing needs and goals.[55] The assumption is that giving groups control over decision making and behavior leads them to better organize and direct their work, more rapidly address problems, and have a stronger sense of commitment.

Much of the discussion about governance in self-managed groups is essentially a consideration of the role of conflict in such systems. There are several types of conflict, and each one may have different implications for governance. Conflict over tasks involves disagreement about the nature of the task or prioritization of tasks. Conflict over relationships pertains to personal differences among participants. Conflict over process relates to tensions about how to address tasks. The literature on conflict within a team suggests that some level of conflict can enhance team performance, but excessive conflict has negative effects.[56]

Power differentials create the need for interaction guidelines that can form a basis for working together in a systems environment. For example, based on a review of the literature and stakeholder research, Cordero-Guzmán identified several key factors for such collaborations in community-based organizations (CBOs), including an explicit mechanism for the selection of participants and concrete criteria for selection.[57] Possible criteria include identification of members who share a stake in both the process and outcome and those who have the ability to compromise and resolve disagreements on goals, programs, and procedures. Development of mutual respect, understanding, and trust is another essential early step. The challenge is how best to promote development of respect.[57] A structured participatory process may be critical in early phases of systems development (e.g., engagement in an active and professionally led planning process that involves significant involvement of participants). Efforts should be made to create opportunities for the collaborating organizations to engage in group activities, discuss common interests, develop clear expectations, and build trust.

Although cross-organizational systems are unlikely to be as structured as organizations themselves are, it is important that roles and policies are clearly defined. Open and frequent communication and established formal and informal communication links are especially important in cross-organizational systems in which opportunities for regular face-to-face exchanges are likely to be less frequent. It is important to be clear and selective in targeting the types and contexts of activities related to the work of the system. Starting an initiative with concrete and visible projects that can show clear and early gains is desirable. This approach enables the systems team to gain experience working as a group and to obtain a quick success that can increase self-confidence. As in any organization, the pressures of day-to-day demands tend to crowd out plans for longer term strategic issues related to the system. Having a process that promotes planning for long-term systems strategies and goals is critical. Finally, and perhaps paradoxically, it is important to manage the exit of organizations from the collaborative group.

Action: From Delegation to Participation

One important concept gained from complex systems research is that interactions of local semiautonomous agents unaware of larger goals can lead to emergent complexity, adaptivity, and self-organization. Using this knowledge, the systems organizing leader must enable individuals to connect their daily objectives and actions (mission) to the larger collective vision of the whole system. One can imagine a system of active agents who are not participating in a larger effort. In everyone's experience, they are people who are very busy but accomplish little. As soon as agents make the link between their local mission and the collective vision, they move from being "active" to being "participatory." When agents are called on to *participate,* rather than merely to take action, they are encouraged to connect their actions to the collective vision of the whole.

One key concept of the systems organizing model is the intimate link between mission and vision—between the action of the parts and the action of the whole. To benefit from a purposeful process, mission must be linked to a collective vision. To benefit from the powers of self-organization and emergence, agents must become participants. Like establishing a vision, establishing a mission is a continuous rather than a discrete process. Agents require time to determine how they can participate and in turn contribute to the collective vision. Many unique gifts and talents of individuals are unknown to their leaders and frequently, even to themselves. However, a systems organizing leader empowers and facilitates a process that helps individuals identify key contributions. Such leaders do not say, "We're going to do X, and I need you to do Y." Instead, they say, "We want to do X. What can you contribute?"

The first step in exploring the concept of facilitative leadership to achieve participant missions is examination of the literature on management for contexts similar to those of complex and dynamic interorganizational systems. One leading candidate is the field of large group interventions (LGIs),[58]

Agents and Missions

When religious missionaries go on a mission, they are active participants in the vision of a larger system. They understand the part their participation plays in serving the vision of the whole. Even though each mission is different, all the missions share abstract or general qualities. The same is true for agents in a system. Each agent may have a mission uniquely suited to him or her, and the collective effect of these missions is attainment of a collective vision. Missions are not "statements" on a boardroom wall. They are collective, distributed, adaptive, and dynamic actions and interactions. Unlike the dissipative structure of visions that makes them dynamically timeless, missions are timely. They change.

collaborative interventions involving the systems, practices, and policies of transorganizational environments. In traditional organizations, such interventions embody strategies to involve both internal and external systems in the change process.[59] These methods are designed to create alignment and consensus around strategic direction and global issues for an organization. Generally, they are processes involving key stakeholders at all levels of the organizational environment. LGIs, also known as critical mass events, large group interactive events, whole systems change, and large-scale organizational change, grew out of the field of organizational development in the 1950s, with the formulation of the theory of sociotechnical systems.[60]

An emerging paradigm of change has arisen to formally challenge and compete with the more traditional sociotechnical systems approaches. LGIs have been embraced by many as the preferred method of change, because they bring a higher level of consciousness and an ecology of the whole system.[61] Whole-systems approaches to organizational change are rooted in the philosophy that organizations act as living

systems or communities and that overall health must be viewed from the perspective of the total system. A whole-systems perspective involves understanding how all parts of the system (e.g., people, resources, knowledge, processes, and leadership) contribute to the successful functioning of the system and how each of the parts relates to each other and to the whole. Other approaches to redesigning organizations to improve productivity, quality, and organizational effectiveness include total quality management and business process reengineering. LGIs can trace their ancestry to a diverse set of approaches including systems theory,[53,60,62] sociotechnical systems and social constructionism,[63,64] values theory,[65,66] social psychology,[67] futuring,[68,69] group dynamics,[70–73] and large group dynamics.[74–78]

Several essential design principles support LGI methodology[58] and are worth consideration in the context of organizing tobacco control. Dialogue among stakeholders is necessary to transform understanding and find deeper meaning, essentially an affirmation of the critical importance of collaborative and participatory approaches in this context. Through powerful and generative dialogue processes, people are capable of extreme change that becomes the source of collective action and collaboration. Community building and relationship formation practices foster interdependence and interconnectedness among the participants in the system. Collective learning increases a system's capacity to produce results that matter. Diversity through shared inquiry promotes system vitality, synergy, resourcefulness, and growth. Self-managing methods build dynamic and synergistic energy that fosters commitment and shared responsibility.

In addition to LGI methods, approaches such as participatory action research are well suited to linking a participatory mission to a collective vision. The systems organizing leader finds that many of the traditional techniques of planning and implementation remain useful in linking this participatory mission. However, these traditional techniques should be reframed in light of these important systems changes to the traditional mission "statement."

Learning: From Discrete Evaluation to Continuous Evaluation

Learning is the adaptive function of societies and organizations. In the traditional management model, learning is most like evaluation. The field of evaluation is undergoing changes parallel to those in science that were discussed in chapter 3 and to the changes in organizational and management thinking discussed earlier in this chapter. The field of evaluation is evolving away from the discrete and linear control model of planning, implementing, and evaluating to more dynamic models that constitute collective adaptive learning. At the cutting edge of the evaluation field, scholars already are moving evaluation criteria from researcher-defined approaches to a participatory, stakeholder-based model consonant with linking theory to practice and evaluation to learning. When evaluation becomes a stakeholder-driven process that integrates both the goals of researchers and the needs of practitioners, the problem addressed is one of the most critical roadblocks in the current science model—the gap between research and implementation of evidence-based practices.

Developing a learning organization[23] means that agents view themselves as both students and teachers in a continuous process in which making mistakes, taking risks, acquiring new knowledge, and sharing that knowledge with others are critical advantages, not just fanciful and occasional reflective indulgences. Individuals in the system must be encouraged not only to *reflect* on what they are doing and adjust their mental models but also to *report* or disseminate what they learn to others.

Evaluation as a conscious empirical endeavor can trace its roots back hundreds or even thousands of years.[79,80] However, evaluation emerged in its modern form primarily as a coherent field, at least in the United States, in the era of the Great Society during President Lyndon Johnson's administration. From the outset, evaluation involved a confluence of many fields, both research based and practice oriented, including most of the applied social sciences and substantive areas of education, health, and social welfare. Thus, it encompassed an eclectic mix of methodologies ranging from experimental and quasiexperimental approaches to qualitative anthropological and field-based strategies and addressed a broad range of concerns from technical and scientific to managerial and practical. Charting the history and evolution of the various strands of evaluation is easily a book in itself.[79-89] Nonetheless, here it is important to identify the most recent directions and how they relate to systems learning in systems organizing.

This section focuses on three broad areas of evaluation methodology illustrating the evolution of systems organizing principles: participatory evaluation, program theory and logic models, and system models for evaluation.

Participatory Evaluation

Participatory evaluation embodies the kind of collaborative, multistakeholder approach envisioned in the four principles of system organizing. Traditionally, the gap between researchers and practitioners has served as one of the major impediments to dissemination and adoption of evidence-based practices. In public health in general, there frequently is a dissonance between research results and the needs of practitioners and other stakeholders, often to the point that community members have a well-documented mistrust of health researchers.[90] There are some key structural reasons for this dissonance.[51] Dissemination of research findings frequently is not by itself an effective tool for initiating behavior change. Best practices, which traditionally result from applied research, often are viewed suspiciously by potential users. Moreover, much of the research that informs the development of guidelines for best practices is conducted in distant places by unknown researchers.

Incorporating the knowledge and expertise of practitioners and community members strengthens the quality of the research.[91] When research questions address issues important to both researchers and practitioners, the data collected are more applicable to the scientific hypothesis under study.[92] Likewise, a close, collaborative relationship between the evaluator and the consumers of the evaluation increases the quality and effectiveness of program evaluation.[93]

Community-based participatory research (CBPR) is an evaluation approach that facilitates collaboration between researchers and community members. The three key elements of participatory research are collaboration, education, and action,[91] which enable the development of effective interventions and address specific community health needs.[94] The involvement of all participants in all aspects and at all stages of the research is essential to CBPR.[49,52,92,94,95] Each participant adds important expertise to any research endeavor and can increase the understanding of factors contributing to poor health outcomes and thus enhance the quality of the research.[90,91,96] To ensure that the voices of community members are heard, the research must involve an active partnership with a CBO, a community

advisory committee, community forums, and public presentations, and must include formative data collection, including interviews with community members.[92]

CBPR can be viewed as an overarching term that encompasses a variety of participatory evaluation methods. Participatory action research is an iterative process of inquiry, reflection, and action, in which a researcher participates with stakeholders to define a problem, generate knowledge, perform research, take action, and evaluate results.[97] The participatory intervention model is a closely related approach that integrates theory and research on interventions that are sensitive to culture and context.[98] This partnership between investigators and communities is designed to promote long-term sustainable involvement of affected stakeholders. Empowerment evaluation[99] is a collaborative approach to the development and use of program evaluation criteria, driven by community stakeholders, as well as investigators. Many of these approaches use the methods described earlier in the section on "vision." They overlap with the emphases described in the discussion of large group interactions in the section on "structure."

Development of a partnership is facilitated by establishing research priorities, funding, and mechanisms for collaboration and decision making early in the collaborative process.[94] Establishing and maintaining trust also are essential to an effective collaboration and require the flexibility and patience of all stakeholders.[49,90,94] To ensure the success of a partnership in research, it is advisable to determine the roles of all stakeholders, define principles of collaboration, and develop a code of ethics before a project is started.[52,90,91,100]

Even though CBPR has many benefits, it does pose challenges, including time constraints, cost-effectiveness issues, and lack of program durability. Funding agencies generally do not provide adequate time for performance of CBPR projects, making detailed community analysis difficult.[52,101,102] In addition, most community research projects primarily are concerned with determining whether the intervention has an effect, not whether the program will endure.[100,102] Despite these concerns, CBPR has much to commend it, especially in the context of open systems.

Program Theory and Logic Models

One of the most important changes in evaluation over the past few decades has been the recognition that good evaluation depends on understanding the underlying theory of how programs or interventions might affect outputs and outcomes, a concept known as *program theory*.[103] Program theory was a reaction to the traditional experimental and quasiexperimental approach[104] that tends to treat the program or intervention as a "black box" and assess causality without concentrating on the processes that bring about effects. Program theory also can be viewed as a transitional step from a more reductionist and hierarchical view of causal relationships toward one that is more dynamic and systems oriented. Paralleling this evolution to program theory were two trends that have implications for systems organizing.

First, methods and processes that would enable comprehensible description and depiction of implicit theories were needed. It was not sufficient for individual scientists and researchers to perform this function alone. Many of the most detailed causal models were likely to be implicitly held in the minds of practitioners and community members who were close to the phenomena. Thus, the problem became one of identifying methods to help groups of stakeholders, including researchers, practitioners, policy makers, and consumers, articulate their implicit models of how interventions work to affect outcomes. Then these models

could be used to perform more sensitive evaluations through methods such as matching of theoretical patterns of expected outcomes with the observed patterns obtained through measurement.[105–107] Not surprisingly, many of the processes that proved useful came from the planning context (see the section on "vision," earlier in this chapter). This is because planners historically used methods to surface implicit models based on the input of heterogeneous groups of stakeholders.

Second, there had been a rise in emphasis on developing visual models that capture the complexity of the program–outcome process, in parallel with the growth of stakeholder-driven models. Perhaps primary among these is the use of *logic models* representing structured evaluation criteria that link outcomes with program activities and processes, as well as the theoretical assumptions and principles of the program.[22] Logic models represent causal models of evaluation in which actions lead to measurable outcomes. As such, they are precursors to the more dynamic analyses with feedback that comes from system dynamics (see chapter 5), where the effects of actions can influence factors, which in turn affect the relationships between actions and outcome.

System Models for Evaluation

The evaluation framework of the Centers for Disease Control and Prevention (CDC; figure 4.4) is a recent example of a participatory evaluation system model that is integrated with use of logic models. This framework illustrates well the shift that is occurring to more collaborative system models for evaluation and systems learning. This model involves a six-step process[108] in which engagement of stakeholders is the initial activity in an evaluation effort, preceding the definition of more formal aspects of the evaluation, such as the program design and logic models used,

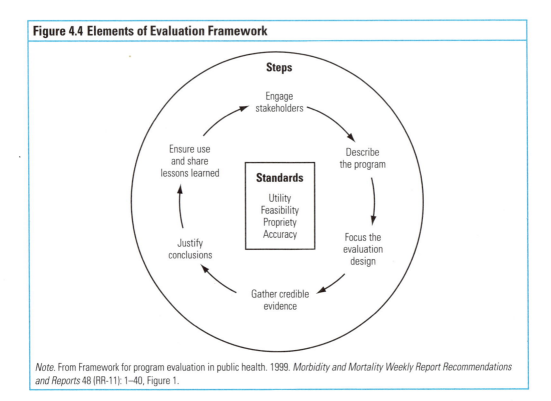

Figure 4.4 Elements of Evaluation Framework

Steps

Engage stakeholders

Describe the program

Ensure use and share lessons learned

Standards
Utility
Feasibility
Propriety
Accuracy

Focus the evaluation design

Justify conclusions

Gather credible evidence

Note. From Framework for program evaluation in public health. 1999. *Morbidity and Mortality Weekly Report Recommendations and Reports* 48 (RR-11): 1–40, Figure 1.

evaluation design, and expected outcomes. This framework also is set in the context of four core standards (figure 4.4, center) that are relevant to the evaluating function of systems organizing:

1. Utility—Degree to which the information needs of intended users are served by evaluation

2. Feasibility—Potential for achievement in terms of project scope, cost, and political factors

3. Propriety—Conformity to legal and ethical standards and acceptable benefit to affected parties

4. Accuracy—Technically accurate information

This framework represents an evolution of evaluation methodology within a large hierarchical organization such as CDC and further evidence of systems organizing

trends combining quantitative and mixed-method techniques with an increased level of stakeholder input.

Summary of Systems Organizing Model

From the perspective of complex systems, the local interactions of semiautonomous agents lead to emergent complex phenomena. To facilitate achievement of purposeful ends in a complex adaptive system, the system as a whole must have a stated goal (*vision principle*) and participatory action of individual agents (*action principle*). Agents also need to connect their actions (missions) to the collective vision and understand that the vision and the mission of the system are in constant feedback with each other; they are distributed, dissipative, dynamic, and adaptive. Structures that afford self-organization rather than simple organization also should be encouraged (*structure principle*). In addition, the culture must be infused with a passion for learning (*learning principle*) and ongoing evaluation. It also is critical that mission be intimately linked with vision and vice versa and that the capacities for self-organization and learning are mapped onto vision and mission. Using these four principles, organizational leaders may choose between more traditional approaches (e.g., leadership, management, delegation, organized structures, and discrete evaluations) and systems approaches (e.g., facilitation and empowerment, self-organizing structures, participatory action, and continuous evaluation).

The leader has the freedom to move between these positions on the continua much like the equalizer on a stereo is tuned, matching the organizational situation and immediate context to a particular style. However, because of their unique and complex interorganizational structures, tobacco control initiatives can benefit greatly from moving toward the systems end of the continua. Numerous methods are available for the systems organizing leader. By linking (mapping) the purposeful principles of vision and action to the emergent principles of structure and learning, a balance between powerful emergent properties and purposeful constitution can be achieved. In addition, because the self-organizing system is participatory and because mission is linked to vision, systems-friendly methods can be used to link semiautonomous and local action and the larger goals and objectives of the whole.

In the discussion of the four systems organizing principles, a wide variety of methods were presented. Table 4.2 shows a matrix that relates the four principles of systems organizing to those methods. Each method is classified in terms of its primary and secondary emphases related to the four principles. This classification is not meant to be definitive; different people would likely classify the methods differently. Some of the methods are ideally suited for one principle; others could be used for several or all of the principles. Excluded from this table and chapter are the great variety of methods relevant to systems organizing that come from the traditions of system dynamics modeling (chapter 5), network analysis (chapter 6), and knowledge management and transfer (chapter 7), because these methods are considered in detail in those chapters.

Collaboratively Constructed Concept Maps for Systems Organizing: Case Studies

A major challenge in systems organizing (of consortia, networks, or partnerships) is the development of methods and processes appropriate for complex interorganizational contexts. Two case studies illustrate incorporation of the ideas of systems organizing into real-world contexts. One study was conducted to improve integration of research and practice in public health, and the other was conducted to develop a conceptual model of the characteristics of strong, cooperative local and state tobacco control programs. Both case studies involve key issues in tobacco control and provide examples of the creation of outcomes through a structured process in a participatory, multistakeholder environment—a system of organizations. At a deeper level, both also produced results that would not have been possible in the absence of organizing a system of stakeholders. The intent is not to argue for a specific methodology but rather to underscore the importance of engaging

Table 4.2 Systems Organizing Methods by Principle

Systems organizing methods	Planning collective vision	Organizing and participatory self-organizing	Facilitating mission leadership	Evaluating and systems learning
Collaborative needs assessment[9]		X		
Brainstorming[10]	X	X	X	X
Nominal groups approach[11]	X	X	X	X
Focus groups[12]	X	X	X	X
Delphi technique[13]	X	X		X
Concept-mapping structured conceptualization[109]	XX	XX	X	X
Concept mapping (mind mapping, idea mapping)[14,15]	X	X		
Strategy maps[20]		X	X	
Cognitive maps[21]		X	X	X
Outcome mapping[25]	X	X		XX
Logic models[22]	X	X	X	X
Future-search conferences[26]	XX	X	X	X
Conference model[27,28]	X		X	X
Large-scale interactive process[29]	X			
Real-time strategic change[30]	X		X	
Participative work redesign[31]		X	XX	
Open-space meetings[32–34]		XX		XX
Appreciative inquiry summit methodology[35]		XX		
Search conference[36]	XX	X	X	
Large group interventions[58]	X	X	X	X
Total quality management				X
Business process reengineering		X		
Community-based participatory research				XX
Participatory action research				X
Participatory intervention model				XX
Empowerment evaluation[99]				XX
Appreciative inquiry as methodology[35]				XX
CDC evaluation framework				XX

Notes. X = method suited for systems organizing function; XX = method especially suited for systems organizing function; CDC = Centers for Disease Control and Prevention.

Managing a Complex National System of Organizational Partners: Notes from the Real World

Systems organizing issues are well illustrated by an example from a field in public health that neighbors tobacco control, the field of obesity control and nutrition. The latter has a much longer history of attempts to coordinate across sectors and organizations. One such effort was a national coalition sponsored by a foundation seeking to mobilize the major national players in nutrition around a campaign called Project Low-Fat Eating for America Now (Project LEAN) in 1988–92. Organizations in the public, private, voluntary, and independent sectors were convened to form a coalition to coordinate their nutrition messages, products, and services around the theme of low-fat eating. The systems organizing issues that needed to be addressed in building a system or coalition of disparate stakeholder organizations were examined by creating vision, structure, action, and learning:

Creating vision. Who is the leader? The first of several caveats on coalitions that one could draw from this example is, "Everybody wants coordination, but nobody wants to be the coordinatee." One corollary is that designation of a chairperson for the meeting of disparate partners in a coalition immediately establishes a perception of imbalance in the partisan positions of the various sectors or organizations. The private sector versus the public sector views of food-labeling policies, for example, would be perceived to be tilted in one direction or the other by the designation of anyone selected to chair the meetings.

Creating structure. The first system problems encountered at the first meeting related to managing the balance of power—governance questions such as who should chair the meetings and what the representation and the voting rights and weights should be of the various organizations. Considering the vastly different sizes and power of the organizations at the table, it was clear that the conveners could treat them equally only at the peril of the cohesiveness of the coalition.

Moreover, a corollary of the coordinator–coordinatee dilemma mentioned here is that large organizations with considerable stake in an issue are loathe to be at the mercy of a coalition's decisions and are the first to break ranks and leave the coalition when they find that their influence is diminished by their membership. The first point at which they may feel diminished is in selection of the chairperson. However, a more compelling reason to bolt arises when they realize that their vote counts equally with the votes of many small partner organizations. They will be even more concerned if they sense that some smaller organizations are or could be ganging up on them in the voting or using the coalition as a platform to berate them or disparage their products or motivations.

Creating action. Another systems issue arises in managing the chain of command in the coalition as the meetings unfold. The first meeting might be attended by many of the chief executive officers of several organizations, and the second and third meetings, by their deputies. By the time of the third meeting and later meetings, depending on the size of the organizations, the people around the table might not be in a position to cut deals or cast a vote that would commit their organization to a plan or an offering of support. Meetings begin to bog down and end in stalemates because many of those present must defer a vote on decisions or withhold support for actions until they can check with superiors.

Creating learning. Finally, following through on the initial vision can be yeoman's work. A set of coalition systems issues arise in the phasing from initial meetings on consensus building and declaration of common purposes, where coalitions are at their best, to later meetings on implementation, where coalitions frequently are at their worst. Coalitions make blunt instruments for micromanagement and often collapse under the weight of their own cumbersome managerial and decision-making structures when they come to the implementation phase.

Over time, there have been a growing number of successful systems organizing efforts in public health practice and literature, ranging from coalition-building efforts such as the Global

Tobacco Research Network[a] to the case studies outlined later in this chapter. At the same time, understanding the kinds of roadblocks that have occurred in past efforts such as Project LEAN can help to inform the kinds of social and organizational issues that must be addressed to make these systems efforts practical and effective.

[a]Research for International Tobacco Control. 2002. Bridging the research gaps in global tobacco control: A synthesis document. Ottawa, ON: Research for International Tobacco Control.

tobacco control from a systems organizing perspective.

These case studies involve the use of concept mapping, one of many systems organizing approaches discussed earlier in this chapter. (For a detailed explanation of concept mapping, see appendix 4A.) Concept mapping, sometimes called structured conceptualization, is a participatory and integrated mixed-methods approach facilitating the collaboration of tens or hundreds of people synchronously or asynchronously on a project, in person or using Web technology, in a manner that enables active involvement of each participant.[16] The primary product of this method is a series of "maps" that summarize the collective thinking of the group, consensus matches to explore the diversity of participant views, bivariate graphs that enable considerable detail to be organized for action planning and implementation, and a broad array of summary data. The method integrates qualitatively based, judgmentally oriented individual and group processes (brainstorming, sorting, rating, and interpretation of results) with a series of multivariate statistical analyses to produce the maps and related outputs. The products enhance the ability of groups or networks to purposefully envision, enact, and manage systems changes that increase the capacities for self-organizing and/or learning.

As one example of systems organizing "friendly" methods, concept mapping is especially useful to build collective vision and the perception that an individual's daily actions are situated in a larger contextual purpose. Metaphorically, concept mapping results in a "you are here" map of the larger system that allows each agent in the system to understand how his or her efforts (mission) are situated in the larger collective action (vision). In addition, methods such as concept mapping provide groups and individuals with a powerful reflective learning process. Finally, any methodology that increases the bonds between agents in a network, especially special types of bonds such as long bonds or a combination of weak and strong ties across diverse networks, can create capacity for desired outcomes. These include phenomena of small worlds, in which small numbers of links bridge any two points within a network,[40] as well as self-organization, adaptation, complexity, and emergence.

There are several reasons for using concept mapping as the vehicle for illustrating systems organizing approaches. First, it is a good exemplar of a structured participatory method, a key feature of systems organizing. Second, it is a hybrid method that integrates well-known qualitative (brainstorming, sorting) and quantitative (multidimensional scaling, hierarchical cluster analysis) methods. In a sense it is a conglomerate of several other systems organizing methods (various group processes and formal modeling methods), and, as a result, the examples illustrate some of the major features of each. Third, it was timely; several projects that were particularly apt illustrations for public health and tobacco control either were in progress or had been recently completed at the time of this project. Despite its advantages as a method for illustrating systems organizing approaches, the use of concept mapping in these examples is not meant to convey any inherent distinction over other systems organizing methods. Many methods are available—this is an extremely dynamic area. Each of them would likely contribute to and complement the results obtainable through concept mapping.

Case Study 1: Closing the Gap between Research Discovery and Program Delivery

The 2001 report of the Institute of Medicine,[110] which determined that the lag time from a scientific discovery to use in practice was typically 15–20 years, drove the motivation for closing the gap between research discovery and program delivery. NCI, the Center for the Advancement of Health, and the Robert Wood Johnson Foundation held a collaborative conference as a foundation for developing a more integrated effort to close the gap between research discovery and program delivery in cancer control.

To make the most of participants' time at the conference, the sponsoring organizations asked them to take part in a preconference collaborative project to help them understand the perspective of experts—practitioners, researchers, and others who work in health promotion, disease prevention, and cancer control. The focus was primary ways for major agencies affiliated with the U.S. Department of Health and Human Services (e.g., NCI, CDC, Agency for Healthcare Research and Quality, Centers for Medicare & Medicaid Services, Health Resources and Services Administration, and National Institutes of Health) and the national, state, and local partners to work together to accelerate adoption of cancer control research discoveries into practice. The results of the conference were then used to develop a logic model and related action plans for implementation. The same framework will subsequently be used to evaluate progress on these plans and to capture the individual and organizational learning that took place.

Thus, the example encompasses both the purposeful (vision and mission) and emergent (self-organizing and learning) principles of the systems organizing framework. Participants were asked to brainstorm online in response to the following focus prompt:

> One thing that should be done to accelerate the adoption of cancer control research discoveries by health service delivery programs is…

Approximately 55 people contributed more than 200 statements that were subsequently synthesized by the steering committee into 98 unique ideas. The statements were sorted by 19 members of the planning committee. The data were aggregated and analyzed with a sequence of multivariate analyses that included multidimensional scaling and hierarchical cluster analysis. The resulting map grouped the 98 ideas into 12 conceptual categories. The participants also were asked to identify clusters of clusters that seemed to belong together and provide a label for each such region of the map. Participants identified four major regions: (1) policy, consisting of policy issues that would enable more integration of research and practice, as opposed to policy that results from such efforts; (2) research; (3) practice; and (4) partnerships and support.

In addition, a broader region of intermediaries, both government and private, was defined by participants, encompassing the regions of policy, research, and practice. Figure 4.5 illustrates the final labeled concept map.

Figure 4.5 can be interpreted meaningfully beginning with the policy region. To enhance the integration of research and practice, begin with "policies" that promote such activities. Then move counterclockwise to "research," especially explicit funding for the integration of research and practice. Continue counterclockwise to "practice," where tools, messages, and dissemination mechanisms are critical. Intermediaries, both government and not-for-profit agencies, provide the "glue" for this process, advocating for policy change, supporting the research community, and helping to translate and disseminate research. This process relies throughout on partnerships and support that provide the network context needed and the input and feedback loop between researchers and practitioners, including the community of relevance.

Participants also were asked to rate each of the statements on importance and feasibility. Figure 4.6 shows the average importance ratings for all participants for each of the 12 clusters. More layers in a cluster signify higher average importance; fewer layers indicate lower importance. The figure shows several clusters with relatively high importance ratings: "diffusion/ dissemination," "strategies," and "service standards." On the other hand, the "training and support" and "barriers" clusters were rated as having relatively low importance. Maps for rating clusters also were produced for different subgroups (e.g., practitioners and researchers) and for the feasibility ratings. Each of these cluster rating maps can be thought of as a "pattern" of the rating across the map.

Figure 4.7 illustrates the pattern match comparing importance and feasibility ratings for these clusters. Importance is depicted on the vertical left axis, and feasibility is shown on the vertical right axis. Each horizontal line represents one of the cluster averages. The point at which the line hits the axis indicates a cluster's average value.

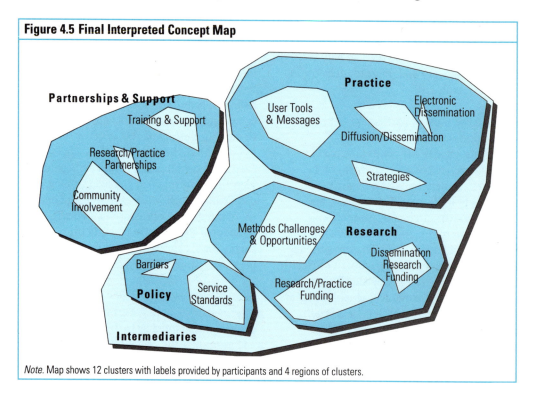

Figure 4.5 Final Interpreted Concept Map

Note. Map shows 12 clusters with labels provided by participants and 4 regions of clusters.

Figure 4.6 Cluster Rating Map

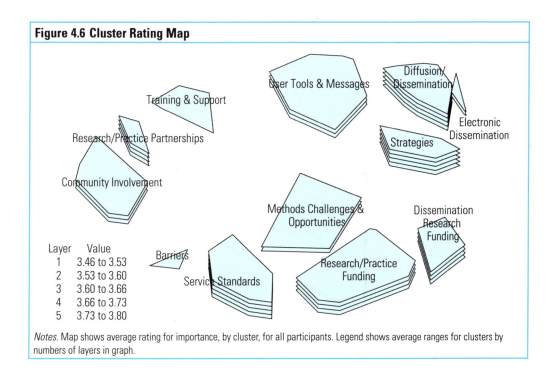

Layer	Value
1	3.46 to 3.53
2	3.53 to 3.60
3	3.60 to 3.66
4	3.66 to 3.73
5	3.73 to 3.80

Notes. Map shows average rating for importance, by cluster, for all participants. Legend shows average ranges for clusters by numbers of layers in graph.

The correlation at the bottom of the pattern matching is a standard Pearson product-moment correlation, indicating the strength of the overall relationship. In a strong positive relationship, the lines would mostly be horizontal. In this case, there are a considerable number of crossover lines, suggesting that the relationship of importance and feasibility is relatively low. The lines that cross over most dramatically are the clusters most different in relative importance and feasibility. For example, "service standards" was considered to be one of the most important clusters and one of the least feasible. In contrast, "electronic dissemination" was judged to be most feasible but relatively low in importance.

The ratings of importance provided by practitioners and researchers are compared in figure 4.8. This match indicates considerable differences in what each group considers to be important. The correlation suggests virtually no relationship between the average importance ratings of these two groups. This result constitutes one

of the most salient findings of this study, a finding with considerable implications for integration of practice and research in this context. It suggests that practitioners and researchers have markedly different priorities and indicates which areas are relatively more important for each group.

A major goal of this project was action planning to improve the integration of research and practice. Because pattern matching revealed fundamental differences in the perspectives of subgroups on the issues, the decision was made to address action planning separately for each major subgroup and to subsequently combine the separate subgroup plans into an integrated action plan. This is an excellent example of identifying individual and/or group needs to establish a mission for their daily action while also understanding the place of that mission among other missions and its linkage to the collective vision. To accomplish action planning, a "go-zone" bivariate plot is often used. Figure 4.9 shows the go-zone plot for the

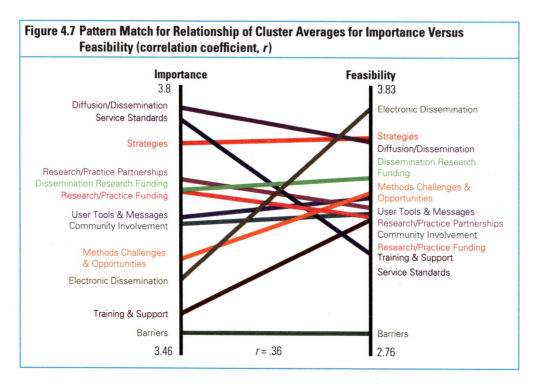

Figure 4.7 Pattern Match for Relationship of Cluster Averages for Importance Versus Feasibility (correlation coefficient, *r*)

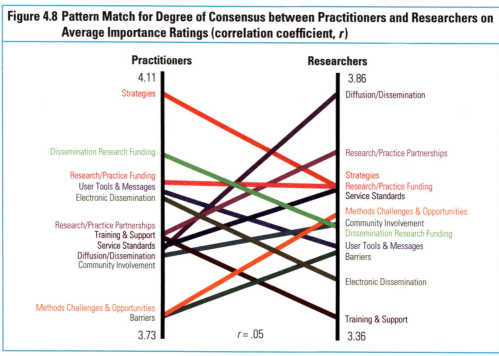

Figure 4.8 Pattern Match for Degree of Consensus between Practitioners and Researchers on Average Importance Ratings (correlation coefficient, *r*)

diffusion/dissemination cluster for the practitioner group. Ideas rated highly on both importance and feasibility are shown in the upper-right quadrant. The go-zone plot shows the data in finer detail, listing actual cluster statements as used in the analysis, and indicating which statements have high importance and feasibility at the statement level as opposed to the cluster level.

The go-zone plot helps point to potential action, but it does not prescribe it. One would not automatically proceed to implementing just the ideas that are in the upper right quadrant. Other factors may be critically important to decisions about action. For example, it is possible that an idea is high in feasibility and only moderately high in importance. Should it be implemented? The answer may very well depend on some other variable, such as cost. If the moderately important action costs almost nothing to implement (probably part of what contributed to its high feasibility rating), it might be implemented

for that reason, even though there are statements that have higher importance ratings. Go-zones, like all of the products in concept mapping, are more useful for their suggestive power than as prescriptive mechanisms.

Across all analyses, results show that each group (researchers, practitioners, and intermediaries) holds different ideas about its own role and the roles of other groups in disseminating and implementing evidence-based interventions. Participants agreed that the responsibility for dissemination must be shared. The concept map acted as the foundation for development of action plans (missions) that would help the participants navigate more effectively toward a more integrated research and practice effort (vision). The ability of each individual or subgroup to establish this important link between mission and vision is critical, because this is the purposeful function of systems organizing. Meanwhile, because it is collaborative, bond forming, inclusive of

Figure 4.9 Bivariate Go-Zone Plot of Importance and Feasibility Ratings of Practitioners, for Diffusion/Dissemination Cluster

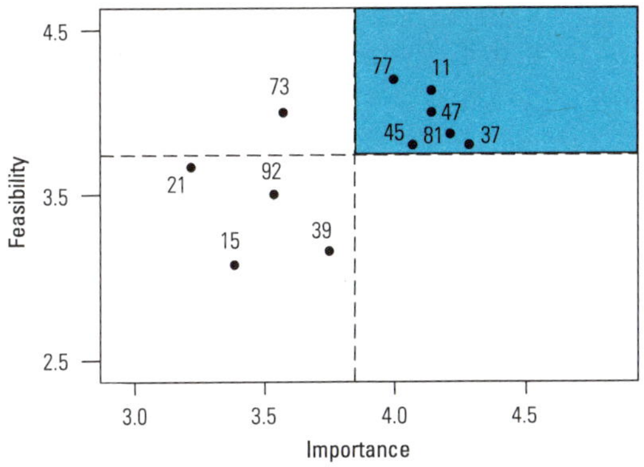

Create mechanisms to distribute practical information (e.g., procedural details) from research discoveries. (11)

Synthesize available research results to reduce the barrage of variable findings from each new "study of the week." (15)

Publish key findings in the form of inserts in targeted magazines. (21)

Develop inexpensive, nontraditional ways to disseminate research findings. (37)

Establish a central clearinghouse to evaluate new discoveries and place them in proper perspective. (39)

Work with the media to disseminate research results in a clear, nonconfusing manner. (45)

Annually publish NCI-funded interventions shown to be effective. (47)

Have NCI hire science writers who can translate research articles into practical advice for practitioners. (73)

Provide best practice examples of how programs adopt evidence-based interventions. (77)

Synthesize and communicate research results in ways that are understandable to practitioners. (81)

Encourage JNCI to publish dissemination studies in each issue. (92)

Note. JNCI = Journal of the National Cancer Institute.

diverse groups and individuals, and process oriented, the concept mapping activity reinforces many of the important qualities of self-organization. The very process is capacity forming.

Participants in the project agreed that ongoing interaction among researchers, practitioners, and intermediaries is essential to improving the effectiveness of activities for cancer control. Participants also noted that there are few incentives and opportunities to focus on these topics in the course of their daily work lives. Several groups suggested strategies to sustain the momentum begun at the meeting, and plans for follow-up were formulated. This result is fairly common in meetings of all kinds, but there often is not enough time to do all that is desired. Instead of developing initiatives, it might be more beneficial to search the system network to find local or small-scale examples of success. By adjusting the flow of resources or information to such initiatives, the systems organizer transfers leadership and planning functions, as well as the collective interests of the group (established in this process), temporarily to one part of the system.

Subsequent to the action-planning conference, a logic model[22] was developed to use the results of the concept-mapping project to integrate research and practice. The logic model is a key mechanism for assessment of both the implementation and outcomes of this effort to integrate practice with research. For each cluster, it is possible to develop one or more measures of performance that can be monitored over time. The map and corresponding logic model can be used to organize all these measures and as a graphic device to display evaluation results. This approach will help to determine whether certain clusters on the map are neglected in action planning or whether certain paths in the logic model are not achieved in practice.

Case Study 2: Empirical Conceptual Model of Strong, Cooperative Local and State Tobacco Control Programs

The objectives of this project were to describe the components of strong tobacco control programs and use the resulting framework to define optimal collaboration between state and local programs. Participants identified themselves as being associated with tobacco control at the state level, local level, or both levels. Participants were asked to respond to a focus prompt for brainstorming:

> One specific component of a strong tobacco control program is...

Two tobacco control experts from the Battelle Centers for Public Health Research and Evaluation and one expert from the Johns Hopkins Bloomberg School of Public Health synthesized the 145 statements into 73 unique ideas. Sorting input from participants was analyzed using concept-mapping analysis,[16] and the results arrayed the 73 statements into a 12-cluster solution. Figure 4.10 displays the final interpreted concept map. First, the map shows a distinct sequence from left to right. More immediate activities and processes are on the left, and longer term services and outcomes are toward the right. The map is divided into four regions (from more immediate to more long term): management, processes, programs and services, and outcomes. The map provides the framework for a process and outcome logic model of the components of process and outcome for strong tobacco control programs.

Second, there is a distinction between an upper and a lower track, from left to right (two arrows). The upper track encompasses more systemic (environmental) change processes, such as policy advocacy and industry monitoring. The lower track

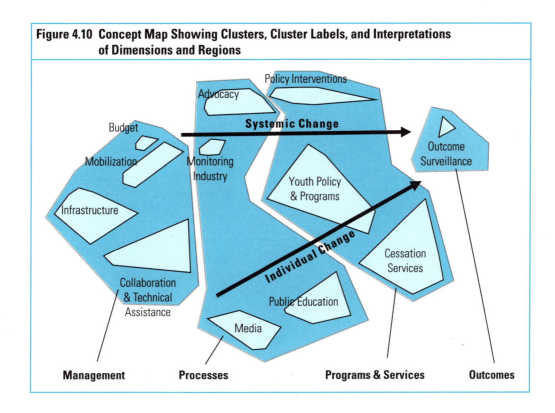

Figure 4.10 Concept Map Showing Clusters, Cluster Labels, and Interpretations of Dimensions and Regions

tends to focus more on efforts to change individual behavior, such as through media and education campaigns and services for smoking cessation. Finally, the cluster for youth policy and programs is in a central position. This position suggests that youth issues were felt to play a central role in tobacco control and that they span the full range of efforts from systemic to individual change.

Describing the components of strong tobacco control programs is a critical first step. However, it is important that the many organizations operating at different levels of the tobacco control system understand their roles and responsibilities relative to each other and to the collective vision. Participants also were asked to rate each of the program components for the degree to which it was a local or state responsibility. Figure 4.11 shows the average responsibility rating for each cluster of components of

tobacco control. More layers signify greater state responsibility, and fewer layers signify more local responsibility. The areas most clearly considered to be the responsibility of the state are budgeting and monitoring industry, followed closely by advocacy, policy interventions, and outcome surveillance. The areas identified most often as local are mobilization, youth policy and programs, and public education. State responsibilities tend to be at the highest levels, with systemic change, and local responsibilities tend to predominate at the lowest levels, with individual change.

A critical question is whether subgroups of raters perceive local and state responsibilities differently. The results of the ratings suggest that there is a high degree of agreement between local and state participants about the relative responsibilities for various program components. A similar consensus is evident

Figure 4.11 Cluster Average Ratings of Responsibility

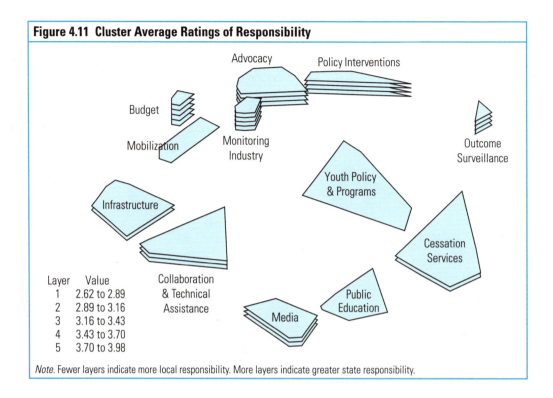

Layer	Value
1	2.62 to 2.89
2	2.89 to 3.16
3	3.16 to 3.43
4	3.43 to 3.70
5	3.70 to 3.98

Note. Fewer layers indicate more local responsibility. More layers indicate greater state responsibility.

regarding ratings from participants who have less experience in tobacco control (≤5 years) and ratings from those who have more experience (>5 years). The results indicate a strong consensus across all subgroups about which components are state responsibilities and which are local responsibilities.

This project summarizes the components of a strong tobacco control program, as identified by the participating state and local stakeholders in the field of tobacco control. The basic map constitutes a conceptual framework categorizing 73 components into 12 categories that, in turn, are grouped into 4 major areas that suggest a natural progression from management and infrastructure, through processes and programs, to outcomes. The framework also identifies how strong tobacco control efforts address both systemic and individual change and that the tendencies are to address systemic change at the state level and individual change at the local level. Finally,

the results show that across all the major identified subgroups (e.g., state and local, front line and research, and experienced and inexperienced), there is consensus about which components are local responsibilities and which are state responsibilities.

These results can be used in several ways. Tobacco control systems can benefit by examination of efforts at the state and local levels to determine whether each sector is addressing components in its respective realm of responsibility. To make such an assessment more feasible, it is essential to develop one or more instruments that can be used at the state and local levels to measure the success of tobacco control programs. Such instruments could build on the strength of tobacco control (SoTC) measure developed as part of the evaluation of the American Stop Smoking Intervention Study.[111,112] The results of the study presented here can inform the local adaptation of this instrument, originally designed to reflect state programs as part of a national study. Furthermore, these results can be used to develop an appropriate short-form assessment instrument for rapid application at the local level that would yield results that can be linked to those of a more comprehensive assessment tool. For example, the map suggests that a simple 12-category assessment instrument may be feasible, highlighting which specific components of the larger domain need to be emphasized in a local SoTC measure.

Summary

This chapter describes a systems organizing approach to systems thinking, an alternative formulation of the traditional management model that, while encompassing it, goes significantly further. In place of the traditional linear progression of processes (planning, organizing, leading, and controlling), the systems organizing model is centered on four principles—vision, structure, action, and learning. These principles are enacted simultaneously and continuously in well-functioning systems. Tobacco control systems can benefit from incorporating these principles and using the many systems organizing methods that embody them.

Two case studies of tobacco control used structured concept mapping[16] to illustrate one of many methods that could be used in a systems organizing approach. The first case study focused on integration of research and practice in a project that was conducted primarily to create a logic model for actions to improve the dissemination of cancer research. The map constitutes a vision for members of the participant group, a model of their collective vision of the overall conceptual terrain for dissemination and integration of research and practice. The details on the map provide the basis for action and help the various participants construe the relationship of their roles to the broader vision. This example shows

the sharp role differentiation between researchers and practitioners, revealing the implicit structure with respect to research dissemination. The map itself provided feedback to the participants, coupled with subsequent action through the logic model, suggesting a step in the evolutionary learning cycle.

The second case study focused on the components of strong tobacco control programs at state and local levels. As in the first project, the map constitutes a conceptual model, a vision of the participants' perceptions. The details of the map differentiate between participant groups, in this case, between state and local roles in the system. In addition, the map links these roles with different change processes, with states primarily responsible for systemic change and local efforts more directly responsible for change at the individual level. The map structure also suggests constructs for evaluation and how they might be organized into measures and collections of measures that can enhance system feedback and learning.

Together, both projects illustrate the integrated quality of the VSAL model. In both, participants left with a better understanding of local, microscale *action* and how it fits into the broader macroscale collective *vision*. Linking the multiple lines of the local participatory action of agents (missions) to the collective and emergent action of the system (vision) is critical in resolving the inherent tension between the purposeful nature and the adaptive nature of such systems. In both projects, the *structure* of the maps emerged from a simple rule-based process (brainstorm, sort, and rate) that was self-organizing. In both, there were clear implications for measurement and evaluation for the next round in an evolutionary cycle of feedback and *learning*. The examples provide working VSAL models that help to balance the tension between purpose and adaptation and between organization and self-organization and to illustrate the link between the model components (vision, structure, action, and learning) and various methods that relate to these components (table 4.2).

Conclusions

1. Systems organizing implies a move away from the classical linear management processes of planning, organizing, leading, and controlling toward a more adaptive, participatory environment expressed here around the concepts of vision, structure, action, and learning:

   ▪ Vision encompasses a move from an environment of leading and managing to one of facilitating and empowering.

   ▪ Structure encompasses a move from organizing to self-organizing.

   ▪ Action encompasses a move from delegation to participation.

   ▪ Learning encompasses a move from discrete evaluation to continuous evaluation.

2. Two concept-mapping projects explored key areas of organizing as a system. One project, examining issues in accelerating the adoption of cancer control research into practice, yielded clusters of action items in areas of research, practice, policy, and partnerships. The other project examined components of strong local and state tobacco control programs and provided the framework for a logic model of process and outcome ranging from near-term to long-term objectives.

Appendix 4A.   Description of Concept-Mapping Methodology

Concept mapping can help describe ideas[16] and represent them visually in the form of a map. The process typically requires participants to brainstorm a large set of relevant statements, sort them into groups of similar statements, rate each statement on one or more scales, and interpret the maps resulting from data analyses. Analyses typically include two-dimensional multidimensional scaling (MDS) of the unstructured sort data, hierarchical cluster analysis of MDS coordinates, and computation of average ratings for each statement and cluster of statements. The maps that result show the individual statements in two-dimensional (x,y) space. More similar statements are located nearer to each other. Statements are grouped into clusters that partition the space on the map. Participants are led through a structured interpretation session designed to help them understand the maps and to label them in a substantively meaningful way.

Procedure

Trochim,[16] who also gives examples of results of several concept-mapping projects,[109] describes the general procedure for concept mapping in detail. The process can be implemented in a variety of ways, taking place in a continuous period as short as a two-day meeting or divided in phases that occur over weeks or months. It can involve as few as 10–15 participants or incorporate input from hundreds or thousands of stakeholders. The procedure described here is for a typical Web-based implementation over several months. All analyses are conducted and maps are produced by using Concept System computer software* designed for this process.

Generation and Structuring of Conceptual Domain

Data are collected over the World Wide Web by using software designed for the purpose. Participants need only a standard Web connection and any standard Web browser. For those who may not have Web access, alternative mechanisms (e.g., manual mail in or faxback) also are made available as appropriate.

During the generation step, participants create statements by using a Web-based, structured brainstorming process[10] guided by a specific focus prompt limiting the types of statements that are acceptable. The focus statement or criterion for generating statements is operationalized as a focus prompt that guides the participants in brainstorming. A typical focus prompt might read:

> One specific issue that needs to be addressed in (insert topic) is…

---

*The Concept System computer software is used to consolidate and edit brainstormed statements, export and print these for sorting and rating, import and enter sorting and rating data, conduct the statistical analysis, including multidimensional scaling and hierarchical cluster analysis, and display a wide variety of map results.[113]

The general rules of brainstorming apply. Participants are encouraged to generate as many statements as possible (upper limit, 200). Because this is a Web-based process, participation is anonymous. Participants cannot challenge or question the statements of others. However, in subsequent steps, they are able to discuss the statements. The process takes approximately 10–15 minutes for each participant. Participants can return to the Web site repeatedly during the brainstorming period. Because participants work on the Web, they type statements directly on the computer and can immediately see their ideas along with everyone else's.

After the brainstorming session, the steering committee reviews the statements, editing them for clarity and grammar but *not* for content and ensuring that the statements are all syntactically "of a kind." In some cases, participants or a designated subgroup are asked via Web/e-mail to review the edited statements and make final revisions.

The structuring step involves three distinct tasks: providing demographic information and sorting and rating the brainstormed statements. As with brainstorming, this information is collected over the Web or through alternative mechanisms for people with no access to the Web. Participants are asked to provide demographic information about themselves or the organizations they represent. These data are used to identify participants for subgroup analysis. For the sorting,[114,115] each participant groups the statements "in a way that makes sense to you." The only restrictions in this sorting task are that there cannot be (1) N groups, with each group having one item; (2) one group consisting of all items; or (3) a miscellaneous group—any unique item is to be put in a separate pile. The Web software enables the participant to create, delete, and name new groups and to move statements from one group to another. Weller and Romney[115] explain why unstructured sorting ("the pile sort" method) is appropriate in this context:

> The outstanding strength of the pile sort task is the fact that it can accommodate a large number of items. We know of no other data collection method that will allow the collection of judged similarity data among over 100 items. This makes it the method of choice when large numbers are necessary. Other methods that might be used to collect similarity data, such as triads and paired comparison ratings, become impractical with a large number of items.[115(p25)]

For the rating task, each participant rates each statement on a five-point, Likert-type response scale. The specific rating variables are determined with the steering committee before the concept-mapping project is started. Typically, participants rate the statements for relative importance, where

1 = relatively unimportant (compared with the rest of the statements);
2 = somewhat important;
3 = moderately important;
4 = very important; and
5 = extremely important (compared with the rest of the statements).

Participants are unlikely to brainstorm statements that are totally unrelated to the focus. Therefore, rating should be considered a relative judgment of the importance of each item in relation to all other items brainstormed. In addition, participants typically also rate the relative feasibility of addressing each issue, where

1 = not at all feasible;
2 = not very feasible;
3 = somewhat feasible;
4 = moderately feasible; and
5 = very feasible.

Other ratings of the statements may be developed and accomplished as the overall project unfolds.

Data Analysis

The concept-mapping analysis is handled automatically by the Concept System program, beginning with construction from the sort information of an $N \times N$ binary, symmetric matrix of similarities, X_{ij}. For any two items, i and j, a 1 is placed in X_{ij} if the two items were placed in the same pile by the participant; otherwise a 0 is entered.[115] The total $N \times N$ similarity matrix, T_{ij}, is obtained by summing across the individual X_{ij} matrices. Thus, any cell in this matrix could take integer values between 0 and the number of people who sorted the statements. The value indicates the number of people who placed the i,j pair in the same pile. The total similarity matrix T_{ij} is analyzed by using nonmetric MDS analysis with a two-dimensional solution. The solution is limited to two dimensions because, as Kruskal and Wish[116] point out:

> Since it is generally easier to work with two-dimensional configurations than with those involving more dimensions, ease of use considerations are also important for decisions about dimensionality. For example, when an MDS configuration is desired primarily as the foundation on which to display clustering results, then a two-dimensional configuration is far more useful than one involving three or more dimensions.[116(p58)]

The analysis yields a two-dimensional (x,y) configuration of the set of statements based on the criterion that statements piled together most often are located more proximately in two-dimensional space and those piled together less frequently are farther apart.

The x,y configuration is the input for the hierarchical cluster analysis using Ward's algorithm[117] as the basis for defining a cluster. Use of the MDS configuration as input to the cluster analysis in effect forces the cluster analysis to partition the MDS configuration into nonoverlapping clusters in two-dimensional space. There is no simple mathematical criterion by which a final number of clusters can be selected. The typical procedure is to examine an initial cluster solution that was the maximum desirable for interpretation in this context. Then successively lower cluster solutions are examined. A judgment is made at each level about whether the merger seems substantively reasonable. The pattern of judgments of the suitability of different cluster solutions is examined. The final number of clusters is selected to preserve the most detail and still yield substantively interpretable clusters of statements.

The Concept System program automatically graphs the MDS configuration of the statement points in two dimensions. This "point map" displays the location of all the brainstormed statements. Statements closer to each other generally are expected to be more similar in meaning. A "cluster map" also is generated that displays the original statement points enclosed by polygon-shaped boundaries for the clusters.

The one-to-five importance and feasibility rating data are averaged across people for each item and each cluster. This rating information is depicted graphically (1) in a "point rating map" showing the original point map with the average rating per item displayed as vertical columns in the third dimension and (2) in a "cluster rating map" that shows the cluster average rating by using the third dimension. The following materials should be available for use in the session on map interpretation:

1. List of brainstormed statements grouped by cluster

2. Point map showing MDS placement of brainstormed statements and identifying numbers

3. Cluster map showing cluster solution

4. Point rating maps showing MDS placement of brainstormed statements and identifying numbers, with average statement ratings overlaid

5. Cluster rating maps showing final cluster solution, with average cluster ratings overlaid

All the graphics are created interactively by the Concept System and projected onto a screen for participants to see.

Interpretation of Concept Maps

A preliminary interpretation of results is conducted by the project facilitation team and used as the foundation for subsequent use. At the meeting itself, the core group participants convene to review and interpret the results directly. This interpretation session follows a structured process described in detail by Trochim.[16] The facilitator begins the session by giving participants the list of clustered statements and reminding them of the brainstorming, sorting, and rating tasks performed earlier. Each participant is asked to read silently through the set of statements in each cluster and generate a short phrase or word to describe or label the set of statements as a cluster. The facilitator leads the group in a discussion, working cluster by cluster to achieve group consensus on an acceptable label for each cluster. In most cases, when people suggest labels for a specific cluster, the group readily comes to consensus. If the group has difficulty achieving consensus, the facilitator suggests hybrid names that combine key terms or phrases from several individuals' labels.

Once the clusters are labeled, the group is shown the point map and told that statements frequently sorted together generally are closer to each other on the map than are statements infrequently sorted together. To reinforce the notion that the analysis placed the statements sensibly, participants are taken on a "tour" of the map by the facilitator, who identifies statements in various places on the map and examines their contents. After becoming familiar with the numbered point map, the participants are told that the analysis also organized the points (i.e., statements) into groups as shown on the list of clustered statements they already have labeled. The cluster map is projected, and participants are told that it is a visual portrayal of the cluster list. The agreed-upon cluster labels are shown on the final projected map.

Participants examine this labeled cluster map to determine whether it makes sense to them. The facilitator reminds them that, in general, clusters closer together on the map should be conceptually more similar than clusters farther apart and asks them to assess whether this seems to be true. Participants are asked to think of a geographic map and "take a trip" across the map, reading each cluster to assess whether the visual structure seems sensible. They are asked to identify interpretable groups of clusters or "regions." These are discussed and labeled on the map. Just as in labeling the clusters, the group arrives at a consensus label for each identified region.

The facilitator notes that all the material presented uses only the sorting data. The results of the rating task are then presented through the maps for point rating and cluster rating. It is explained that the height of a point or cluster represents the average rating for that statement or cluster of statements. Again, participants are encouraged to examine these maps to determine whether they make intuitive sense and to discuss possible implications of information on the maps in relation to the focus issue. Figure 4A.1 shows a concept map from a previous project.

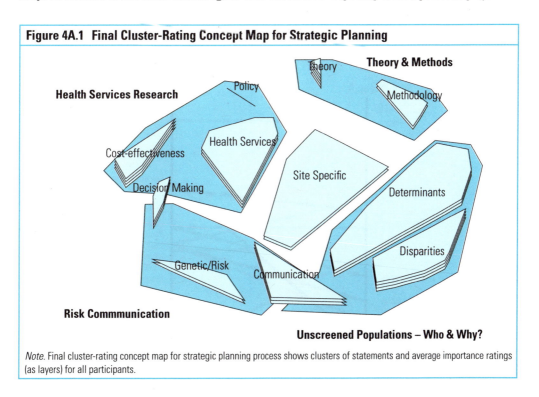

Figure 4A.1 Final Cluster-Rating Concept Map for Strategic Planning

Note. Final cluster-rating concept map for strategic planning process shows clusters of statements and average importance ratings (as layers) for all participants.

Consensus Analysis

Pattern matching[105,106] is used for a number of purposes in this process. The most immediate use is exploration of consensus across different stakeholders or stakeholder groups. Pattern matching is both a statistical analysis and a graphic analysis. Graphically, a pattern match is portrayed by using a "ladder" graph consisting of two vertical axes (one for each "pattern"). The vertical axes are joined by lines indicating average values for each cluster on the concept map for any variable specified. Statistically, the two patterns are compared with a Pearson product-moment correlation displayed at the bottom of the ladder graph. Figure 4A.2 illustrates a pattern match describing the degree of consensus between two stakeholder groups.

In a "ladder" graph, strong agreement between patterns results in a set of near-horizontal lines that look like a ladder. The match in figure 4A.2 highlights discrepancies in cluster importance ratings between these groups. In addition, the pattern match enables immediate identification of cluster areas showing the greatest consensus or lack of agreement. Participants explore a number of such matches to ascertain the degree of consensus among stakeholders.

Action Planning

For detailed action planning, it is useful to partition the results graphically by cluster. Typically, go-zone plots of the type shown in figure 4A.3 are used. The bivariate plot displays the relative importance and feasibility of each statement in the cluster.

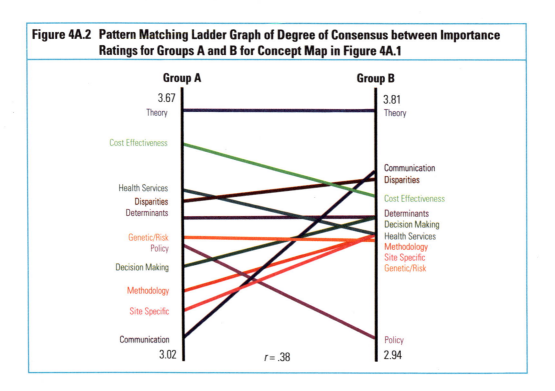

Figure 4A.2 Pattern Matching Ladder Graph of Degree of Consensus between Importance Ratings for Groups A and B for Concept Map in Figure 4A.1

Figure 4A.3 Go-Zone Plot of Feasibility Versus Importance for Methodology Cluster in Concept Map (Figure 4A.1)

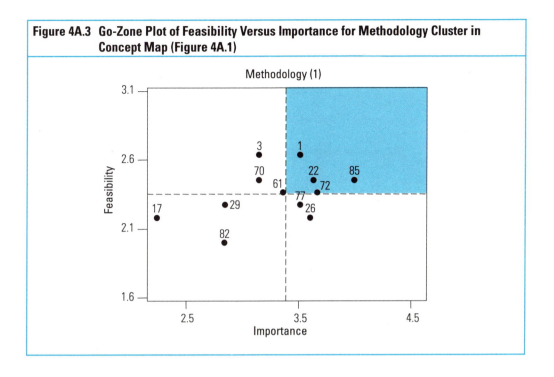

Each point represents a brainstormed issue. Each statement is shown with its identifying number. The upper-right quadrant indicates statements that have relatively high importance and feasibility. The plot takes its name from this quadrant, which is sometimes called the go-zone to indicate that these are the first issues one should "go" to when thinking about action planning. The participants review these plots and use them as the basis for an initial discussion about action planning.

References

1. Trochim, W. M., F. A. Stillman, P. I. Clark, and C. L. Schmitt. 2003. Development of a model of the tobacco industry's interference with tobacco control programmes. *Tobacco Control* 12 (2): 140–47.

2. Griffin, R. W. 2002. *Management.* 7th ed. Boston: Houghton Mifflin.

3. Daft, R. L. 2004. *Management.* 6th ed. Mason, OH: Thomson/South-Western.

4. Taylor, F. W. 1923. *The principles of scientific management.* New York: Harper and Brothers.

5. Veney, J. E., and A. D. Kaluzny. 1984. *Evaluation and decision making for health services programs.* Englewood Cliffs, NJ: Prentice-Hall.

6. Cabrera, D. 2001. *Knowledge Age Operating System: Four principles of project design.* Version 1.0. Loveland, CO: Project N Press.

7. Mintzberg, H. 1994. The fall and rise of strategic planning. *Harvard Business Review* (January–February): 107–14.

8. Nutt, P. C. 1984. *Planning methods: For health and related organizations.* Wiley Series in Health Services. New York: John Wiley and Sons.

9. Witkin, B. R., and J. W. Altschuld. 1995. *Planning and conducting needs assessments: A practical guide.* Thousand Oaks, CA: Sage.

10. Osborn, A. F. 1948. *Your creative power: How to use imagination.* New York: C. Scribner's Sons.

11. Delbecq, A. L., A. H. Van de Ven, and D. H. Gustafson. 1975. *Group techniques for program planning: A guide to nominal group and Delphi processes.* Management Applications series. Glenview, IL: Scott, Foresman.

12. Stewart, D. W., and P. N. Shamdasani. 1990. *Focus groups: Theory and practice.* Applied Social Research Methods series 20. Thousand Oaks, CA: Sage.

13. Linstone, H. A., and M. Turoff, eds. 1975. *The Delphi method: Techniques and applications.* Reading, MA: Addison-Wesley.

14. Novak, J. D. 1998. *Learning, creating, and using knowledge: Concept maps as facilitative tools in schools and corporations.* Mahwah, NJ: Lawrence Erlbaum.

15. Buzan, T., and B. Buzan. 1993. *The mind map book: Radiant thinking; The major evolution in human thought.* London: BBC Books.

16. Trochim, W. M. K. 1989. An introduction to concept mapping for planning and evaluation. *Evaluation and Program Planning* 12 (1): 1–16.

17. Delaware Cancer Consortium. 2004. *Turning commitment into action: Year-one accomplishments.* Cancer Consortium Reports. Dover: Delaware Health and Social Services, Division of Public Health.

18. Trochim, W. M., B. Milstein, B. J. Wood, S. Jackson, and V. Pressler. 2004. Setting objectives for community and systems change: An application of concept mapping for planning a statewide health improvement initiative. *Health Promotion Practice* 5 (1): 8–19.

19. Stokols, D., J. Fuqua, J. Gress, R. Harvey, K. Phillips, L. Baezconde-Garbanati, J. Unger, et al. 2003. Evaluating transdisciplinary science. *Nicotine & Tobacco Research* 5 Suppl. 1: S21–S39.

20. Kaplan, R. S., and D. P. Norton. 2003. *Strategy maps: Converting intangible assets into tangible outcomes.* Boston: Harvard Business School Press.

21. Axelrod, R. M., ed. 1976. *Structure of decision: The cognitive maps of political elites.* Princeton: Princeton Univ. Press.

22. W.K. Kellogg Foundation. 2001. *Logic model development guide: Using logic models to bring together planning, evaluation and action.* Battle Creek, MI: W.K. Kellogg Foundation.

23. Senge, P. M. 1990. *The fifth discipline: The art and practice of the learning organization.* New York: Currency Doubleday.

24. Richardson, G. P. 1991. *Feedback thought in social science and systems theory.* Philadelphia: Univ. of Pennsylvania Press.

25. Earl, S., F. Carden, and T. Smutylo. 2001. *Outcome mapping: Building learning and reflection into development programs.* Ottawa, ON: International Development Research Centre.

26. Weisbord, M. R. 1992. *Discovering common ground.* San Francisco: Berrett-Koehler.

27. Axelrod, D. 1992. Getting everyone involved: How one organization involved its employees, supervisors, and managers

in redesigning the organization. *Journal of Applied Behavioral Science* 28 (4): 499–509.

28. Axelrod, R. 2000. *Terms of engagement: Changing the way we change organizations.* San Francisco: Berrett-Koehler.

29. Dannemiller, K. D., and R. W. Jacobs. 1992. Changing the way organizations change: A revolution of common sense. *Journal of Applied Behavorial Science* 28 (4): 480–98.

30. Jacobs, R. W. 1994. *Real time strategic change: How to involve an entire organization in fast and far-reaching change.* San Francisco: Berrett-Koehler.

31. Emery, F. 1995. Participative design: Effective, flexible and successful, now! *Journal for Quality and Participation* 18 (1): 6–9.

32. Owen, H. 1992. *Open space technology: A user's guide.* San Francisco: Berrett-Koehler.

33. Owen, H., ed. 1995. *Tales from open space.* Cabin John, MD: Abbott.

34. Owen, H. 2000. *The power of spirit: How organizations transform.* San Francisco: Berrett-Koehler.

35. Cooperrider, D. L., and D. Whitney. 2000. *Collaborating for change: Appreciative inquiry.* San Francisco: Berrett-Koehler.

36. Emery, M., and R. E. Purser. 1996. *The search conference: A powerful method for planning organizational change and community action.* San Francisco: Jossey-Bass.

37. Darwin, C. 1988. *The origin of species, 1876.* New York: New York Univ. Press.

38. Koch, R. 2001. *The natural laws of business: Applying the theories of Darwin, Einstein, and Newton to achieve business success.* New York: Currency/Doubleday.

39. Raup, D. M. 1991. *Extinction: Bad genes or bad luck?* New York: W. W. Norton.

40. Watts, D. J. 1999. *Small worlds: The dynamics of networks between order and randomness.* Princeton: Princeton Univ. Press.

41. Gray, B. 1989. *Collaborating: Finding common ground for multiparty problems.* San Francisco: Jossey-Bass.

42. Chisholm, R. F. 1998. *Developing network organizations: Learning from practice and theory.* New York: Addison-Wesley.

43. Nishiguchi, T., and A. Beaudet. 1998. The Toyota group and the Aisin fire: Case study. *MIT Sloan Management Review* 40 (1): 49–59.

44. Weick, K. E. 1976. Educational organizations as loosely coupled systems. *Administrative Science Quarterly* 21 (1): 1–19.

45. Orton, J. D., and K. E. Weick. 1990. Loosely coupled systems: A reconceptualization. *Academy of Management Review* 15 (2): 203–23.

46. Perrow, C. B. 1981. Normal accident at Three Mile Island. *Society* 18 (5): 17–26.

47. Meyerson, D., and J. Martin. 1987. Culture change: An integration of three different views. *Journal of Management Studies* 24 (6): 623–47.

48. Deal, T. E., and L. D. Celotti. 1980. How much influence do (and can) educational administrators have on classrooms? *Phi Delta Kappan* 61 (7): 471–78.

49. Lantz, P. M., E. Viruell-Fuentes, B. A. Israel, D. Softley, and R. Guzman. 2001. Can communities and academia work together on public health research? Evaluation results from a community-based participatory research partnership in Detroit. *Journal of Urban Health* 78 (3): 495–507.

50. Wallerstein, I. M. 1999. *The end of the world as we know it: Social science for the twenty-first century.* Minneapolis: Univ. of Minnesota Press.

51. Green, L. W., and S. L. Mercer. 2001. Can public health researchers and agencies reconcile the push from funding bodies and the pull from communities? *American Journal of Public Health* 91 (12): 1926–29.

52. Krieger, J., C. Allen, A. Cheadle, S. Ciske, J. K. Schier, K. Senturia, and M. Sullivan. 2002. Using community-based participatory research to address social determinants of health: Lessons learned from Seattle Partners for Healthy Communities. *Health Education and Behavior* 29 (3): 361–82.

53. Katz, D., and R. L. Kahn. 1978. *The social psychology of organizations.* 2nd ed. Hoboken, NJ: John Wiley and Sons.

54. Locke, E. A., K. N. Shaw, L. M. Saari, and G. P. Latham. 1981. Goal setting and task performance: 1969–1980. *Psychological Bulletin* 90 (1): 125–52.

55. Manz, C. C. 1992. Self-leading work teams: Moving beyond self-management myths. *Human Relations* 45 (11): 1119–40.

56. Wall Jr., J. A. and R. R. Callister. 1995. Conflict and its management. *Journal of Management* 21 (3): 515–58.

57. Cordero-Guzmán, H. R. 2001. Interorganizational networks among

community-based organizations. http://www.newschool.edu/Milano/cdrc/pubs/r.2002.1.pdf.

58. Griffin, T. J. 2004. Large group interventions for organizational change: Towards a generative theory of wholeness. PhD diss., Benedictine Univ.

59. Bunker, B. B., and B. T. Alban. 1997. *Large group interventions: Engaging the whole system for rapid change.* San Francisco: Jossey-Bass.

60. Emery, F. E., and E. L. Trist. 1965. The causal texture of organizational environments. *Human Relations* 18:21–32.

61. Ray, M. 1995. Community building as a metaphor for worldwide paradigm shift. In *Community building: Renewing spirit and learning in business,* ed. K. Gozdz. Santa Cruz, CA: Vision Nest Publishing.

62. von Bertalanffy, L. 1952. *Problems of life.* New York: John Wiley and Sons.

63. Berger, P., and T. Luckmann. 1966. Society as a human product. In *The social construction of reality: A treatise in the sociology of knowledge,* ed. P. L. Berger and T. Luckman, 51–61. Garden City, NY: Anchor Books.

64. Gergen, K. J. 1994. *Realities and relationships: Soundings in social construction.* Cambridge, MA: Harvard Univ. Press.

65. Maslow, A. H. 1943. A theory of human motivation. *Psychological Review* 50:370–96.

66. McGregor, D. 1960. *The human side of enterprise.* New York: McGraw-Hill.

67. Lewin, K. 1951. *Field theory in social science: Selected theoretical papers,* ed. D. Cartwright. New York: Harper and Row.

68. Lippit, R. 1983. Future before you plan. In *NTL manager's handbook.* Arlington, VA: NTL Institute.

69. Schindler-Rainman, E., and R. Lippitt. 1980. *Building the collaborative community: Mobilizing citizens for action.* Riverside: Univ. of California.

70. Bion, W. R. 1961. *Experiences in groups: And other papers.* London: Tavistock.

71. Bennis, W. G., and H. A. Shepard. 1956. A theory of group development. *Human Relations* 9 (4): 415–37.

72. Tuckman, B. W. 1965. Developmental sequence in small groups. *Psychological Bulletin* 63:384–99.

73. Smith, K. K., and D. N. Berg. 1987. *Paradoxes of group life: Understanding conflict, paralysis, and movement in group dynamics.* San Francisco: Jossey-Bass.

74. Alford, C. 1990. *Melanie Klein and critical social theory: An account of politics, art, and reason based on her psychoanalytic theory.* New Haven, CT: Yale Univ. Press.

75. Turquet, P. 1975. Threats to identity in the large group. In *The large group: Dynamics and theory,* ed. L. Kreeger. London: Karnac Books.

76. Pasmore, W. A., and M. R. Fagans. 1992. Participation, individual development, and organizational change: A review and synthesis. *Journal of Management* 18 (2): 375–97.

77. Gilmore, T. N., and C. Barneyt. 1992. Designing the social architecture of participation in large groups to effect organizational change. *Journal of Applied Behavioral Science* 28 (4): 534–48.

78. Kreeger, L., ed. 1975. *The large group: Dynamics and theory.* London: Karnac Books.

79. Shadish, W. R., T. D. Cook, and L. C. Leviton. 1991. *Foundations of program evaluation: Theories of practice.* Thousand Oaks, CA: Sage.

80. Weiss, C. H. 1997. *Evaluation.* 2nd ed. New York: Prentice Hall.

81. Berk, R. A., and P. H. Rossi. 1990. *Thinking about program evaluation.* 2nd ed. Thousand Oaks, CA: Sage.

82. Chelimsky, E., and W. R. Shadish, eds. 1997. *Evaluation for the 21st century: A handbook.* Thousand Oaks, CA: Sage.

83. Royse, D., and B. A. Thyer. 1996. *Program evaluation: An introduction.* 2nd ed. Belmont, CA: Wadsworth.

84. Guba, E. G., and Y. S. Lincoln. 1989. *Fourth generation evaluation.* Thousand Oaks, CA: Sage.

85. Rossi, P. H., and H. E. Freeman. 1993. *Evaluation: A systematic approach.* 7th ed. Thousand Oaks, CA: Sage.

86. Cronbach, L. J. 1982. *Designing evaluations of educational and social programs.* San Francisco: Jossey-Bass.

87. Mark, M. M., G. T. Henry, and G. Julnes. 2000. *Evaluation: An integrated framework for understanding, guiding, and improving policies and programs.* San Francisco: Jossey-Bass.

88. Posavac, E. J., and R. G. Carey. 1992. *Program evaluation: Methods and case studies.* 4th ed. Englewood Cliffs, NJ: Prentice Hall.

89. Worthen, B. R., and J. R. Sanders. 1987. *Educational evaluation: Alternative approaches and practical guidelines.* New York: Longman.

90. Higgins, D. L., and M. Metzler. 2001. Implementing community-based participatory research centers in diverse urban settings. *Journal of Urban Health* 78 (3): 488–94.

91. Macaulay, A. C., L. E. Commanda, W. L. Freeman, N. Gibson, M. L. McCabe, C. M. Robbins, and P. L. Twohig. 1999. Participatory research maximises community and lay involvement. North American Primary Care Research Group. *British Medical Journal* 319 (7212): 774–78.

92. O'Fallon, L. R., and A. Dearry. 2002. Community-based participatory research as a tool to advance environmental health sciences. *Environmental Health Perspectives* 110 Suppl. 2:155–59.

93. Schnoes, C. J., V. Murphy-Berman, and J. M. Chambers. 2000. Empowerment evaluation applied: Experiences, analysis, and recommendations from a case study. *American Journal of Evaluation* 21 (1): 53–64.

94. Metzler, M. M., D. L. Higgins, C. G. Beeker, N. Freudenberg, P. M. Lantz, K. D. Senturia, and A. A. Eisinger. 2003. Addressing urban health in Detroit, New York City, and Seattle through community-based participatory research partnerships. *American Journal of Public Health* 93 (5): 803–11.

95. Minkler, M. 2000. Using participatory action research to build healthy communities. *Public Health Reports* 115 (2–3): 191–97.

96. Eisinger, A., and K. Senturia. 2001. Doing community-driven research: A description of Seattle Partners for Healthy Communities. *Journal of Urban Health* 78 (3): 519–34.

97. Reason, P., and H. Bradbury, eds. 2000. *Handbook of action research: Participative inquiry and practice.* Thousand Oaks, CA: Sage.

98. Nastasi, B. K., K. Varjas, S. L. Schensul, K. T. Silva, J. J. Schensul, and P. Ratnayake. 2000. The participatory intervention model: A framework for conceptualizing and promoting intervention acceptability. *School Psychology Quarterly* 15 (2): 207–32.

99. Fetterman, D. M., S. J. Kaftarian, and A. Wandersman. 1995. *Empowerment evaluation: Knowledge and tools for self-assessment and accountability.* Thousand Oaks, CA: Sage.

100. Potvin, L., M. Cargo, A. M. McComber, T. Delormier, and A. C. Macaulay. 2003. Implementing participatory intervention and research in communities: Lessons from the Kahnawake Schools Diabetes Prevention Project in Canada. *Social Science and Medicine* 56 (6): 1295–1305.

101. Riley, P. L., R. Jossy, L. Nkinsi, and L. Buhi. 2001. The CARE–CDC Health Initiative: A model for global participatory research. Editorial. *American Journal of Public Health* 91 (10): 1549–52.

102. Thompson, B., G. Coronado, S. A. Snipes, and K. Puschel. 2003. Methodologic advances and ongoing challenges in designing community-based health promotion programs. *Annual Review of Public Health* 24:315–40.

103. Chen, H. T. 1990. *Theory-driven evaluations.* Thousand Oaks, CA: Sage.

104. Campbell, D. T., J. C. Stanley, and N. L. Gage. 1963. *Experimental and quasi-experimental designs for research.* Boston: Houghton Mifflin.

105. Trochim, W. M. K. 1985. Pattern matching, validity, and conceptualization in program evaluation. *Evaluation Review* 9 (5): 575–604.

106. Trochim, W. M. K. 1989. Outcome pattern matching and program theory. *Evaluation and Program Planning* 12 (4): 355–66.

107. Trochim, W. M. K., and J. A. Cook. 1992. Pattern matching in theory-driven evaluation: A field example from psychiatric rehabilitation. In *Using theory to improve program and policy evaluations,* ed. H. Chen and P. Rossi, 49–69. Westport, CT: Greenwood.

108. Centers for Disease Control and Prevention. 1999. Framework for program evaluation in public health. *Morbidity and Mortality Weekly Report Recommendations and Reports* 48 (RR-11): 1–40.

109. Trochim, W. M. K. 1989. Concept mapping: Soft science or hard art? *Evaluation and Program Planning* 12 (1): 87–110.

110. Institute of Medicine. 2001. *Crossing the quality chasm: A new health system for the 21st century.* Washington, DC: National Academies Press.

111. Stillman, F., A. Hartman, B. Graubard, E. Gilpin, D. Chavis, J. Garcia, L. M. Wun, W. Lynn, and M. Manley. 1999. The American Stop Smoking Intervention Study: Conceptual framework and evaluation design. *Evaluation Review* 23 (3): 259–80.

112. Clark, P. I., F. A. Stillman, W. J. Strauss, W. Trochim, and C. L. Schmitt. 2001. Strength of tobacco control: Escaping the black box of program evaluation. Paper presented at the 129th annual meeting of the American Public Health Association, Atlanta. http://apha.confex.com/apha/129am/techprogram/paper_31740.htm.

113. Concept Systems. 2006. Company Web site. http://www.conceptsystems.com.

114. Rosenberg, S., and M. P. Kim. 1975. The method of sorting as a data-gathering procedure in multivariate research. *Multivariate Behavioral Research* 10 (4): 489–502.

115. Weller, S. C., and A. K. Romney. 1988. *Systematic data collection.* Qualitative Research Methods series 10. Thousand Oaks, CA: Sage.

116. Kruskal, J. B., and M. Wish. 1978. *Multidimensional scaling.* Quantitative Applications in the Social Sciences series 11. Thousand Oaks, CA: Sage.

117. Everitt, B. 1980. *Cluster analysis.* 2nd ed. New York: Halsted Press and John Wiley and Sons.

5

How to Anticipate Change in Tobacco Control Systems

Systems methods represent an evolutionary step in the ability to solve complex problems, moving from simple cause-and-effect models to more realistic scenarios in which causes and effects influence each other with dynamic, evolving feedback. This chapter provides examples of the application of one systems thinking approach, system dynamics modeling, to current tobacco control issues. System dynamics has a rich research heritage, emphasizes use of simulation models for anticipating dynamic change, and has the potential to provide a more sophisticated understanding of key issues in tobacco control, especially factors that influence smoking prevalence. This chapter also presents the results of a research project by the Initiative on the Study and Implementation of Systems (ISIS) to explore the use of system dynamics to develop

- *A causal map of tobacco control variables, based on participatory input from expert stakeholders;*

- *Formal simulation models based on factors derived from these causal maps; and*

- *Simulations of tobacco use prevalence and consumption across an aging chain of smokers.*

The systems that fail are those that rely on the permanency of human nature, and not on its growth and development.

—Oscar Wilde (1854–1900)

Introduction

Today's tobacco control environment represents a complex and dynamic interrelated system of issues and stakeholders. In this dynamic environment, change is continuous and poses significant challenges for those who would anticipate change and prepare for its consequences. There is growing recognition that systems approaches need to be able to address this challenge of dynamics and to anticipate change. System dynamics modeling is one of the most prominent and promising approaches for addressing such problems and, in doing so, helping to achieve more effective integration of research knowledge and its practical implications.

ISIS developed a detailed illustration of how system dynamics modeling could be applied to tobacco control to demonstrate the potential of this approach. The goal is to encourage further interest in and exploration of the promise of systems thinking and, ultimately, to provide new insights into how to reduce tobacco use. As demonstrated in the overview of systems thinking in chapter 3 and the following chapters in this monograph, system dynamics is only one systems thinking approach to tobacco control. Other methods offer different insights, and there is considerable potential to develop new thinking about tobacco control through the skilled application of a range of systems approaches.

System dynamics facilitates an understanding of feedback processes, especially how self-reinforcing or "vicious" cycles can arise. These often are unintended negative consequences of interventions. Simple illustrative examples of such counterintuitive thinking include the following:

- Building highways to ease traffic congestion eventually fails because less congestion invites more cars and drivers, thus clogging the highways again.

- Large-scale crackdowns and violent responses to terrorist acts kill and harm innocent people. Surviving friends and family join the terrorists, so the violence escalates.

- Corporate efforts to gain advantage in the competition for executive talent lead to raises in total compensation packages. Other firms respond in kind, negating the first firm's momentary advantage and creating an overall self-reinforcing structure of raises and counterraises. Ultimately, this structure drastically increases executive compensation packages across the nation.

- Tobacco control efforts intended to reduce smoking prevalence cause market pressures that force tobacco companies to defend their interests with advertising and product promotion, strategic pricing, new product design, and target marketing, which tend to increase smoking prevalence.

At the same time, system dynamics is more than an attempt to quantify vicious cycles and unintended consequences. The conceptual and quantitative models are tools to enhance the ability to think about the dynamics of systems, leading to better decisions. The models can demonstrate effects that might not otherwise be envisioned or that might be counterintuitive. These approaches can highlight areas of uncertainty, helping to set priorities for future research or demonstrating that some things are simply unknowable. At a deeper level, they also can be used to simulate change to help in predicting what lies ahead and in shaping a more desirable future. Early system dynamics efforts have been undertaken to address different aspects of promoting or controlling tobacco use, such as

- Individual and family factors, such as genetics, personality traits, and parental role modeling

- Community-level interventions, such as smoking restrictions in public places and restrictions on advertising and promotion of tobacco products in retail stores

- State and national policies and practices, such as laws governing the purchase of tobacco products by minors, subsidies to tobacco growers, and research funding for the public health effects of active and passive smoking

- Global policies and practices, such as how multinational corporations maintain profitability by exploiting weaknesses in the policies of some countries, in trade agreements, and in the international Framework Convention on Tobacco Control, the first international health treaty[1]

Current best practices in areas ranging from prevention of smoking and smoking cessation programs to policy interventions have led to impressive short-term gains in factors such as reduced prevalence and consumption and morbidity and mortality.

At the same time, these successes often carry within them the seeds of future problems, such as reduction in funding for tobacco control, shifting of public health priorities, and the counterefforts of the tobacco industry. As a result, poorly anticipated problems frequently loom, ranging from higher prevalence of smoking among groups such as young women, increased global marketing of tobacco, and fragmentation of efforts among tobacco control stakeholders—issues that ultimately could negatively affect overall public health. In areas such as these, in which traditional tools have proved insufficient, system dynamics modeling can provide a way to extend cause-and-effect models to include the dynamics of feedback and thereby provide more accurate models on which to base future policy.

System Dynamics

Computer simulation is used to assist thinking about complex dynamic systems. This approach grew out of (1) advances in computing technology, (2) an improved understanding of strategic decision making, and (3) developments in understanding the

---

Definitions: System Dynamics Versus Systems Thinking

System dynamics approaches such as those outlined here constitute one of many methods to treat behavior as a system. However, definition of the broader term *systems thinking,* which is at the core of this monograph, is the subject of considerable dispute. To some, systems thinking is the broad discipline of exploring and modeling system behavior. To others, systems thinking is more narrowly defined, constituting their essential approach to systems. Those involved in ISIS have taken a broad-based and more inclusive stance on the definition. This chapter provides background on this issue, especially as it relates to the field of system dynamics.

Systems investigator Barry Richmond felt strongly that systems thinking had a narrow, specific meaning (i.e., making inferences about behavior based on its underlying structure), which encompassed the modeling approach inherent in system dynamics.[a] He represents this "operational definition" of systems thinking by using a Venn diagram, arguing that system dynamics modeling forms a large part of the broader discipline of systems thinking. He contrasts this approach with other views, such as that of systems pioneer Jay Forrester of the Massachusetts Institute of Technology.[b] Forrester contends that systems thinking served as a small part of the overall system dynamics approach. The figure that follows is adapted from Richmond's paper.[a]

Forrester's View (left) versus Richmond's View (right) on System Dynamics and Systems Thinking

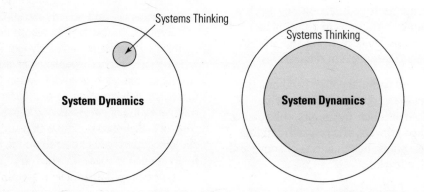

In comparison, many people, including those involved in ISIS, now see system dynamics modeling as one of the broad range of tools and methods encompassed by systems thinking. The best representation of this relationship may be that system dynamics modeling is one of several components within the broader context of systems thinking.

System Dynamics Modeling as One Approach to Systems Thinking

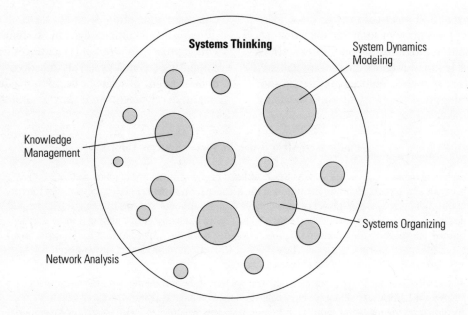

The debate about system dynamics and systems thinking terminology becomes particularly significant in light of other methodologies that adopt the "systems" label. One such methodology is Peter Checkland's soft systems methodology.[c] It counters the emphasis that systems thinking is a modeling and measurement endeavor, seeing it instead as a learning process that takes a phenomenological rather than deterministic stance. Checkland views systems thinking as an evolving process driven by the purposeful activities of its stakeholders, in which all voices are represented and boundaries between divergent views are free to shift. This approach, in turn, has become part of the critical systems thinking approach espoused by Flood and Romm[d] and Midgley,[e] in which systems thinking is seen as a stakeholder-driven process. In his classic book *Systems Thinking, Systems Practice: Includes a 30-Year Retrospective,* Checkland himself defines systems thinking as a process that "makes conscious use of the particular concept of wholeness captured in the word 'system' to order our thoughts."[c(p4)]

The argument presented here is against the parochial or narrow view of systems thinking and in favor of viewing it as a broad range of approaches that examine behavior as a system. In addition to approaches described in other chapters (systems organizing, network analysis, and knowledge management), there are other strategies that provide different lenses for examining systems. These include but are not limited to the following:

- System dynamics modeling, which seeks to create mathematical simulation models incorporating stocks, flows, and feedback, defined later in this chapter

- "Soft" systems approaches that focus on processes and people, such as Checkland's soft systems methodology,[c] Midgley's participatory stakeholder-driven approaches,[e] and Senge's concept of a learning organization.[f] Compared with traditional system dynamics, these strategies examine the evolution of a system as an ecological process, poorly or imperfectly reflected through mathematical simulation

- Chaos and complexity approaches that examine behavior as systems of autonomous agents following simple rules, such as a flock of birds that take flight by following a leader and maintaining a specific distance from their neighbors, or a tobacco control intervention modeled on agents who create effects and countereffects

A continuing part of the evolution of the systems community, which can be seen itself as a system, is an evolution over time from the modeling of simple cause-and-effect relationships, such as logic models, to complex real-world interrelationships that are depicted iteratively over time with feedback. This depiction allows examination of effects, such as side effects, edge effects, and unintended consequences. The systems community ultimately represents an evolution from the "black box"—used in an attempt to understand reality—toward more detailed and realistic models of the dynamics of reality.

This evolution mirrors trends in science and technology that in turn enable more accurate representation of reality. These trends range from simple problems that can be solved as single equations to more complex problems that must be solved adaptively with evolving feedback. Today, this evolution continues from simple feedback to broader concepts such as neural networks, cybernetics, complex adaptive systems, and other self-learning physical phenomena.

[a]Richmond, B. 1994. System dynamics/systems thinking: Let's just get on with it. Paper presented at the 1994 International Systems Dynamics Conference, Sterling, Scotland. Reprinted with permission from ISEE Systems. http://www.intraxltd.com/Downloads/Files/SystemDynamicsSystemsThinking.htm.

[b]Forrester, J. W. 1961. *Industrial dynamics.* Cambridge, MA: MIT Press.

[c]Checkland, P. B. 1999. *Systems thinking, system practice: Includes a 30-year retrospective.* Chichester, UK: John Wiley and Sons.

[d]Flood, R. L., and N. R. A. Romm, eds. 1996. *Critical systems thinking: Current research and practice.* New York: Plenum.

[e]Midgley, G. 2000. *Systemic intervention: Philosophy, methodology and practice.* Contemporary Systems Thinking series. London: Springer.

[f]Senge, P. M. 1994. *The fifth discipline: The art and practice of the learning organization.* New York: Currency.

role of information feedback in the dynamics of complex systems. System dynamics practitioners seek to frame system behavior in terms of endogenous components with definable and self-contained behaviors, which in turn interact with each other to produce an evolutionary outcome.

Some abbreviate this idea as the "system as cause." Explaining the behavior of a system in terms of self-contained components that interact over time can force causal influences to double back on themselves, forming feedback loops of circular causality. The feedback concept empowers this component-level point of view and gives it structure. Thus, the system dynamics approach is partly characterized by its heavy use of a feedback perspective.

This viewpoint is so important that system dynamics practitioners and others might define systems thinking succinctly as the mental effort to uncover integral sources of

system behavior. Much of system dynamics can be thought of as *computer simulation in support of systems thinking*. The power of the system dynamics approach comes from this component-level, feedback-rich viewpoint, in which all purposeful action takes place in the classic cybernetic loop that includes

- Goals for the system

- Current state of the system

- Perceptions of that current state

- The gap between goals and perceptions

- Action intended to reduce the gap, resulting in a new state of the system

- Revised perceptions, leading to further actions

Unfortunately, the world that analysts attempt to simulate is more complicated than that, as figure 5.1 suggests. The

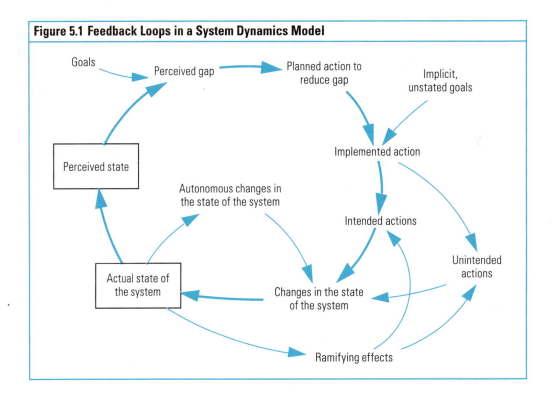

Figure 5.1 Feedback Loops in a System Dynamics Model

Goals

Perceived gap

Planned action to reduce gap

Implicit, unstated goals

Implemented action

Perceived state

Autonomous changes in the state of the system

Intended actions

Unintended actions

Actual state of the system

Changes in the state of the system

Ramifying effects

bold loop in the figure is the classic cybernetic loop, striving to bring the state of the system toward some set goal. However, unstated goals often intervene and unintended effects are triggered. The system changes from its own forces, and all sorts of effects feed back to alter the actions of the actors. (In a system dynamics perspective, there are no "side" effects, only effects.) Moreover, complex systems have many actors, each with personal or organizational goals, so this structure is repeated countless times in real systems. The result is that actions one group takes to reach toward its goals disturb the system and prompt other groups to implement counteraction, striving to reassert the status quo or lead to a different status quo. In contrast, the simpler cause-and-effect behavior can result when these factors are held constant. Thus, a system often will *compensate* for changes and weaken or even negate them, much as a price cut can stimulate competitive forces that negate its original goal of increasing sales. This phenomenon is referred to as *policy resistance*.[2]

In complex systems, this natural policy resistance can be seen as a pattern of dynamic behavior formed by individual events and decisions and a conscious effort to perceive in this stream of decisions the persistent policy structure producing them. System dynamics models strive to capture that policy structure as a part of system structure and produce, as output, graphs over time that represent this aggregate view of events and decisions. For example, the destruction of the World Trade Center on September 11, 2001, clearly was a significant event in the contemporary world. Without diminishing that significance, a systems view would place that event in its dynamic context, looking back in history to trace the slow accumulation of pressures that gave rise to the event itself and the extent of the nation's capacities to deal with it.

One example of system dynamics modeling can be seen in a welfare reform study[3] that was conducted in three counties in New York State. The study was an attempt to help the diverse agencies providing social services to the poor cope with the threat of persistently rising costs when some families would begin timing out of welfare benefits under reform. The mapping and modeling work was performed with groups of welfare stakeholders and social service providers in each county. This work eventually yielded a formal model of more than 600 equations used (1) to examine a number of "what if" scenarios and policy options and (2) to create an environment in which stakeholders could learn from exploring the structure and behavior of the complex system.

One key finding was a classic "better before worse" scenario commonly seen in complex dynamic systems (interventions work in the short term; compensating feedback involves a delay). As more families come off assistance, they strain employment resources intended to match job seekers with stable jobs. This increases the number of marginally employed families who may fall back into the need for assistance. The result is that fewer families make it to stable jobs and more flow back into assistance, eventually increasing the population at risk for needing assistance.

These findings suggest the need to invest more resources in areas such as job coaching, job maintenance, child care, transportation, and other interventions intended to keep people employed. These areas are not the traditional purview of social services. They rely heavily on coordinated efforts of the private sector and nongovernmental service providers. These types of insights led two of the three counties to implement strategies to increase resources for these efforts. It is noteworthy that the welfare reforms have been a huge success. While the role of such modeling in the success has not been documented, this example illustrates how such modeling influenced at least some policy makers. The system dynamics approach, particularly when used in a group context with multiple stakeholders and diverse viewpoints, has seven characteristics:

1. *Engagement.* Key stakeholders are involved as the model evolves, and their own expertise and insights drive all aspect of the analysis.

2. *Mental models.* The model-building process uses the language and concepts participants bring with them to explain the assumptions and causal mental models managers use in decision making.

3. *Alignment.* The modeling process benefits from diverse, sometimes competing, viewpoints, as stakeholders have a chance to wrestle with causal assumptions in a group context. Often these discussions realign thinking and are among the most valuable portions of the overall group modeling effort.

4. *Determination of behavior by structure.* The formal simulation models resulting from this approach show how system structure influences system behavior. This leads to insights based on familiar system stocks and flows, and reveals understandable but initially counterintuitive tendencies such as policy resistance or "better before worse" behavior.

5. *Refutability.* The formal model yields testable propositions, enabling managers to determine how well their implicit theories match available data about overall system performance.

6. *Empowerment.* By using the formal model, participants can envision how actions under their control can change the future of the system.

7. *Estimation of parameters.* The model can help to estimate useful parameters

that are not otherwise available, such as model factors that lack an empirical base of values.

System Dynamics Application to Tobacco Control

A demonstration project to illustrate the modeling of factors in tobacco prevalence and consumption by using a system dynamics approach was undertaken as part of ISIS, incorporating heuristic data from participants in the ISIS innovation team. This model was designed both as a proof-of-concept project for system dynamics simulations of macrolevel tobacco issues and as a starting point for discussions on integration of such methods with other transdisciplinary aspects of a systems thinking environment.

Brainstorming Components of Tobacco Control Systems

During initial ISIS workshops in Washington, DC, participants helped form the concepts for the model presented here through a group brainstorming exercise. Workshop participants listed ideas, one per sheet, and then ideas were arranged on a wall, as a base for facilitated discussions on clusters of model issues. Building on the insights and data gained through these workshops, the facilitator constructed a causal map and simulation model based on factors in tobacco prevalence and consumption. The primary purpose of this model was to use it as a learning tool to attempt to create a simulation environment in which tobacco control stakeholders can experiment and theorize. Although the model was based on heuristic input from ISIS participants, its concepts serve as a prototype for future analyses using validated models and accurate data sources.

Path to System Dynamics Approaches to Tobacco Control

The system dynamics simulation model in this chapter, examining tobacco consumption and prevalence, is part of a growing tradition of efforts to use systems methods for policy simulation to address issues in tobacco control and public health. Initial projects in this area range from a 1980s systems study at the Massachusetts Institute of Technology projecting an accelerated decline in tobacco use[a] to the comprehensive tobacco policy model developed at the University of California at Irvine,[b] as well as proof-of-concept work undertaken at the National Cancer Institute before the efforts of ISIS.[c] More recent efforts detailed by Levy and associates[d] include the following:

- SimSmoke, funded by the Substance Abuse and Mental Health Services Administration's Center for Substance Abuse Prevention and the Robert Wood Johnson Foundation, models smoking rates and smoking mortality over a 40-year period. This model bases its projections from historical data on factors such as smoking prevalence, consumption, initiation, cessation, and mortality, as well as the influence of policy factors such as laws, taxes, and tobacco control activities. SimSmoke's projections range from a status quo scenario gradually reducing prevalence from 18.5% to 15.4% by 2040, with rising annual mortality during much of the period because of population trends, to proportionately lower prevalence based on the impact of specific policy interventions.

- A system model funded by the Substance Abuse Policy Research Program of the Robert Wood Johnson Foundation used age-specific rates for initiation and cessation of smoking. It demonstrated that smoking prevalence will continue to fall under current trends. However, it also established the implausibility of the goals for prevalence set for the *Healthy People 2010* initiative.

- GlaxoSmithKline sponsored a dynamic model for smoking control designed to project demand for its products for nicotine replacement therapy. The model focuses on the decision to stop smoking based on the "stages of change" model and uses empirical data about population demographics and behavior involved in quitting smoking. Its findings include the observation that lowering barriers to aids for smoking cessation, such as nicotine replacement therapy, increased cessation rates.

[a]Roberts, E. B., J. Homer, A. Kasabian, and M. Varrell. 1982. A systems view of the smoking problem: Perspective and limitations of the role of science in decision-making. *International Journal of Biomedical Computing* 13 (1): 69–86.

[b]Tengs, T. O., N. D. Osgood, and L. L. Chen. 2001. The cost-effectiveness of intensive national school-based anti-tobacco education: Results from the tobacco policy model. *Preventive Medicine* 33 (6): 558–70.

[c]Leischow, S. 2003. Social network analysis in tobacco control. Presentation at the National Cancer Institute, Bethesda, MD.

[d]Levy, D. T., F. Chaloupka, J. Gitchell, D. Mendez, and K. E. Warner. 2002. The use of simulation models for the surveillance, justification and understanding of tobacco control policies. *Health Care Management Science* 5 (2): 113–20.

Grouping Components into Sectors

The initial data used to form this model were derived from discussions, exercises, and a series of graphs created by ISIS conference participants (figure 5.2). Participants were asked to draw rough sketches or graphs showing how they thought the brainstormed components evolved over the past few decades and how they might be projected into the future. The graphs from these experts were grouped

---

Figure 5.2 Sample of Graphs on Tobacco Use Factors from Expert Participants at 2003 Conference on ISIS

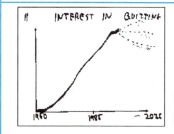 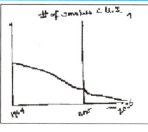 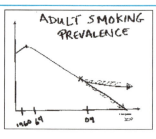

Note. These images were hand-drafted by participants in the exercise.

---

into substantive sectors to create a series of composite pictures, collapse the issues to a more manageable size, and provide useful talking points as the team progressed to modeling. Examples of sectors resulting from this exercise included the following:

Tobacco use. The sector on tobacco use examined the relationship between people and tobacco—whether they smoke and rates for starting, stopping, or resuming tobacco use. For this sector, participant graphs were supplemented with compiled data showing the fractions of the U.S. population who were current or former smokers or who never smoked during 1965–2000.[4] Some of the original hand-drawn graphs were generated by the experts for the sector on tobacco use. As part of the exercise, participants drew a graph to show changes for each key variable over time. Dotted or shaded lines represent alternative future scenarios.

Tobacco industry. The sector on the tobacco industry examined the influence and lobbying efforts of the industry, combining participant graphs of these factors with data from the Economic Research Service of the U.S. Department of Agriculture showing variations in the tobacco supply from 1950 through 2000.

Tobacco control and government intervention. The sector on tobacco control

and government intervention examined trends in tobacco control efforts over time. These included the measure for strength of tobacco control that was developed to measure state-level tobacco control resources, capacity, and efforts, as well as factors such as resources and funding, regulation of tobacco by the U.S. Food and Drug Administration, and percentage of restaurants with a smoking ban in place over time.[5] The data compiled from these ISIS participants, supplemented with historical data on tobacco-related factors from official sources, contained many observed trends, such as a clear plateau in the historical decline in tobacco use, increasing near-term tobacco sales, and a rise and fall of tobacco control efforts over time, tied to recent decreases in funding for tobacco control.

Developing a Causal Model

A causal map typically consists of the following elements:

- *Stocks* are accumulated or integrated quantities with values or levels (e.g., number or proportion) that do not change instantaneously. Stocks accumulate in response to flows. Stocks are the written words on a causal map (e.g., tobacco revenues or people smoking), and stocks that are central to specific causal loops are highlighted in boxes.

- *Flows* are varying quantities that create the dynamics in the system by increasing or decreasing stocks. Flows (e.g., production of tax revenues by smokers) are represented by the arrows on a map.

- *Loops* are linked, directional relationships between model parameters.

- *Delays* are built-in characteristics of any system, providing more realistic linkages of cause and effect that may be difficult to observe. For example, it takes time to introduce new legislation or develop a new marketing campaign. A delay can be seen as a property of a stock.

These brainstormed components, organized by sector, formed the basis for construction by the project facilitator of an overall causal loop model of factors in tobacco prevalence and consumption, as a precursor to the development of a formal system dynamics model. A causal loop model (presented later in this chapter) was built step-by-step as outlined in this section.

Causal loop diagrams are an integral part of system dynamics modeling, helping to foster group knowledge and understanding and providing a concise view of an enormous amount of complexity and a starting point for simulation. In ISIS, such diagrams act as a bridge, drawing information from participants and data sources, and resulting in a "map" that helps stakeholders define and, more important, discuss the fundamental hypotheses and connections leading to more formal modeling. (The final causal map shown later in this chapter was developed heuristically and is meant to be illustrative rather than authoritative.)

One group of participants created the causal map and used the brainstormed components organized by sector and the graphs of functions over time to draft the initial flow diagram. To better explain development of the overall causal model, the model is examined a section at a time and the logic is described. The final causal loop model shown later in this chapter presents the full map, and figure 5.3 shows the segment examining social norm and tobacco growing issues.

In the diagram, "smokers" represent the pool of people who smoke. As the number of smokers increases, the revenue generated

Figure 5.3 Causal Map Segment, Incorporating Social Norm and Tobacco Grower Factors

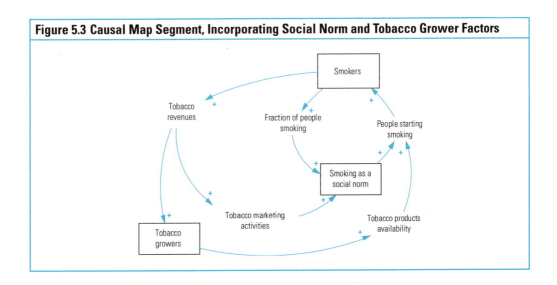

by their purchase of tobacco products also increases, which is indicated by the plus sign next to the line that connects "smokers" and "tobacco revenues." This increase has two effects: it enables the tobacco industry to increase tobacco production (tobacco growers) to meet the demand of increased smoking, and it generates more money for "tobacco marketing activities."

Following the inside loop, the increase in "tobacco marketing activities" creates greater acceptance of smoking and tobacco use. Marketing activities tend to normalize smoking as a behavior rather than simply capture more market share. Marketing, for the tobacco industry, is a source of new smokers. Following the outside causal loop, as the capacity for tobacco production increases, there is an increased availability (e.g., discounted cost) of tobacco products. The establishment of "smoking as a social norm," complemented by the increased availability of tobacco products, results in an increase in the number of "people starting

to smoke," and consequently, an increase in the "fraction of people smoking."

If this initial model segment is expanded to a slightly larger segment (figure 5.4), it becomes apparent that research on the health effects of smoking leads to growing awareness of health risks from tobacco use, which eventually disseminates to the general public and helps build pressures and motivations for people to stop smoking. As the "fraction of people smoking" increases, the "researchers' awareness of tobacco as a health risk" becomes clearer. This increased awareness prompts researchers to formulate new questions and apply for "funding for research on tobacco as a health risk." Their work eventually finds its way to "public awareness of tobacco as a health risk." Reports on the negative effects of smoking and exposure to secondhand smoke filter from research to a broader awareness. As individuals process this information, they choose to stop smoking in greater numbers.

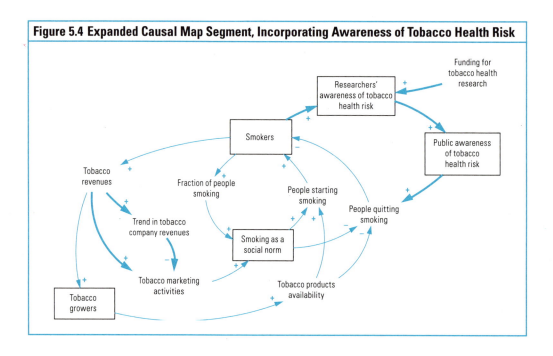

Figure 5.4 Expanded Causal Map Segment, Incorporating Awareness of Tobacco Health Risk

The new causal path captures the idea that the "trend in tobacco company revenues" is a decrease because as the number of smokers decreased, tobacco companies would increase spending on "tobacco marketing activities." The minus sign next to the line between "trend in tobacco company revenues" and "tobacco marketing activities" depicts the negative relationship that as tobacco revenues *decrease,* marketing is *increased.* By an increase in marketing, tobacco companies would try to compensate for the successes of the research community in prompting people to try to stop smoking.

"Antitobacco constituencies" represent those who advocate against support for the tobacco industry. As both "researchers' awareness" and "public awareness of tobacco as a health risk" increase, the number of people and organizations opposing tobacco use tends to grow. The map expanded as shown in figure 5.5 suggests that these antitobacco constituencies can move more funding to tobacco research and control, leading to further growth (1) in awareness of tobacco

as a health risk and (2) in efforts to control or reverse the growth of tobacco production and use.

The outside loop highlights some of the effects of tobacco control programs. As "funding for tobacco control programs" increases, "pressure on tobacco companies to reduce marketing activities" increases (e.g., via legislated bans on certain forms of advertising). This pressure is an additional factor but only one of many that determine levels of tobacco company marketing.

A segment on government awareness of tobacco as a health risk is added in figure 5.6. The government draws from three sources of information to understand the risk posed by tobacco use. First, government depends on "researchers' awareness of tobacco as a health risk" to provide information on the health risks of tobacco. Second, government relies on "public awareness of tobacco as a health risk" to gain a better understanding of the degree to which tobacco use is an issue among its constituents. The higher the public awareness of tobacco risks, the

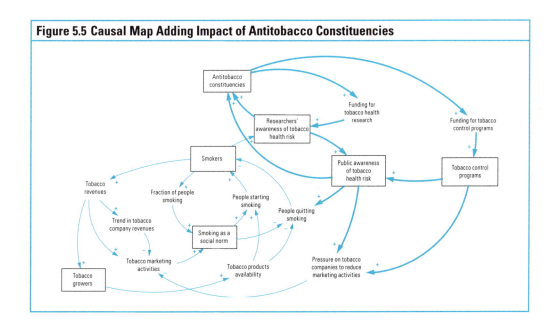

Figure 5.5 Causal Map Adding Impact of Antitobacco Constituencies

Figure 5.6 Causal Map Adding Government Awareness of Tobacco as a Health Risk

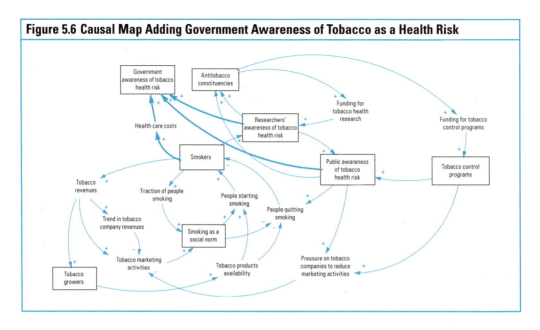

Figure 5.7 Causal Map Adding Impact of Protobacco Constituencies

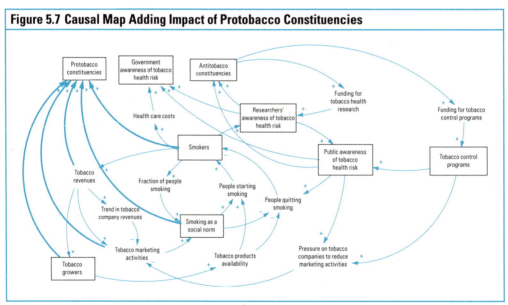

more motivated people are to pressure their legislators to act. Finally, government experiences a direct feedback loop in the "health care costs" associated with tobacco use. As the number of smokers increases, the health care costs associated with smoking also increase. The government directly bears many of these costs through Medicare. However, such costs also are

indirectly affected by the public debate over the general cost of health insurance.

The influence of protobacco constituencies is added in figure 5.7. Protobacco constituencies represent those who advocate in favor of tobacco products and their increased availability. Tobacco companies, smokers, and those who

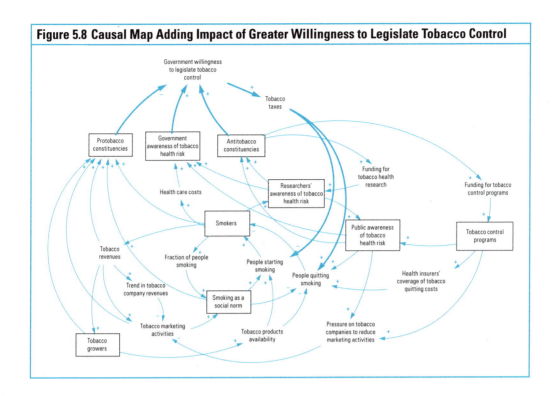

Figure 5.8 Causal Map Adding Impact of Greater Willingness to Legislate Tobacco Control

accept smoking as a social norm generate the ability to provoke action against tobacco control measures. From a social and psychological perspective, smokers play an important role in the protobacco constituency, because they often are interested in ease of availability and few limitations on smoking behavior.

Tobacco revenues create an obvious incentive for people to protect tobacco. Shareholders in tobacco companies desire increased revenue, and companies have a vested interest in the success of their product. Consequently, the tobacco industry takes steps to protect their investment.

The willingness of government to take actions against tobacco interests depends on the balance of forces created by the protobacco and antitobacco constituencies and the government's perceptions of health risks associated with tobacco use. Segments showing the forces influencing willingness to legislate are added in figure 5.8. Increased

taxes on tobacco are an early result of this growing government willingness to act against tobacco interests. The impacts of taxes on individual motivation to start or stop smoking create a number of feedback loops in the system, countering the growth of the population of smokers and contributing to its eventual decline.

Some effects of government legislation to control tobacco use are added to the model in figure 5.9. For example, as government receives more money from tobacco taxes, it is more willing to increase that revenue stream. However, this loop also works in reverse. As government revenues from tobacco taxes decrease, the government may actually become less willing to act against tobacco interests because it would be threatening its own revenue stream.

Tobacco tax revenue is dependent on the taxes associated with tobacco use, as well as the number of people who smoke (figure 5.9). As either increases, one would expect

Figure 5.9 Causal Map Adding Impact of Government Tax Revenues and Funding for Tobacco Control

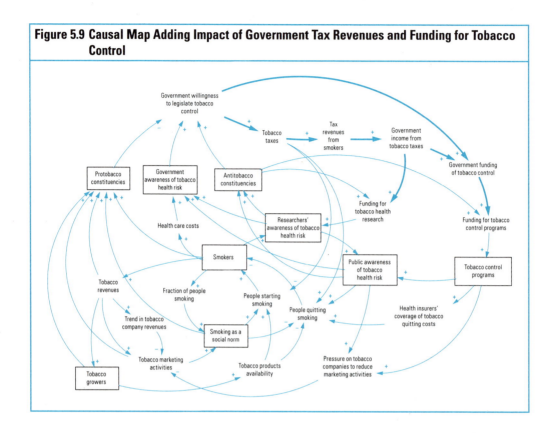

that tax revenue would also increase. These increased revenue streams increase government income. The model suggests that more money moving into the system from tobacco taxes results in increased funding of both basic research and tobacco control.

Finally, government willingness to legislate tobacco control ultimately leads to policy interventions such as antismoking legislation, which in turn has effects on the marketing of tobacco products and their availability. Both of these factors are affected directly by legislative restrictions, as well as by side effects such as counterefforts by the tobacco industry. Adding the impact of these factors leads to the final causal map (figure 5.10) drafted for this pilot project.

The building of this map, as outlined in figures 5.3 through 5.10, was based on participant identification of components,

grouping of these components into sectors, and descriptions of the dynamic patterns of the variables over time. The facilitator used this information to construct the causal map and provided it to the participant group for feedback and potential revision. The causal map would doubtless benefit from input from a broader range of stakeholders, such as tobacco growers. This would likely add additional stocks and flows and open some current model elements to debate. The causal map, in turn, was used to inform the development of segments of the formal system dynamics model discussed in the next section.

The tobacco system articulated by this causal map is but a system within a larger system. For example, there have always been competing public health priorities, most recently exemplified by the focus on obesity. In many ways, playing tobacco against obesity competitively is a zero-sum game. With finite

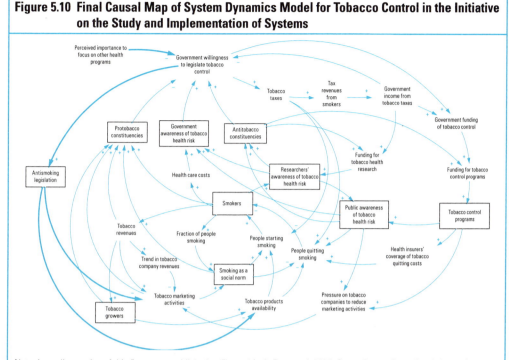

Figure 5.10 Final Causal Map of System Dynamics Model for Tobacco Control in the Initiative on the Study and Implementation of Systems

Note. An earlier version of this figure was published as Figure 1 in A. Best et al. 2006. Systemic transformational change in tobacco control: An overview of the Initiative for the Study and Implementation of Systems (ISIS). In *Innovations in health care: A reality check,* ed. A. L. Casebeer, A. Harrison, and A. L. Mark, 189–205. New York: Palgrave Macmillan. Reproduced with permission of Palgrave Macmillan.

resources, the public health community must set priorities. If the importance of obesity as a health risk increases relative to that of tobacco use, the government's willingness to act and the direction of funding for tobacco control and research may be affected. Issues such as these point to the importance of continuing the use of system dynamics models and the evolution of these models from original assumptions based on changes in the environment.

Developing System Dynamics Models

How does a system dynamics modeler move from hand-drawn graphs, empirical data, and the causal map to a formal system dynamics model? This section presents selected model segments that were used in a larger formal simulation of factors in tobacco use over time.

Compared with the earlier causal maps showing relationships among model factors, these "shards" of system dynamics models form the detailed basis for the estimated parameters used for simulation. They constitute the basic structure of the formal model, showing how causal elements discussed here were translated into a simulation. However, there is not a one-to-one correspondence between segments of the causal map described previously and these model shards. For the purposes of this demonstration project, the simulation model was informed by the overall content of the causal map, and adaptations were made according to the judgment of the analyst and feedback from participants. Only some of the

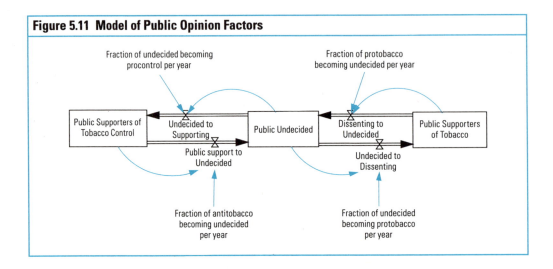

Figure 5.11 Model of Public Opinion Factors

Public Opinion Sector

The model shown in figure 5.11 relates to the "smoking as a social norm" portion of the causal maps shown in figures 5.3–5.10. That segment of the maps was translated into part of the simulation model by building a closed set of stocks, linked by inflows and outflows in which it is assumed that opinion moves through this closed chain in response to pressure. For example, every year, some fraction of the undecided population moves from the undecided stock to public support of tobacco use or public support of control of tobacco use.

Tobacco Use Sector

Figure 5.12 depicts several "aging chains" used in the formal model to track the inflows and outflows of current and former smokers and people who never smoked, from birth to death. Formulation in this

formal model shards are described here to illustrate how this part of the modeling process works in the context of this example. (The figures shown for these shards are taken from program output from the VENSIM software used for this simulation.)

manner is consistent with historical monitoring of tobacco use and enables substantial comparison. If it is assumed that all people are born nonsmokers, one of five behavior scenarios takes place:

1. Youths start to smoke tobacco products or age into adulthood as nonsmokers.

2. Adult nonsmokers start to smoke or continue as nonsmokers until they die.

3. Youths who smoke stop smoking, becoming former youth smokers, age into adulthood as former smokers, or resume smoking after stopping.

4. Youths who age into adulthood as smokers die as smokers or stop smoking and become former adult smokers.

5. Former adult smokers resume smoking or remain former smokers.

Proximate drivers of flows are built into the formal model in figure 5.12. As shown earlier in this chapter, the state of current opinion affects the rates at which adults and youths begin and stop tobacco use. For example, as public opinion builds in support of tobacco control, rates of initiation of smoking decline. As public opinion builds in support of tobacco use, rates of initiation increase.

Figure 5.12 Model of Aging Chains of Smokers (Birth to Death)

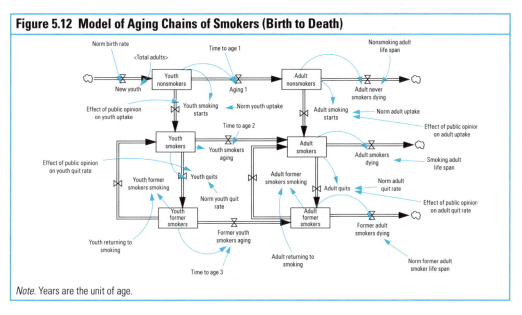

Note. Years are the unit of age.

Figure 5.13 Model of Research and Dissemination Factors

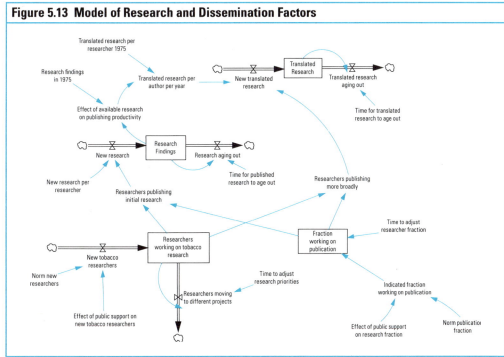

Research and Dissemination Sector

The simulation model in figure 5.13 illustrates research and dissemination (education) factors. These factors play an important role in influencing public health awareness, as described in figure 5.5. This model assumes there are *x* numbers of researchers performing research on tobacco use and control who create initial research (e.g., published in peer-reviewed journals) or translate initial research into information

Playing "What If" Games with Smoking Prevalence

If the number of children who start smoking were suddenly cut in half, how would it affect the number of smokers 40 years from now? As part of the ISIS system dynamics model described in this section, a simulation was performed by using the model for the aging chain of smokers (birth to death) that shows the impact of rates for smoking initiation and cessation at specific ages on the prevalence of tobacco use. This model was then used to test the effect of dramatic changes in these initiation rates, in different age groups, on prevalence over a 40-year period.

The simulation results show that cutting smoking initiation in children under age 12 years in half had minimal impact downstream. However, similar decreases in adolescent (ages 12–20 years) and adult smoking initiation produced much greater declines. Factors behind these results ranged from the relatively small number of child smokers to the cascading effects of each group on subsequent rates for smoking initiation and cessation.

Effect of 50% Declines in Child, Adolescent, and Adult Smoking Initiation in Longitudinal Studies of Smoking Prevalence

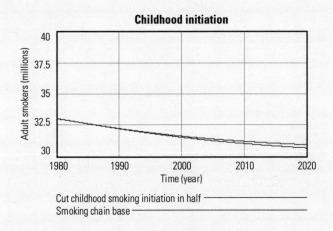

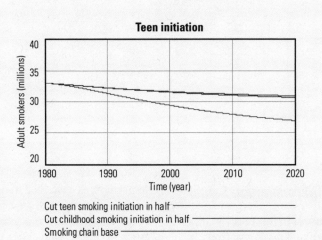

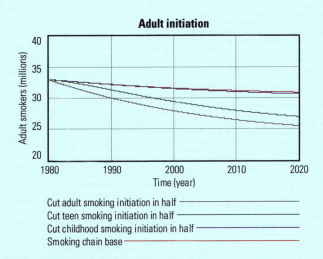

Adult initiation

Cut adult smoking initiation in half ─────────────
Cut teen smoking initiation in half ─────────────
Cut childhood smoking initiation in half ────────
Smoking chain base ─────────────

Perhaps an even more important outcome from this simulation was the reaction of other tobacco control stakeholders, many of whom felt that this simulation would not necessarily reflect long-term outcomes in real life. Some people, particularly those involved with tobacco use issues among young people, thought that a sharp decline in youth smoking could become a powerful agent in other factors. These include social and culture change, which could in turn create conditions for much greater reduction in prevalence.

Although this simulation was designed only as a proof of concept project with limited data, it brought two important points to life for ISIS participants: that system dynamics models often can reveal unexpected outcomes and that the results depend strongly on the assumptions behind the model. These factors highlight a key limitation in system dynamics modeling, which is that the modeling cannot easily be validated. When surprising results occur, it is not clear whether they have arisen from one or more unwarranted assumptions. The second key limitation is the great difficulty in parameterizing system dynamics models. These limitations reinforce the point that system dynamics models are aids to thinking about complex issues, not tools for delivering "truth."

available for dissemination to the public (e.g., tobacco fact sheets available for download on many public health Web sites or television news pieces on recent tobacco-related health warnings).

Several effects of public opinion are built into this model. The model assumes that the rising tide of public support may increase the demand for researchers engaged in tobacco-related projects and, likewise, increase the demand for materials on awareness of risk for dissemination to the public.

Not all of the causal map has been explicitly included in the model. Sometimes factors in the causal map are handled differently in formal modeling. This was the case for factors related to the tobacco industry. Instead of separately modeling the influence of these factors, this model considers the rate at which research translated for dissemination reaches the population as a net gain, after subtracting for an effect of counterresearch and propaganda from the tobacco industry.

Government Sector

Figure 5.14 examines government intervention. The hypothesis is that government intervention grows in response to public support for tobacco control. This segment of the formal model illustrates the idea of a delay, labeled "time to change government intervention." This is interpreted as the time it takes to create new legislation or repeal existing legislation, as the support for tobacco control rises and falls.

Public Opinion Revisited

With the assumption of basic understanding of the tobacco use, research and dissemination, and government sectors, figure 5.15 shows the effects of the public opinion sector on tobacco control.

Changes in public opinion are influenced by the number of smokers and nonsmokers in a population. This hypothesis is based on the assumption that, for example, a firmly established social norm in favor of smoking tends to produce more smokers, who tend to support the existence of the social norm.

Translated research will tend to "push" public opinion toward control of tobacco use, because the assumption is that a more informed population chooses reduction of tobacco use. The model indicates a weak "backlash" effect in response to increasing government intervention. This is based on the presumption that government constraints on personal behavior may draw some opinion away from support.

These segments of simulation models illustrate how causal maps and other factors such as experience and expertise in subject matter are translated into more formal simulations. Such simulations enable researchers and practitioners to change different parameters in efforts to explore the likely effects of these changes throughout the dynamic system. Based on those trials and how appropriate the results appear, the simulation itself might be revised. In this manner, the act of simulation constitutes

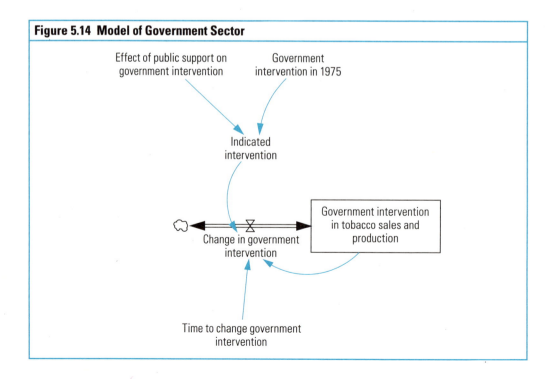

Figure 5.14 Model of Government Sector

Effect of public support on government intervention

Government intervention in 1975

Indicated intervention

Change in government intervention

Government intervention in tobacco sales and production

Time to change government intervention

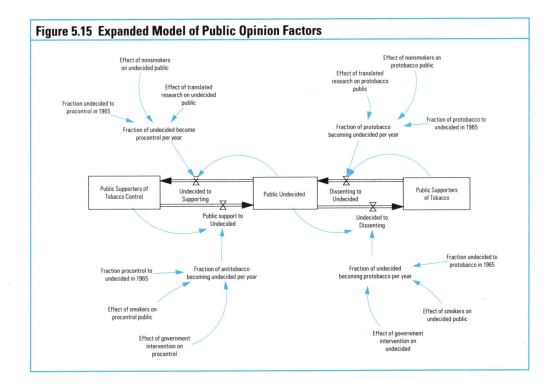

Figure 5.15 Expanded Model of Public Opinion Factors

a type of dynamic laboratory for trial-and-error efforts to better anticipate the effects of different conditions.

Validating Simulation of System Dynamics Models

Simulation of system dynamics models means allocating numbers to the "stocks" in the model and activating the "flows" so that changes in behavior over time are simulated. An example of the behavior of the model is presented here through text description and graphical representation. This section highlights causal loops to provide supplementary explanations for important model dynamics and shows how simulation models are set against real-world data in an ongoing process of revising and validating the models.

The results in the initial simulation model are compared with outcome data in figure 5.16. Data from the Centers for Disease

Control and Prevention,[6] represented by the short lines in the model, are compared with the simulation projections, represented by the long lines. The test model fits existing data well over time. However, the simulation model has the advantage of allowing projections into the future, represented by the extension of the long line over the short line.

System dynamics modeling does not simply assume that projections into the future are accurate or valid because of a correspondence of simulation estimates with historical data. A multitude of simulation models might correspond just as closely with historical estimates. Modeling is done primarily for its probative value, as a tool for exploring possible effects, but modeling of this type can be a basis for more confident projections. For instance, multiple models that predict similar longer term outcomes, all making differing assumptions, form a stronger basis for validity than any one model alone would.

The historical data progressively diverge from the simulation data during 1990–2000 (figure 5.16, graph on right). This finding suggests that important parameters influencing more recent projections were either not included or were not properly weighted in the simulation. This finding might be used to start a series of trial-and-error revisions to the simulation model to explore possible reasons for such a discrepancy.

Estimating Parameters

An additional advantage of the model is that it allows exploration of sectors for which no data exist. Modelers use intuition to decide whether the model "makes sense." For example, the stocks for public opinion are visible in figure 5.17. The initial parameters for the public opinion stocks are a function of the smoking rates in a population. For example, those who smoke are assumed to be proponents of tobacco use. Those who have used tobacco and stopped smoking are assumed to be supporters of tobacco control. These assumptions are open to challenge, but they are useful for illustrative and probative purposes.

Support for tobacco control has been increasing, although not necessarily at a predictable or constant rate. In this model, the reason public support fails to establish a linear positive trajectory at its end point is

Figure 5.16 Model Data Versus Actual Data on Population Fractions of Current and Former Smokers

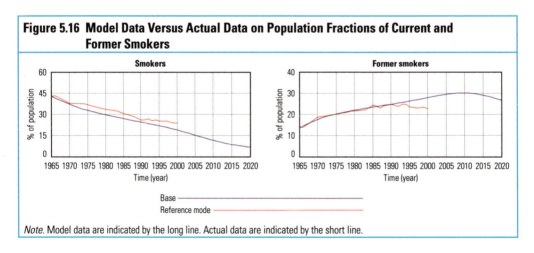

Note. Model data are indicated by the long line. Actual data are indicated by the short line.

Figure 5.17 Stock Values for Public Opinion over Time (Baseline)

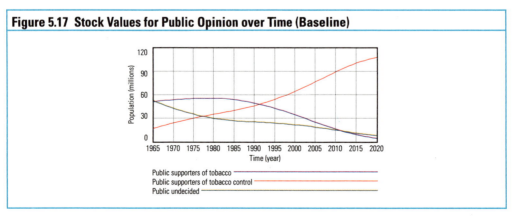

based on several important feedback loops, shown in figure 5.18.

Because the model begins in 1965 with a substantial number of current smokers, the size of the smoking population allows support of tobacco use to continue to grow for several years. It is bolstered slightly by the effect of government intervention in the wake of the 1964 Report of the Advisory Committee of the Surgeon General on smoking and health.[7] Until regulations on tobacco product warnings became institutionalized by the Federal Cigarette Labeling and Advertising Act in 1965,[8] the government warning about tobacco use as a health risk had an effect opposite to that intended on the tobacco-using population.[9] This result was in keeping with the modeling assumptions discussed earlier on the effects of this intervention on public opinion (figure 5.19).

Momentum to control tobacco use builds slowly, as rates of the decline in smoking and public interest in intervention and research grow. Eventually, the stock of support for control overtakes the stock of tobacco use.

Simulation Results

Examination of the effects of changing various model parameters and their effects can lead to a better understanding of the system. These effects are grouped by model sectors. For each grouping, the most relevant scenarios are discussed, although they represent only a small fraction of all possible scenarios.

Tobacco Use Sector

An informative initial test is to evaluate the following proposition: the effect of public support for tobacco control on tobacco use has been underestimated. The blue baseline in figure 5.20 represents the original effect of public opinion on the adult rate of starting to smoke. The x axis indicates the input, that is, the level of public support for tobacco control. The y axis indicates the impact of this support on the current adult rate for smoking initiation. The shape of the blue baseline changes with changes in the

Figure 5.18 Feedback Loops Affecting Public Opinion

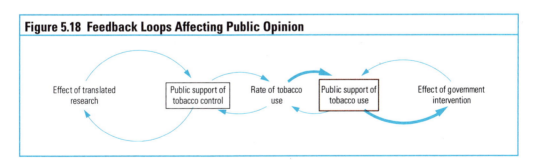

Figure 5.19 Feedback Loops with Change in Feedback Levels

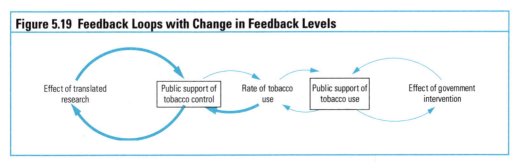

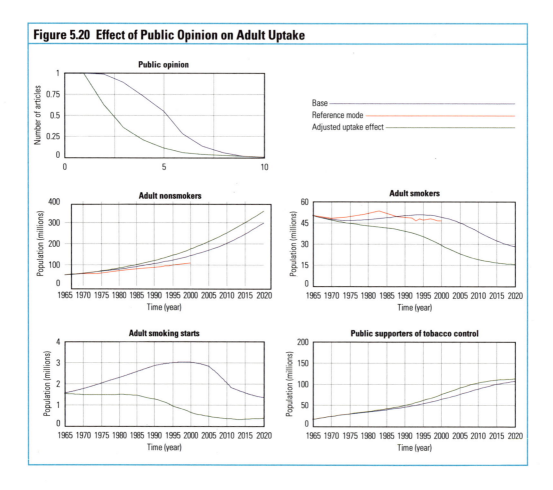

Figure 5.20 Effect of Public Opinion on Adult Uptake

parameter of public opinion. The graph of new data shown by the green line suggests that a change in public opinion yields a much greater change in the rate of smoking initiation among adults.

The largest impact of the change is indicated in the graphs for adult smokers, because the rate of smoking initiation declines much more quickly than in the baseline simulation, which consequently reduces the number of former smokers. The number of supporters of tobacco control also is slightly higher, but this effect moderates quickly.

The effect of public opinion on the rate for smoking cessation among adults also may be different from that at baseline. The original base assumption and an altered

assumption are both expressed in figure 5.21. The altered assumption suggests that public opinion has a more significant impact on smoking cessation than the original assumption.

When the effect of public opinion is amplified, predictably, fewer people are smoking, and a much higher percentage of people have stopped using tobacco. After 1995, the percentage of people who never smoked also is significantly higher. As shown in the causal loops in figure 5.22, this increase is due to the feedback effect of public opinion on the rate of smoking initiation.

Change in the smoking cessation rate directly affects the numbers of smokers and former smokers. This model shows that the growing

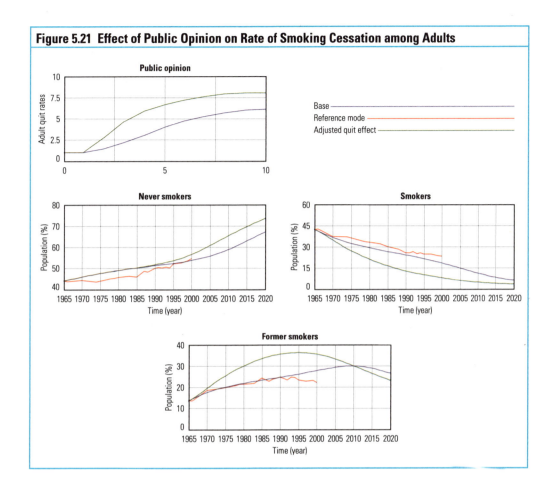

Figure 5.21 Effect of Public Opinion on Rate of Smoking Cessation among Adults

contingent of nonsmokers also has an effect on the number of adults who never smoked (figure 5.22). As public opinion grows, the rate at which adults initiate smoking declines. In this way, the model captures what might be hypothesized as an elusive shifting of the social norm regarding tobacco use. These effects have only begun to become visible during the more recent decades. Should the model capture the dynamics of the system accurately, it can provide useful details about its behavior in coming years.

Research and Dissemination Sector

Additional tests can be designed to explore the dynamic effects of public opinion in the research and dissemination sector. For example, figure 5.23 shows the results of simulation of the effect that public support for tobacco control has on altering the research fraction. This is the proportion of researchers conducting basic research versus the proportion translating research into information that can be disseminated to the public. Based on the assumptions of the model, the greater the public support for tobacco control is, the more emphasis is placed on funding basic research (figure 5.23, top). Paradoxically, more public support may mean less translational research. The amount of funds for all research (basic plus translational) is growing because of public support. However, it does not grow as rapidly as the proportion for basic research that appears to be responsive to the public. The

Figure 5.22 Causal Loops for Public Opinion and Support of Tobacco Control

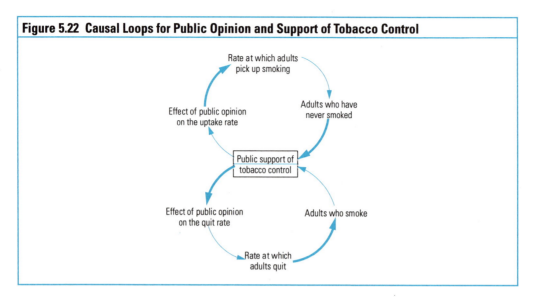

Figure 5.23 Effect of Public Support for Tobacco Control on Research Fraction

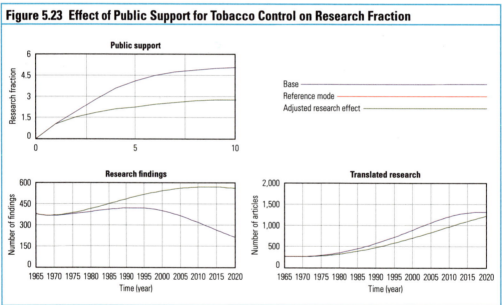

model suggests that the effect of public support is weaker than it was at baseline (figure 5.23, graph at lower left). Despite the shift to more initial research, the simulation shows that the amount of translated research does not decline as much as might be expected (figure 5.23, graph at lower right).

A compensating loop in this model addresses the publishing productivity of those who translate research. With more public support for tobacco control, the research fraction is altered to favor more basic research, a higher volume of such research is accumulated, and consequently, the publishing productivity of researchers working on translational research is affected negatively (figure 5.24). The change in translated research is significant enough to alter the stock of tobacco use (figure 5.25).

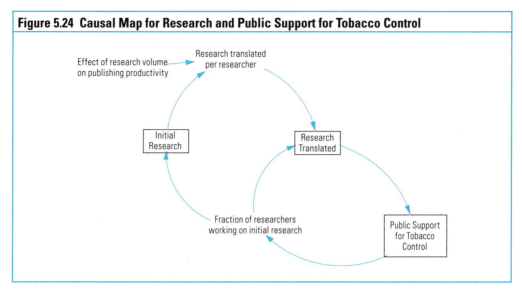

Figure 5.24 Causal Map for Research and Public Support for Tobacco Control

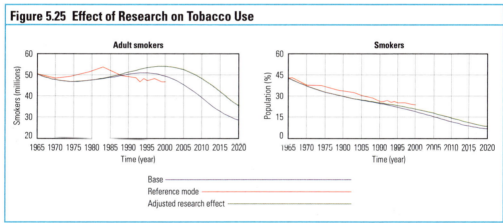

Figure 5.25 Effect of Research on Tobacco Use

However, the effect moderates toward the end of the simulation, and one suspects that this effect would disappear over time.

Public Opinion Sector

Previously, a test was performed to determine how significantly public opinion affects the amount of research being performed. For the next test here, this assumption is reversed and the impact of relevant and timely research on public opinion is explored. As has been mentioned during ISIS workshops, providing such data to the general public is a vital component of a tobacco control policy.

A simple test explores the sensitivity of translated research by changing the time it takes to "age out" of the public's awareness. The baseline assumption is that the public's memory of awareness about tobacco use as a health risk is fairly long; the time until the research ages out is set at 25 years. The results of changing that parameter to 15 years are shown in the graphs in figure 5.26.

Because translated research flows through this stock more quickly and thus remains in the public's mind for a shorter period, less of it accumulates. Less accumulation of research directly and negatively affects

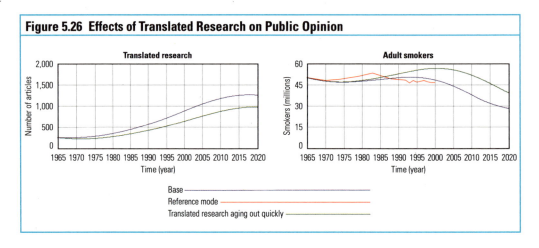

Figure 5.26 Effects of Translated Research on Public Opinion

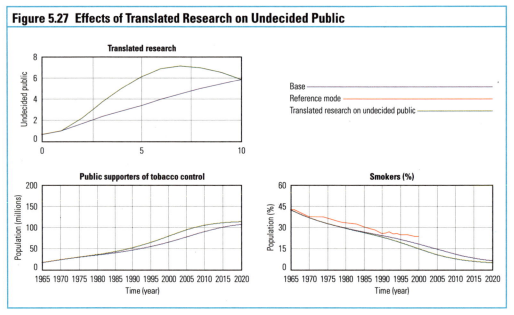

Figure 5.27 Effects of Translated Research on Undecided Public

the shifting social norm, and a higher stock of current smokers results. The life span of relevant tobacco research is an important concept, even though it may be difficult to accurately measure. Although it is beyond the scope of this simple model, it is clearly worthwhile to consider the quality of translated material. This is because quality undoubtedly affects the durability of tobacco research and education.

This simulation environment offers other ways to explore the effects of research. A

new assumption suggests that, as in the baseline run, more translated research yields a greater effect (figure 5.27). In this new run, however, the model also reveals that there is a point at which more research does not yield greater impact but leads to less movement into the stock for tobacco control. Practically speaking, if the volume of antitobacco information available far exceeds the public's ability to integrate it into the current social consciousness, it will likely be filtered out. A slight gain in support for tobacco control and, consequently, a decline

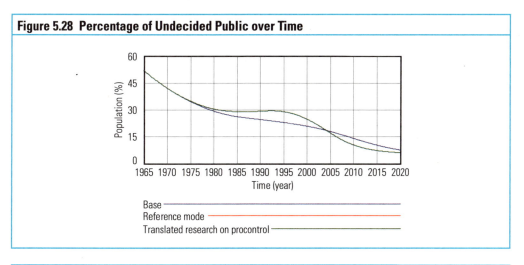

Figure 5.28 Percentage of Undecided Public over Time

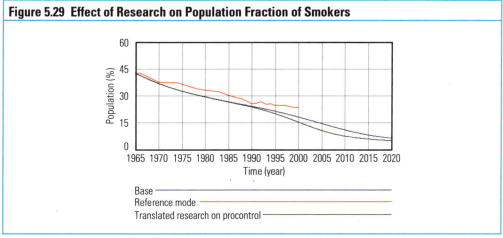

Figure 5.29 Effect of Research on Population Fraction of Smokers

in the fraction of people using tobacco are shown in figure 5.27 (lower graphs). If translated research has a greater effect than that in the baseline run, the simulations result in a predictable gain for the stock for the undecided public (figure 5.28).

The "gain" illustrated in figure 5.28, practically, means that 30% of the public has been undecided on the issue of tobacco control for more than two decades. Those without a keen eye on the long-term behavior of the system may be tempted to consider this finding as something other than progress. Based on this model, the absence of a dramatic gain for tobacco control could be interpreted as the natural

evolution of the system. As the undecided public begins to shift toward support of tobacco control, a drop in rates of tobacco use will become apparent, as shown in figure 5.29.

Government Sector

A final example simulation experiment toggles the impact of government intervention. This model includes an assumption that government intervention may have the unintended effect of producing a backlash against tobacco control. In New York State, for example, laws regulating smoke-free restaurants and bars have produced a solid and well-funded campaign against tobacco regulation. This campaign threatens to weaken not only the law but also the movement to protect nonsmokers from the health effects of tobacco use.

The effects of government intervention on the shift from support for tobacco control to

an undecided position and from undecided to a protobacco position are shown in figure 5.30 (top left and top right, respectively).

As expected, the decreased strength of the effect leads to more tobacco control advocates and fewer supporters of tobacco. Over a longer period, the impact of the

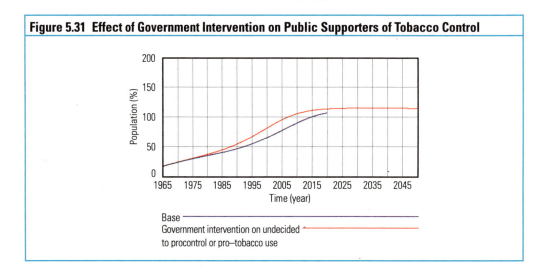

Figure 5.30 Effects of Government Intervention on Shift from Support for Tobacco Control to Undecided and from Undecided to Support for Tobacco Use

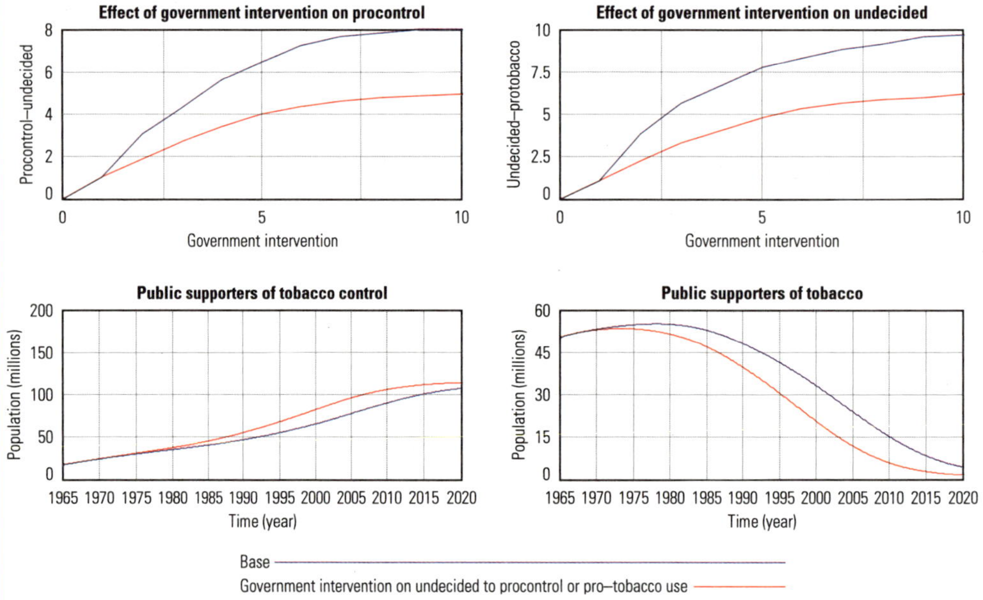

Figure 5.31 Effect of Government Intervention on Public Supporters of Tobacco Control

effect does not yield a significant change in behavior. The reaction of a population to a series of government regulations, all else being held constant, does not have a long-standing influence on the changing social norm (figure 5.31).

This model presents a simplified view of factors in tobacco prevalence and consumption, which were developed for illustrative purposes. Although the model represents only one iteration, it provides a base from which further modeling work, corrections, additions or subtractions, and enhancements could be easily accomplished as part of a more accurate simulation. Meanwhile, it serves as a mechanism for raising questions, provoking discussion, and gaining a deeper understanding of the complexity of this dynamic system. It also opens a valuable dialogue among stakeholders in tobacco control and other disciplines in the ISIS project.

Summary

This chapter examines the potential for using system dynamics modeling in tobacco control and public health and presents a case study of developing and using a system dynamics model to explore trends in tobacco use over time. It demonstrates use of a modeling approach to represent the interrelationships among key factors in tobacco use and their evolution over time. The project developed here can be considered a heuristic and preliminary model, but many of the results compare well with actual outcome data. Overall, this project serves as a valuable proof of concept for future systems-level modeling efforts.

This case study project was designed to develop clearer ideas about system dynamics and about the range of approaches that can contribute to more effective tobacco control and public health in general. The system dynamics approach arose, at least partly,

from dissatisfaction with the limitations of simple cause-and-effect approaches that have no feedback for tackling the challenges of tobacco control. These approaches are effective in improving understanding of individual causal mechanisms or small clusters of mechanisms. However, they cannot provide much assistance in addressing the dynamic complexity of tobacco control.

The ISIS project used the rubric of systems thinking to establish a starting point for investigating the world of dynamic modeling and its application to tobacco control. Many approaches to systems thinking exist, sometimes with tensions evident among them. Nonetheless, the research outlined in this chapter provides a clear sense of how one systems approach, system dynamics, can help the tobacco control community to understand, model, and react to the complexities of the current tobacco control environment. System dynamics is an aid to thinking differently about the tobacco control world—to characterizing it in terms of feedback, stocks and flows, and structure and behavior. System dynamics elucidates the role of feedback, which keeps the system in balance and leads to change that may or may not be advantageous. System dynamics modeling also has the potential to work in concert with the other areas under study in ISIS, including the following:

- Management of organizations as a system, with an understanding of the macrodynamics of planning, implementation, and evaluation and how these constitute a feedback mechanism that is both driven by system forces and drives them (chapter 4)

- Network methods, encompassing the development and management of stakeholder groups that define the system of interest and its dynamics (chapter 6)

- Knowledge management and knowledge transfer, which facilitate the use and management of explicit and tacit knowledge (in the form of both data and people) that helps to describe and evolve system models (chapter 7)

System dynamics methods, in conjunction with other systems thinking approaches, are a useful tool for probing, exploring, understanding, simulating, and interacting with future issues in tobacco control. Many issues remain to be investigated to build on the foundations established here. At the same time, the concepts presented in this chapter represent a starting point toward developing a more systemic approach. This new approach would underpin the ability to work with increasingly complex, multifaceted tobacco control issues. It also would provide the foundation for transforming knowledge about a range of public health issues into effective policy and practice.

Conclusions

1. Tobacco control consists of dynamic relationships over time and requires approaches, such as system dynamics modeling, that can address such dynamics.

2. Understanding of tobacco control and public health issues has evolved from simple cause-and-effect studies and logic models to more complex, ecological problems that involve feedback and evolving behavior.

3. System dynamics uses mathematical simulation approaches based on stocks, flows, and feedback loops, which can model system structures and simulate future system behavior, including possible unintended consequences and long-term effects.

4. Demonstration projects, such as the system dynamics simulation of tobacco prevalence and consumption developed for the Initiative on the Study and Implementation of Systems, show the potential to model and simulate future tobacco issues to design more effective interventions.

5. Opportunities are likely to surface for integrating system dynamics modeling and other systems thinking approaches at epistemological and methodological levels. Systems approaches can and should integrate within a larger systems thinking environment encompassing components such as systems organizing, networks, and knowledge management.

Appendix 5A.   Detailed Development of a System Dynamics Model

This section outlines the specific system dynamics model sectors created for a demonstration model of tobacco prevalence and consumption from 1965 to the present. This model was designed to simulate the effects of specific changes to model variables on prevalence and consumption of tobacco over time. Specific model segments are shown in detail in this appendix.

Figure 5A.1 Tobacco Use Sector

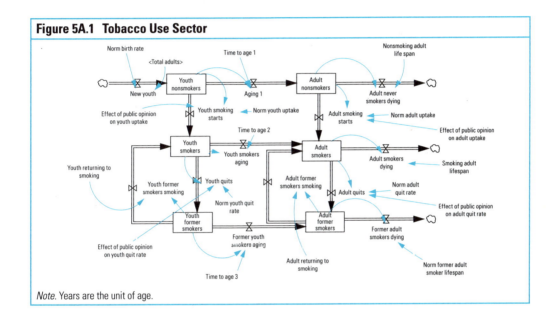

Note. Years are the unit of age.

Figure 5A.2 Tobacco Research and Education Sector

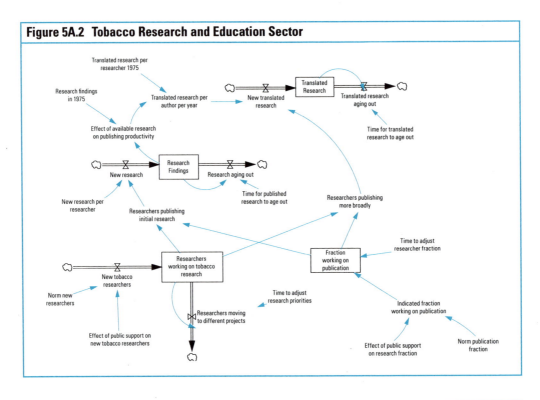

Figure 5A.3 Government Sector

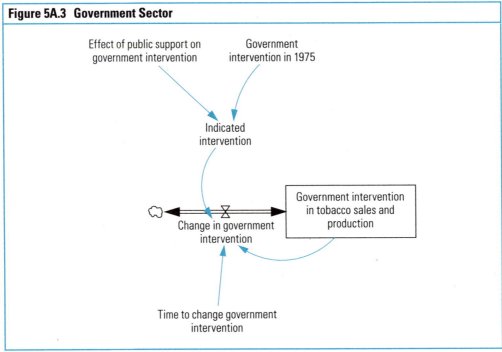

Figure 5A.4 Public Opinion Sector

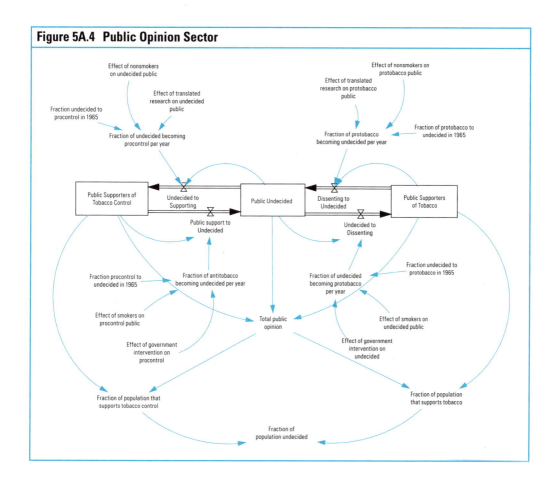

References

1. Framework Convention Alliance for Tobacco Control. 2005. The WHO Framework Convention on Tobacco Control: A public health movement. http://www.fctc.org.

2. Sterman, J. D. 2000. *Business dynamics: Systems thinking and modeling for a complex world.* New York: McGraw-Hill/Irwin.

3. Zagonel, A. A., J. Rohrbaugh, G. P. Richardson, and D. F. Andersen. 2004. Using simulation models to address "what if" questions about welfare reform. *Journal of Policy Analysis and Management* 23 (4): 890–901.

4. Centers for Disease Control and Prevention. 2004. *Percentage of adults who were current, former, or never smokers, overall and by sex, race, Hispanic origin, age, and education. National Health Interview Surveys, selected years—United States, 1965–2000.* Atlanta: U.S. Department of Health and Human Services, Centers for Disease Control and Prevention, National Center for Chronic Disease Prevention and Health Promotion, Office on Smoking and Health. http://www.cdc.gov/tobacco/research_data/adults_prev/adstat1print.htm.

5. National Cancer Institute. 2006. *Evaluating ASSIST: A blueprint for understanding state-level tobacco control* (Tobacco control monograph no. 17, NIH publication no. 06-6058). Bethesda, MD: National Cancer Institute. http://cancercontrol.cancer.gov/tcrb/monographs/17/index.html.

6. Centers for Disease Control and Prevention. 2004. Cigarette smoking among adults—United States, 2002. *Morbidity and Mortality Weekly Report* 53 (20): 427–31.

7. U.S. Department of Health, Education, and Welfare. 1964. *Smoking and health: Report of the Advisory Committee of the Surgeon General of the Public Health Service* (PHS publication no. 1103). Washington, DC: U.S. Department of Health, Education, and Welfare, Public Health Service, Center for Disease Control.

8. Federal Cigarette Labeling and Advertising Act. 1965. Pub. L. No. 89–92, 79 Stat. 282 (1965).

9. Hyland, M., and J. Birrell. 1979. Government health warnings and the "boomerang" effect. *Psychological Reports* 44:643–47.

Understanding and Managing Stakeholder Networks

The current environment for tobacco control consists of many "silos" of organizations and expertise, with connectedness within disciplines but few clear linkages between disciplines and among stakeholder groups. There may be a future for the tobacco control field in which linked, interdependent resources are used collaboratively to build synergy, share expertise, and reduce duplication of effort. The processes of creating, analyzing, and maintaining networks of tobacco control stakeholders are key to functioning in a systems environment.

This chapter provides an overview of network theory and analysis methods and approaches for using knowledge to provide a deeper understanding of strategies to promote collaboration of people and organizations in a public health context. The chapter explores issues involved in applying networks to tobacco control and implications for research in the field. Finally, findings are presented from a case study using network analysis for evaluation of the tobacco control process.

Society must be reconceptualized as a complex network of groups of interacting individuals whose membership and communication patterns are seldom confined to one such group alone.

—Diana Crane, Invisible Colleges (1972)

Introduction

The complexity of tobacco use is such that no one person or organization is likely to "solve" the problem. Effective tobacco control programs are comprehensive and have components that attack the problem at individual, organizational, community, and societal/environmental levels. For example, intervention programs aimed at the individual (e.g., offering advice on smoking cessation) are more likely to reduce smoking in the population if they coincide with interventions at the organizational level (e.g., smoking bans in the workplace and at home) and at the environmental level (e.g., increased price of cigarettes through increases in excise taxes or passage of minimum price laws). Comprehensive tobacco control programming requires collaboration among a mix of individuals and organizations with varied interests, talents and skills, knowledge, and resources.

Similarly, because of the complex and multidimensional determinants of tobacco use, no one scientific discipline is likely to solve the problem either. Instead, a high degree of transdisciplinary collaboration is required, leading to development of new research tools and conceptual models and, finally, to interventions that take into account the full spectrum of biobehavioral and environmental aspects of tobacco use.

This complexity requires collaboration among tobacco control practitioners and scientists. In addition, the work of the scientists must be made accessible to practitioners, and the experiential knowledge of the practitioners must be accessible to scientists. This will ensure that the appropriate research questions relevant to tobacco control are being asked and answered.

This chapter examines the questions of "who works with whom" in a system and how organizations and individuals are brought together. The approach here focuses on the concepts in network analysis theories and the applications of network analysis that can be used to improve collaboration among and between the communities of public health practice and science.

Overview of Network Theory

In their recent book, *Social Networks and Organizations,* Kilduff and Tsai[1] provide a useful introduction to the importance of networks. They cite the example of Paul Revere and his famous "midnight ride" in 1775 to alert local townspeople near Boston, Massachusetts, of the imminent arrival of British soldiers. Most Americans know this story, thanks to Longfellow's poem. It is not so well known that on the same night, another rider, William Dawes, carried the same message and rode the same number of miles to other towns in the Boston area. Thanks to Revere, the message that the British were arriving spread rapidly. For Dawes, however, the message went largely unheeded, so most people, including the local militia leaders, were unprepared. Why was there such a difference? The answer, according to Kilduff and Tsai, is that Revere knew very well the communities he visited that night, and thus, he knew which individuals to contact so his message would spread rapidly. Because Dawes did not know many people in the communities he rode through, he contacted very few of the right people. Those he did contact were not well connected to others who could both spread the word quickly and initiate action to prepare for the coming invasion.

This example, whether apocryphal or not, demonstrates the importance and value of networks. Despite good intentions, similar resources, and high motivation, success in getting things done is often highly dependent on having an effective social network. Most people by now understand this point, at least regarding the importance of their personal network for such things as obtaining a desired job, achieving a promotion, or accomplishing politically sensitive tasks. The role networks play in society has been popularized through the movie *Six Degrees of Separation* and by the work of Watts,[2] who discusses "small-world" properties of networks. He argues that small-world networks, which exhibit only a few degrees of separation between any two nodes, can be used to explain the operation of both social and physical systems and the connection between seemingly random actions. It is far less well known how the study of networks, through network analysis, can be a valuable tool for organizational administrators and policy officials, in their efforts to address complex health and social problems through multiorganizational collaboration. Networks are critical to organizational life. However, attempts to apply what scholars know about networks to enhance the effectiveness of multiorganizational efforts in complex areas such as tobacco control, obesity, and chronic disease have been extremely limited.

Networks have been defined in a variety of ways, and no single definition is widely accepted. Even the term *network* is not always used. Many who study community and other organizational networks prefer to talk about partnerships, strategic alliances, interorganizational relationships, coalitions, or collaborative agreements.[3] Many also focus only on dyads (relationships between two persons or two organizations). Despite differences, nearly all definitions refer to certain common themes, including social interaction, relationships, collaboration, collective action, trust, and cooperation. Here, a network is defined as a group of three or more individuals, groups, or organizations connected in ways that are believed to facilitate achievement of a common goal. The relationships among network members are primarily

nonhierarchical and have partial and often substantial operating autonomy. Network members can be linked by many types of connections and flows, such as information, materials, economic resources, services, and social support. Examination and analysis of a network include relationships, the absence of relationships, and the implications of both for achieving outcomes.

No single, grand "theory of networks" exists. Instead, scholars in a wide range of disciplines, including anthropology, communication, economics, management, psychology, political science, and sociology, have used a number of theories over the years to help explain network structure and processes in interpersonal networks and organizational networks. Because the focus of this chapter is interorganizational networks, the theories, concepts, and measures are discussed, whenever possible, as they apply to organizations. To use the terminology of network analysis, organizations are considered as the "nodes" of the network. The primary caveat is that organizations consist of individuals. Social interaction among organizations ultimately occurs primarily between individuals acting on behalf of organizations.

Network Perspectives from Two Levels of Analysis

Network theory can be thought of as coming from two different but complementary perspectives: the view from the individual (actor) level and the view from the network level of analysis. Wasserman and Galaskiewicz[4] also make this distinction, referring to a microlevel versus a macrolevel network focus.

Individual-level theories have a long tradition in social research and have guided most of the knowledge about networks. Individual-level views, often considered to be egocentric, are concerned with trying to explain how involvement of an individual or organization in a network affects its actions and outcomes. For example, some individual-centered theories focus on an organization and its "embeddedness"[5] in a network. Prominent examples in the organizational literature include work by Burkhardt and Brass,[6] Burt,[7] and Uzzi.[8] Frequently, the focus of this research is dyadic relationships between organizations.[9] Dyads are the basic building blocks of networks. However, dyad-focused research is limited in that the network is primarily seen as a collection of two-party relationships, rather than as a unique, multiorganizational social structure in its own right.

Individual-level theories and related research can help to answer questions such as (1) which types of links are most or least beneficial to individual network members; (2) which network positions might be most or least influential; and (3) how the position of organizations in a network might shift over time in response to changes within and outside the network.

Structural issues that are typically examined and used to explain networks and network outcomes on an individual level include the following:

- *In-degree and out-degree centrality.* Does an organization occupy a central position or a more peripheral position in the network based on the number of networking ties it sends to or receives from other organizations? Degree centrality is based on the number of *direct* links maintained by an organization. Calculation of in-degree and out-degree centrality is based on the balance of assets such as resources, information, and clients coming *into* an organization from others in the network versus those being sent *out* to other organizations.

- *Closeness centrality.* Is an organization in a structural position to discern or spread information that might reside

in any organization in the network, even through indirect ties? Central organizations have short "paths" (connections) to all other organizations in the network. Closeness centrality is thus calculated by considering the shortest path connecting an organization to all other organizations in the network. Direct connections, where A is connected to B, are shorter than indirect ones, where A is connected to B only indirectly through ties to C, which is tied directly to B. Unlike the case with degree centrality, in closeness centrality, *indirect* connections are viewed as valuable conduits of exchange.

- *Betweenness centrality.* Does an organization serve as a gatekeeper within the network? If so, it must maintain intermediary links between organizations that are not directly connected with one another. Hence, the organization's betweenness centrality is calculated by considering the extent to which an individual's position in the network lies "between" the positions of other individuals.

- *Multiplexity.* What is the strength of the relationship an organization maintains with network partners, based on the number of types of links (e.g., joint programs, referrals, and research) connecting them? Multiplex ties are thought to be an indicator of the strength and durability of links, because they enable the connection between two organizations to be sustained even if one type of link dissolves.

- *Broker relationships and structural holes.* To what extent does an organization span gaps (structural holes) in a network, and what are the implications of this for the organization? Organizations that span structural holes are considered to be brokers, often occupying positions of considerable influence.

- *Cliques.* Cliques are clusters of three or more organizations connected to one another. The level of connectedness in a clique affects organizational outcomes in ways that are different from the effects of dyadic involvement.

Network-level theories draw on and use many of the ideas and measures developed by individual researchers. However, the focus is not on the individual organization but on explaining properties and characteristics of the network as a whole. The key consideration is outcomes on the network level, rather than on the organization level. For instance, instead of examining how organizational centrality might affect the performance or influence of individual member organizations, the network-level perspective would focus on overall network structures and processes. Network-level characteristics would be determined, compared across networks, and then used to answer questions such as how overall sustainability or absorptive capacity of the network could be enhanced or how the multiorganizational services provided to a client group might be strengthened. This perspective presumes that a network involves many organizations working collaboratively toward a common goal and that the success of one network organization may or may not be critical to the success of the entire network and its client group. The preference is for optimization of the network even if it comes at the cost of local maximization for any node or group of nodes in the network.

Work at the network level has blossomed over the past decade, but it has primarily been conceptual, anecdotal, or based on single case studies performed at one point in time. Networks have been used in studies of mental health,[10–13] and comparative empirical work has been done in other settings.[14–17] These and other studies used many of the structural issues discussed previously in this section for individual-level networks. Typically, these structural issues are aggregated across an entire network and then compared with those of other networks providing similar services. Unique network-level properties also are considered in those studies, including the following:

- *Density.* What is the overall level of connectedness among organizations in the network? Are some networks more fully connected than others? How much density is beneficial versus detrimental to the effectiveness of the network?

- *Fragmentation.* Are all or most network members connected, either directly or indirectly (i.e., through another organization), or is the network broken into fragments of unconnected organizations, dyads, and cliques? Fragmented networks have many structural holes.

- *Governance.* What mechanism is used to govern and/or manage the overall network? This mechanism can range from self-governance, with network members collectively running the system, to lead-agency models governed by a single organization that also provides critical core services, to a network administrative organization model. In this model, a separate entity is established for the sole purpose of facilitating network activity.

- *Degree, closeness, and betweenness centralization.* To what extent are a small proportion of the organizations in the network considerably more central in terms of degree, betweenness, or closeness centrality, as opposed to a network in which most organizations have relatively similar levels of centrality? Highly centralized networks may be organized in a manner approximating a hub-and-spoke pattern, popularized recently as "scale free" networks. Decentralized networks are far more dispersed, with links spread more evenly among members.

- *Cliques.* What is the clique structure of the network? How many cliques exist? Which types of organizations are involved? How large are the cliques? Are they connected to other cliques or fragmented? How much overlap is there across cliques, depending on the type of link involved (e.g., shared information or joint programs)?

Theories of Social Networks and Network Behavior

As previously noted, there is no single, unified theory of networks. Some researchers[18,19] even argue that there is no network theory at all. Rather, they claim that the study of networks is, at this point, more of an attempt to study social relationships by using a particular set of analytic methods and concepts (e.g., centrality). Most who study networks, however, do draw on one or more of a number of theories developed to explain networks and network behavior. These theories are discussed in considerable depth in two recent books: one by Monge and Contractor[20] on communication networks and the other by Kilduff and Tsai[1] on organizational networks. A brief overview of the major categories of theories that have been used to explain network behavior is provided here.

- *Self-interest.* Self-interest theories, drawing on economic principles of maximization of individual value, explain network behavior based on the self-interest of those involved in the network. In its simplest form, this explanation contends that organizations seek network links with other organizations if and only if it is in their interest to do so. For instance, one organization might want to create a network link to another organization from which it seeks to draw knowledge, skills, or resources. Network members can build their own social capital and thus enhance their outcomes by acting as social entrepreneurs and brokers, spanning structural holes.[7] Transaction cost economics also has

been used to explain networks based on self-interest. Using this approach, network members seek connections that allow them to operate most efficiently by minimizing the cost of transactions (e.g., overhead, distance, and accessibility) and maximizing the gains from transactions (gross value of services or materials being sought). Theories of self-interest are most useful in understanding networks in which the organization with the self-interest has the ability to coerce other organizations to be a part of its network.

- *Exchange and resource dependence.* A more viable network explanation is premised on theories of exchange and resource dependence. According to this perspective, organizations seek and form network ties with other organizations to reduce uncertainty and attract needed resources. The nature of these interorganizational ties is based on implicit consideration of the relative terms of exchange. The primary issue is power or its reciprocal, dependence. One organization may develop strong ties to another based on resource needs (e.g., money and information). However, it also seeks to balance this dependence through mutual dependencies with its linkage partner (i.e., exchange of needed resources) or through the influence and power this relationship provides for dealing with others in the network.[21,22] Decisions to be part of a network thus involve a complicated set of exchange relationships between and among all network members.

- *Collective action.* The two previous approaches are based on individual organizations structuring their network to draw resources from one another. Theories of collective action, on the other hand, explain situations in which organizations create network links with other organizations, not to seek or exchange resources with one another, but to maximize their joint ability to seek resources from or provide them to third parties. For instance, organizations might choose to share information to mobilize more effectively in a campaign to promote smoking cessation. Theories of collective action explain the viability of network links based on the mutual interest and benefits associated with joint action by the two organizations. These theories build on public goods theory[23] with the idea that individuals and organizations are motivated to join and work in networks to reap the benefits of collective action. The benefits presumably could not be obtained by acting through motives of self-interest or social exchange, even in a network context. Theories of collective action are broadly useful for explaining why organizations might form and sustain a network. Researchers[24] have explored reasons behind the formation of particular network structures and which structures might be most effective under particular conditions.

- *Social contagion.* The perspective of social contagion focuses on the impact of network involvement on subsequent behaviors. Contagion occurs as a result of interacting with network members and being "infected" by their attitudes and behaviors. In general, greater involvement (embeddedness) results in greater contagion, leading to similar attitudes, beliefs, and behaviors among network members. In the organizational literature, network involvement has frequently been used to explain why some organizations mimic the behavior of others, such as adopting total quality management; other "trendy" solutions to management problems;[25] or certain attitudes, innovations, or ideas.

- *Homophily.* The approach of homophily provides relatively simple but compelling reasons for why networks form and to a lesser extent, why they are sustained. Homophily is based on the assumption that individuals and organizations are more likely to create links with one another if they are similar. It is the "birds of a feather flock together" argument.[26] The underlying contention here is that there is a "comfort zone" associated with maintaining links with like-minded individuals or organizations. Although such networks may be attractive, it is reasonable to infer from research on group decision making that homogeneous networks also are likely to be less creative and innovative.

- *Proximity.* Like homophily, proximity provides a simple but powerful explanation for the maintenance of network links. Early research in organizational settings indicates that the frequency of face-to-face dyadic communication drops precipitously after the first 75–100 feet.[27,28] Proximity is based on the concept that physical closeness is likely to result in more opportunities for a social relationship than is separation by longer distances. More recent studies[29] considered the effect of communication technologies (e.g., e-mail and instant messaging) on the impact of physical proximity. Findings suggest that the effects of higher levels of interactions via electronic channels have a bimodal distribution. The impact is highest among those with the closest physical proximity and those who are the greatest distance apart.

- *Change and evolution.* Theories of organizational change and evolution have focused nearly exclusively on internal change or on the evolution of organizational populations.[30] However, some researchers have made efforts to extend what is known about change and evolution to networks by examining the influence of network involvement on organizational survival and on evolution of the network itself. The work on network involvement addressed network life-cycle stages and the importance of building legitimacy if the network is to be sustained.[31] A central assumption is that organizations create network links to maximize the "fitness" of the entire network and thereby to be "selected" from an ecology of other networks in the community. This perspective might explain why organizations involved in the tobacco control network might strategically create ties that help to preserve the long-term viability of the tobacco control community relative to other networks in health care communities, such as those focusing on obesity control.

Researchers have used all of these theoretical approaches to explain key aspects of network behavior. In some sense, they are competing theories, because all are attempts to explain the same basic phenomenon. However, networks are complex mechanisms, and an explanation of the actions and structures of network members and the network as a whole cannot be boiled down to one simple theory. Individuals and organizations typically join and sustain their involvement in networks for multiple reasons. The theories merely reflect this complexity. Indeed, there is a compelling case for the use of multitheoretical, multilevel models for explaining, simulating, and designing real-world networks.[17,20]

Effective Organizational Networks

Drawing on these theories, researchers have studied many networks in a broad range of settings. On the basis of research at the network level of analysis, a number of tentative conclusions can be drawn about criteria for an effective network. This list is not exhaustive, but it provides a brief overview of much of the existing knowledge about organizational networks. It also forms the basis of the subsequent discussion about application of network analysis to build and strengthen tobacco control efforts.

- *Multiple levels of collaboration.* Collaboration should occur at multiple organizational levels. Having network ties at only one organizational level (e.g., top-level administrators) minimizes commitment to the network by lower-level organizational participants. This reduces the chances of successful implementation of network strategies. Involving multiple people in an organization also increases the likelihood that network links will be maintained when someone leaves the organization.

- *Focused integration.* Extremely dense networks are inefficient, requiring a great deal of time and energy to maintain. Effective networks should have moderate levels of integration among members, with some fragmentation and structural holes.

- *Strong links.* The strength of linkages (multiplexity) among network members should be varied, depending on critical network needs. Some organizations should be connected through multiple ties, but other network members can and should maintain weak ties.

- *Network governance.* Governance of the network should be based on the size and complexity of the network and on its stage of evolution. Generally, small networks can be self-governed, but larger networks are most effective when governed through a lead agency or network administrative organization.

- *Involvement.* Most network relationships should be based on trust and commitment to network goals, even when contractual ties (e.g., funding) are present. Trust and commitment generally need to be built gradually, often first through low-intensity ties.

- *Legitimacy.* Networks must build legitimacy as they grow, both internally (through network members) and externally (e.g., through outside funding and the media). Legitimacy helps to build commitment to the network and its goals and is critical for sustaining the network.

- *Resources.* Effective networks have sufficient resources to work on network-level goals and activities, rather than focusing solely on internal organizational issues. Resources can come from network members or from outside sources. Minimally, resources are needed for basic business necessities, such as staffing, telephones, and a newsletter.

- *Knowledge repositories.* Organizations that publish materials in digital knowledge repositories (e.g., Web sites) are more likely, not less likely, to be targeted for direct communication from other organizations. Organizations use published information in digital repositories to identify "who knows what" and "who knows whom." Then, rather than being content to download the published information in these repositories, they seek out the "who" directly for further clarification and collaboration. In essence, a knowledge repository serves as an effective signal of the organization's knowledge but not as an effective substitute for disseminating knowledge to other organizations within the network.

- *Dedicated network alliance function.* Nodes in effective networks have developed an in-house dedicated network alliance function as part of human resources activities. The purpose is to help build "learning" about how to grow the network more effectively and to monitor for action cues to dissolve some network links.

- *Exploration, exploitation, and mobilization.* Organizations use "dense" (highly connected) networks to effectively exploit resources. This practice may contribute to incremental innovation. However, organizations use sparse small-world networks to explore novel ideas. This approach is most appropriate

for identifying disruptive technologies and might contribute to disjunctive innovations. In addition, organizations use "star" networks to enable mobilization. This strategy is most appropriate for formulating and implementing standards, policies, or procedures.

- *Goals.* Long-term goals such as improved health status are important, but results are frequently not apparent for many years. Thus, networks must have goals that are specific, attainable, and appealing to a broad range of network members. To build commitment and legitimacy, network members must have a sense of accomplishment. Such goals can focus on network structure, processes, and short-range outcomes.

- *Stability.* Although networks are designed for flexibility, major system upheavals are not conducive to the effectiveness of networks, especially after early formation and growth. Major system change can disrupt established, trust-based relationships that have evolved over a long period.

Value of Organizational Networks

Use of cooperative networks of organizations has become a key strategy for addressing the public's most pressing health and human services needs. These networks have become important mechanisms in many states and communities, as well as nationally and internationally. Their functions are as follows:

- Building capacity to recognize complex health and social problems

- Planning strategies systematically to best meet critical public health needs

- Developing and implementing policy related to public health needs

- Mobilizing, leveraging, and obtaining scarce resources

- Facilitating the flow of knowledge and information to address complex problems

- Delivering needed services

By working together as a network, organizations can improve both their efficiency and the effectiveness of the services and programs they offer.[32,33] Potential benefits of network involvement are substantial. They include improved services, better access to services, less duplication of effort, better communication and access to information, improved innovation, and ultimately, more sensitive and reliable indicators of health status. Research has demonstrated that networks are especially valuable for nonprofit and public organizations working to address a broad range of problems in community and regional health and human services.[12,34] Organizational networks offer the following benefits to health care providers:

- *Provide a team approach to complex public health issues.* Networks are especially helpful for addressing problems that are complex and seemingly intractable.[32] The magnitude of many problems in health and human services is simply too great for any one organization to resolve single-handedly. Such problems require a "fishing net" approach—a structure of organizations that is agile, flexible, easily reconfigured, and yet robust, and that can rapidly bring together the set of diverse skills, resources, and expertise required to address these problems effectively.

- *Address multiple needs.* Networks can work with clients who have multiple needs (e.g., education, disease prevention, treatment, and referral), as well as requirements to treat combinations of illnesses (e.g., substance abuse and mental illness or cancer and depression).

- *Counteract fragmentation of multiple-provider organizations.* Despite the multiple needs of clients, health care providers usually offer a limited range of services. Such fragmentation may be cultural or it may be based on differing treatment philosophies and methods, traditions, or funding streams. When services are fragmented, clients generally suffer, receiving only partial treatment or being forced to deal with multiple providers on their own. When organizations establish a network, however, fragmented services can be integrated across providers, enabling clients to enter a *system* for delivery of services that meets a broad range of needs across multiple organizations.

- *Ease problems related to geographic dispersion.* Organizations in large cities, rural areas, or different states, regions, or countries often can benefit immensely by sharing information, ideas, and resources. However, geographical dispersion often keeps them isolated. Networks provide a formal mechanism to encourage and facilitate collaboration, even when face-to-face contact is not possible.

- *Optimize use of resources.* Networks are efficient mechanisms for providing needed services under the constraints of limited resources. When provided through a network, scarce resources can be shared and duplication of services can be minimized through the coordinated efforts.

- *Facilitate transfer of knowledge and enhance learning.* Organizations have considerable knowledge and expertise, but that information frequently stays within the organization or is shared only sparingly. To address complex health care problems, however, the broad sharing of knowledge is critical. By establishing formal mechanisms to facilitate information transfer and by creating the framework for more informal interactions, networks can enhance the flow of knowledge across organizations. This improves both the amount and speed of learning by participants in the organization. In addition, networks can be used to build "transactive memory systems"[35] in which highly differentiated but easily accessible pockets of specialized knowledge are distributed across the network. Such networks can enhance the efficiency (speed) and effectiveness (quality) of learning across a broad range of areas, including client needs, delivery of services, advocacy, research, policy, and funding.

Networks also have shortcomings that can seriously undermine their effectiveness, even resulting in dissolution. Challenges to building and maintaining a successful network are numerous, but several factors affecting networks stand out as being most common, based on the research conducted.

- *Undermining of autonomy in decision making.* The downside of collaboration in any setting is that participants can no longer focus solely on their own needs. In organizational networks, members must consider the interests and expectations of other network members, thereby limiting their autonomy in decision making. The problem is most acute for network members who cooperate very closely, because decisions made by one member have a major impact on the other member(s). In addition, most contemporary organizations are confronted with the dilemma of having to cooperate with many of the same organizations they compete with in other contexts. A generic form of this dilemma occurs when organizations cooperate to provide complementary health services in a local community but compete for resources from local, state, and federal agencies to provide these services. This phenomenon of cooperation and competition[36] in the network further undermines autonomy in decision making.

- *Generation of conflicting loyalty and commitment.* Even in organizational networks, the key links are among

---

Putting Network Analysis to Work on Rural Chronic Disease

A team led by University of Arizona professor Keith Provan[a] explored the impact of community networks on management of chronic disease in a rural county of southern Arizona, using classic network analysis measures and self-assessment by participants.

This project, with support from a Turning Point grant funded by the W.K. Kellogg and Robert Wood Johnson Foundations, involved creation of a participatory coalition led by the Cochise County department of health to address issues of chronic disease. This group included stakeholders such as local politicians, law enforcement groups, faith-based organizations, and service providers. The work of the group was repeatedly evaluated during the two-year study, through data-collection efforts and participation in focus groups.

Results include a higher level of collaboration over an increased number of channels, including a near doubling in the number of nonredundant referrals and a broad perception (>90% of the 22 respondents) that collaboration had enhanced the agency's ability to serve its clients. At the same time, key issues for future network efforts were identified, including the need for strong leadership and continued funding.

[a]Provan, K. G., L. Nakama, M. A. Veazie, N. I. Teufel-Shone, and C. Huddleston. 2003. Building community capacity around chronic disease services through a collaborative interorganizational network. *Health Education and Behavior* 30 (6): 646–62.

individuals. These individuals are employed by, trained by, and socialized in one organization. Network involvement means going beyond the employing organization, in effect, becoming a multiorganizational participant. Often, however, loyalty and commitment to the organization are stronger than those to the network, even though organizational goals may best be accomplished through network collaboration. Some also may have internal conflicts, advocating network goals in their organization but encountering resistance from those who do not share this view. In general, having a narrow, organizational perspective can severely limit the achievements of a network.

- *Requirements for additional time and resources.* One of the main benefits of networks is that they can overcome deficiencies in systemwide resources. Nevertheless, they do require resources to become established and to operate. These resources may come from external sources, such as government agencies or foundations, or they may consist of contributions from network members. In either case, however, network members may feel that these resources could best be spent on their own organization and its clients. This problem is especially true considering the contribution of time required to participate in maintaining the network and its management. Directors of health and human service agencies generally embrace the network concept but not necessarily the time, effort, and money required to build and maintain an effective network. This is one of the reasons some effective organizations have invested in the creation of a "dedicated network alliance function" to nurture the network.

- *Need to manage collaboratively rather than hierarchically.* Traditional bureaucratic forms of control may not be widely accepted in most health and human service settings. However,

organizational employees still work in hierarchical settings governed by rules, procedures, and the decisions of supervisors and top management. This mechanism is efficient and well understood. In contrast, networks are mostly not hierarchical. Some organizational members may clearly be more influential than others, and some networks are constructed around funding and/or regulatory relationships. Yet, members can always withdraw from the network, despite consequences. As a result, network decisions can be messy, time consuming, and often frustrating, especially to those accustomed to working in a hierarchy. Some networks are designed to only share information, which limits this problem. However, many others are designed to coordinate delivery of services and programs, requiring significant agreement from participants. Although network decisions need not be consensual, they do need to be based on trust and reciprocity if the network is to be successful over an extended period.

These shortcomings are very real and can limit the accomplishments of networks. Nonetheless, most health and human services professionals recognize the advantages of networks, at least generally, and they believe strongly in the value of the collaborative process. However, many of those involved in networks, especially network leaders, may have difficulty recognizing and demonstrating progress in building the network. In light of the potential problems mentioned here, it may be relatively easy to conclude that the potential of the network is not being fully realized. The apparent lack of progress and tangible outcomes can be frustrating, especially for those who played a leadership role in building the network and are strongly committed to its success.

One problem is that most health leaders do not feel equipped to take steps to examine the quality and functioning of their network. This can best be accomplished through an objective and systematic process, but most network participants do not have the tools to do this. In addition, most tend to view the network from the perspective of the effect on their organization of network relationships. This view limits an objective understanding of the network as a whole. If collaborative efforts are to be effective, participants must look beyond their own needs, interests, and perspectives and consider how a multiorganizational network might be structured and governed to maximize its capacity to address critical health and human service problems.

In the academic and research literature of the past two decades, a great deal of knowledge about organizational networks has been generated.[3] Unfortunately, very little of this work has reached the world of health practice, except in a very general way.[37,38] Nonetheless, network analysis, as developed in the scholarly literature, can be used in a very applied way to help public and nonprofit organizations build and sustain networks across a broad range of health and human services, including control of tobacco use, chronic diseases such as diabetes and HIV/AIDS, obesity control, child and youth health, mental health, and substance abuse. Network analysis techniques offer four key benefits to these efforts:

1. They offer a global view, which helps participants understand the network and its components and how the network operates.

2. They help stakeholders to see exactly where their organization fits in the structure of the network, based not just on their own impressions but on the actual experiences of the other network participants.

3. They give managers access to data that they can use to shift priorities

and resources to become more or less involved either in the network as a whole or with certain key organizations that may be critical to their own effectiveness and the effectiveness of the network as a whole.

4. They provide members of the network with the tools to visually navigate the network and seek out relevant partners to help them solve specific problems. In this way, network analysis techniques help people involved in tobacco control to learn more about "who knows what" and where to go to obtain needed information.

Application of Network Analysis

As described previously, network analysis is a method of collecting and analyzing data from multiple individuals or organizations that may be interacting with one another. Unlike more traditional methods, the unit of analysis is the relationship between organizations, not the organization itself. Network analysis allows for examination and comparison of the relationship between one organization and another (dyads), among clusters or cliques of three or more organizations, and among all the organizations that constitute the network as a whole. Depending on the type of data collected, it is possible to examine a range of issues across these organization groupings. Issues include the following:

- Overall level of involvement among organizations in the network

- Pattern or structure of involvement

- Number of other organizations to which any one organization is linked

- Specific organizations and types of organizations to which any organization is connected

- Types of interactions between organizations (e.g., client referrals, shared resources, and shared information)

- Organizational level of the relationship (e.g., administrative or service level)

- Extent to which network ties are narrow (e.g., relationship between two individuals) or broad (e.g., relationships among multiple individuals in each organization)

- Extent or strength of each relationship (e.g., through referrals only or referrals and shared resources)

- Level of trust each organization has in its dealings with every other organization

- Perceived benefits and drawbacks of network involvement

Because network analysis focuses on relationships across and among all network members, once collected, data generally are displayed and analyzed by using a matrix reflecting each organization's links with every other organization in the network. Typically, data are collected from every network member (e.g., agency head or program director) by using questionnaires or structured interviews. The next section presents details about network data-collection methods focused specifically on tobacco control. Monge and Contractor[20] provide a more comprehensive description of techniques for measurement of communication networks.

Once network data are collected and analyzed, this information can be used in a variety of ways to assist leaders in understanding the structure and condition of the network and to facilitate strategic planning to strengthen the network. A recent publication of Provan and associates[39] offers a series of guidelines for this process. Their work forms the basis of a set of practical research questions that are developed at the

end of this chapter to guide the study and use of network analysis in tobacco control.

Even though network analysis can be extremely helpful for building the "capacity" of a stakeholder community[40,41] to address its most critical health needs through enhanced collaboration, it is certainly not a panacea. Network analysis is useful to demonstrate connections and relationships among agencies, reflecting the structure of the network. However, structure alone provides only a partial understanding of the reason(s) a network may or may not be effective. Networks having few and/or weak ties based on low trust are unlikely to be effective. Having many structural ties does not, in itself, guarantee the success of the network. Network goals must still be clearly established and collectively addressed, and effective network leadership is critical to the process.

Use of Network Methods for Tobacco Control

Once the applicability and value of network analysis are established for critical issues in health care, particularly within a tobacco control context, the question becomes one of defining the key issues in conducting a network study. What information should be collected? How should data be collected? What might be the results of data analysis? This section addresses these questions, focusing specifically on networks in tobacco control.

The discussion is guided by knowledge of two emerging but very different networks in tobacco control—the North American Quitline Consortium and the Global Tobacco Research Network (GTRN).

- *North American Quitline Consortium.* On February 3, 2004, the U.S. Secretary of Health and Human Services announced a plan to establish a nationwide toll-free telephone number (1-800-QUIT NOW) that will serve as a single access point to a national network of "quitlines" (hotlines for obtaining help to stop smoking). At the time of the announcement, 38 states had independent quitlines to deliver information, advice, support, and referrals to smokers or their surrogates. Telephone counselors at the Cancer Information Service, National Cancer Institute (NCI), were charged with providing assistance to individuals in states with no quitlines until those states could develop their own systems. The launch of the nationwide access number triggered a need for closer collaboration among the previously independent state-sponsored quitlines, which used different technologies, offered different services, and received funding and technical support from different sources. Working toward a national capacity to deliver quitline services will require collaboration among state and provincial health departments, quitline vendors, researchers, and national organizations.

- *Global Tobacco Research Network.* GTRN was started with the goal of enhancing research by promoting collaboration and partnerships, providing information, facilitating training, and sharing research tools among investigators around the world. The network is being developed around three core concepts: global network consolidation, global knowledge management, and global knowledge sharing. It aims to consolidate the weakly interlinked multisector community of researchers and institutions involved in the broad spectrum of research addressing the determinants, consequences, and control of tobacco production; promotion and consumption of tobacco products; and exposure to tobacco smoke. The NCI-funded initiative is timely, because of the need to implement the World Health Organization-sponsored Framework Convention on Tobacco Control, a

framework for consistent global tobacco control policy and legislation.

Information Needed for Network Analyses

Network studies must address certain fundamental questions about the type of information to be collected—Who? What? How? Where? When? The question of "who?" is probably the most basic. It refers to which organizations, groups, or individuals are involved or should be involved in the network for provision of tobacco control services. These are the *nodes* of the network. The nodes may vary from network to network (e.g., from one state to another). Therefore, a key first step is to determine who is and who should be involved in the network being studied. For example, in the Quitline network, relevant organizations might include the following:

- Tobacco control advocacy groups

- Research groups (e.g., government agencies, universities, nonprofit organizations, and drug firms)

- Sources of funding (e.g., governments and foundations)

- Agencies and groups disseminating information

- Providers of technical services (e.g., state and provincial health departments)

- Providers of treatment services

- Health insurers and health maintenance organizations

- Mental health agencies and institutions treating substance abuse

The list may seem daunting at first. A critical problem in network analysis research has been to determine who qualifies to be included in the network (i.e., the problem of "network bounding"). Most network researchers prefer to cast a

Global Network for Tobacco Control

Far too often, "silos" of information and knowledge in tobacco control exist within the borders of countries and organizations. To address this problem, the Global Tobacco Research Network (GTRN)[a] has evolved as a Web-based portal for linkage and knowledge sharing in the international tobacco control community. Current features include the following:

- Contact directories, opportunities, and event calendars related to global tobacco control
- Access to country profiles and industry documents
- Research resources ranging from youth programs to epidemiology, including both source materials and presentations
- A searchable database of tobacco control literature
- Employment and learning opportunities
- An ambitious Tobacco Atlas of statistics and information
- A Research Assistance Matching project linking researchers in developing countries with appropriate experts in the network

GTRN is administered by the Bloomberg School of Public Health, Johns Hopkins University, Baltimore, Maryland, with a technology infrastructure provided by GLOBALink. GTRN itself operates in a network environment, through the governance of a steering committee. Members include NCI, the American Cancer Society, and tobacco control research and advocacy organizations.

[a]Global Tobacco Research Network. 2006. Web site. http://www.tobaccoresearch.net.

relatively wide net initially—for example, including all organizations that might be involved in tobacco control in a particular state or region in a state quitline network. Once data collection begins, many of these organizations may "self-select" out of the process, informing researchers that they have little or no involvement in tobacco control efforts. In addition, the actual analysis of the network data ultimately collected determines which organizations are central, which are peripheral, and which are not involved at all.

On the other hand, researchers conducting a network study must be adequately informed *before* data are collected so that all relevant organizations are included. Decisions on which organizations to include and which to exclude from the study often are based on a procedure known as reputational "snowball" sampling. In this procedure, people who are known to be centrally involved in the network are asked to identify organizations and individuals active in tobacco control in

a particular community, state, or region or in a certain domain of policy or research. This process is continued with other key informants until no new names are generated.

The second question for network data collection is "what?" This question involves more deeply examining the services offered by each of the types of organizations identified here as relevant to quitlines. These services are in a broad range of areas including but not limited to education, language (e.g., translation), referral, clinical treatment, funding, counseling, research, pharmacy, policy and advocacy, training and technical assistance, and outreach. These areas also may include categories that focus on target communities to which these services are offered—for example, low-income children in minority groups and older single women.

In their work in mental health, Provan and Milward[12] identify the concept of a "service implementation network," which is highly relevant here. This concept refers to involvement of parts of an organization, rather than the entire organization, in a program effort. In tobacco control, the organizations identified by answering the question "who?" may be only partially involved in tobacco control, through a single service, or they may provide multiple tobacco control services. In either case, to understand fully how the network is structured and operates, it is essential to collect data on services, not just data on organizations.

This concept helps to provide a better understanding of the importance of the "what?" question. In most states or cities, for example, a public health department manages many programs, including but certainly not limited to tobacco control. Thus, the connection of a public health department to 10 other agencies has relevance to tobacco control only if the connection is based on tobacco control services and activities. Furthermore, it is critical to know whether the department is involved in only one aspect of tobacco control efforts or in multiple aspects. Thus, to know that a public health department is a node in a state quitline network may be interesting, but only a more thorough understanding of the network reveals its value to tobacco control efforts. Some examples are presented here.

- The public health department in one state may be linked to other organizations in the quitline network through funding, treatment, referrals, and technical support. In contrast, in another state, the department may be linked to the same number of other quitline network organizations, but solely through the technical support it provides. This difference in level of involvement may be critical for explaining why the first network is effective and the second is struggling.

- By obtaining a full range of specific types of tobacco control services, it is possible to tell, for example, how certain types of services and activities are clustered in the network, if certain types of services and activities are underrepresented or are being duplicated, and which other organizations' network members might seek to acquire needed advice, expertise, and treatment for clients.

- In the case of GTRN, knowledge of which organizations are involved in the network and the types of information that are differentially exchanged would help to reveal the pattern of knowledge transfer among different types of members (e.g., health agencies and research centers) and whether such patterns differ across geographic regions.

The third question for network data collection is "how?" This question refers to the type and frequency of network relationships. These may be either formal or informal and ongoing or intermittent. Formal relationships are specifically constructed with a strategic purpose in mind. Examples are joint programs, funding contracts, and memoranda of agreement. Most of these relationships are established by organizational directors and administrators, and they tend to be governed by enforceable contracts and/or operating guidelines.

Such relationships may be highly cooperative and may be used to solidify the ties between two or more organizations. On the other hand, the relationship may be somewhat distant (at arm's length) and may involve considerable monitoring. The formal relationships described here are mostly ongoing, because they typically establish the framework for a relationship that occurs regularly over an extended period. More intermittent formal relationships might include meetings among network members. Such meetings would be formalized to ensure that network members have a specific opportunity to share ideas, concerns, or issues with each other. However, such meetings generally would occur only occasionally, particularly when difficulties are involved in bringing all members together at one time or place.

Informal relationships also are common. They represent the real "glue" that holds any network together. Ring and Van de Ven[42] discuss the relationship between formal and informal aspects of interorganizational relationships. If network members are bound together only through formal mechanisms, they frequently do not develop the trust that enables a network to operate effectively as a network, as opposed to a loose collection of organizations with a more or less common goal. Informal relationships also can be ongoing or intermittent. However, like any social relationship, the less frequently the tie is used, the more likely the relationship is to dissolve.

The most common type of informal relationship is likely to be shared information. Information can be shared through channels such as e-mail, telephone calls, and personal meetings. Many of these activities may initially be based on friendship. Yet, when people try to construct a viable network to improve health outcomes, the evolution of informal ties can be encouraged through use of more formal mechanisms such as electronic mailing lists and conferences. GTRN provides a good example of how ties based on informal information sharing can be encouraged and formalized to establish a mechanism for building global understanding of research on tobacco control. The mechanism itself has been formalized. However, the flow of information on research and policy is informal, based on the needs, interests, and expertise of the network members operating in many different countries throughout the world.

In the area of services delivery, an important additional source of informal relationships

is client referrals. Referrals typically are based on an informal understanding among organizations that clients/patients can be served most effectively through the efforts of multiple, interconnected providers. In tobacco control, this might mean that a patient enters the system through a quitline but is referred to several other agencies for services such as treatment, counseling, or education. Each agency involved is part of a knowledge network and therefore has a more or less accurate understanding of the expertise and capacities of the other organizations in the network. Each agency refers patients accordingly, on a trust-based assumption that other agencies in the knowledge network will do their part to help the patients.

The fourth question is "where?" This question refers to the location of the levels of involvement that constitute a network. Essentially, networks can form either vertically or horizontally, and often both forms are involved. Vertical networks might include relationships between organizations operating at the community level and those operating at the state or provincial level. They could also include the interactions between state and national organizations or between community and national organizations. Vertical networks are frequently formal, involving ties between funding sources and recipients, technical service ties, and connections between policy formulation and implementation.

Horizontal relationships are network ties that occur within a community, state, province, or nation, or internationally, as is the case with GTRN. Horizontal relationships can be formal or informal. Informal, trust-based ties usually make up a large part of most successful horizontal networks. At the same time, however, the network could have a formalized governance structure, designed to facilitate network collaboration and interactions, attract funding, and act to resolve conflicts. Horizontal relationships are most common when organizations recognize the need to cooperate to achieve common goals and interests. However, the services and activities they perform are complementary, rather than competitive.

The fifth and final question is "when?" The vast majority of research on networks is cross-sectional, focusing only on data collected at one point in time. However, networks are constantly evolving as new organizations enter and old ones leave and as network members change their partners and mode of interaction. The theorizing[42,43] and limited longitudinal research on network evolution clearly point to differences in the ways in which relationships develop.[44] Identifiable stages of evolution are even suggested, from initial formation and early growth, through maturity, to sustainability or ultimate demise.[31] When data are collected from multiple networks, caution must be exercised so comparisons are made only across networks at relatively similar stages of development. In addition, network data collected at one point in time should be interpreted with the knowledge that conclusions drawn may be unique to that particular stage of network evolution.

To summarize, in studies of networks in tobacco control, five types of data are needed for full understanding of network structure and processes.

- "Who?"—Which organizations are and should be involved in the network?

- "What?"—What specific services and activities are exchanged by each network member?

- "How?"—How are relationships among network members constructed (i.e., what types of ties)? How frequently do these relationships occur?

- "Where?"—Where do the relationships among network members occur? Do these relationships involve vertical and/or horizontal ties?

- "When?"—When do different kinds of network relationships develop? How do they change over time?

Conducting Research on Tobacco Control Networks

Despite the lack of previous research on tobacco control networks, the case made thus far is that networks offer valuable mechanisms for building the strength of the tobacco control system at multiple levels (i.e., community, regional, national, and international). However, to maximize the impact and benefit of networks, one must fully understand them both conceptually and analytically. Thus, network analysis can be a powerful and important tool for strengthening tobacco control efforts. The previous section discusses types of information needed to conduct such an analysis. Details of data collection are presented here. Again, discussion of methods focuses on the quitline networks and GTRN.

The quantitative analysis of organizational networks is not more common in health care in general and in tobacco control in particular for two reasons. First, most social scientists are trained in traditional data-collection methods, especially random sampling and data analysis with use of inferential statistics. These methods generally are not appropriate for network analysis, although more and more researchers have become familiar with network methods in recent years. Second, network analysis is not more common because the research can be costly and time consuming. This is true especially if data are collected over multiple periods, across multiple networks, and using both quantitative and qualitative methods. This sort of research is critical for advancing knowledge about the operation and evolution of networks, and it can contribute to the solution of complex health problems. Typically, little or no data are available from secondary sources on relationships between and among organizations involved in a network, except perhaps through formal ties such as contracts. As a result, most network data must be collected from primary sources. Longitudinal data collection performed across multiple networks requires large-scale grant funding from federal agencies or private foundations.

In view of the importance and prevalence of networks in most areas of health, the time has come to apply what is known about both the theory and methods of networks to help strengthen tobacco control efforts. To that end, a number of sequential steps can be followed to collect the data described in the previous section. The approach used by Provan and colleagues[14,31,45,46] in multiple network studies is outlined here, but it can be adapted for use in a variety of settings. Presentation of this comprehensive approach is followed by several more streamlined alternatives that can be used if time and cost considerations are paramount.

- Select the network(s) that will be the focus of investigation (e.g., quitline networks, GTRN, or national networks for tobacco control policy).

- Ascertain whether the study focus will be a single network (i.e., the quitline network or GTRN) or comparison of multiple networks with similar focus— that is, a study examining and comparing networks of researchers in each of the Transdisciplinary Tobacco Use Research Centers, based at eight major universities across the United States.

- Talk with key network leaders to build an initial understanding of what the network is doing, which organizations are involved, and at which levels (e.g., community, regional, or national; see "where?" question in previous section).

- Try to determine the types of involvement critical to the network (see "what?" question)—for example, patterns of information sharing or research capacity in GTRN or referrals, contracts, shared information, or technical support for quitline networks. The "how?" question also may be addressed at this point, especially to limit the types of involvement to be studied—for example, deciding not to consider intermittent referrals.

- Develop an inclusive list of network organizations that use "reputational" sampling techniques (see "who?" question). Reputational sampling[19,47] is an iterative process relying on cumulative knowledge of network participants about who is involved in the network. The procedure starts with questioning those who are presumed to be the most central network members and then moving outward, depending on who is named.

- Determine (e.g., through telephone calls) the key individuals at each organization who are most likely to be knowledgeable about the network activities and involvement of their organization. Decide whether only one or several of these "key informants" should provide data on the network involvement of their organization. Because individuals in the same organization, especially a large organization with diverse services, often interact with outside organizations, responses of multiple informants about network involvement should be aggregated to form a single organizational response. Some of these key informants may have helped to define the network initially (i.e., the "who?" question). However, in the absence of objective data on which organizations are included in the network (e.g., an official membership list) or on specific network activities and ties, some cross-contamination is likely to be unavoidable.

- Develop broad cooperation and support from network participants for conducting the network analysis. If possible, make one or more presentations to the members of each network studied, demonstrating the type of data to be collected; how data will be collected; what is expected of them as respondents; how results will be reported to them;[39] and how the findings might be used to strengthen tobacco control efforts for their organization, their network, and other tobacco control networks.

- To achieve the best response rate, obtain one or more letters of support/endorsement of the study from the most important and/or influential network members, especially from key funding agencies such as NCI or the Centers for Disease Control and Prevention (CDC).

- Create a survey instrument that addresses who, what, how, and where and that provides sufficient information to develop a comprehensive understanding of the network (see list in previous section on "Application of Network Analysis"). One member of the Initiative on the Study and Implementation of Systems (ISIS) team[14] recently used this questionnaire in a study of a broad-based community coalition addressing chronic disease prevention and treatment. The organizations in the network are listed on the survey, so that every organization responds to an identical and complete list of network participants. Additional questions can and should be added to obtain specific data on individual organizations and respondents. Such data might include organizational funding, involvement with tobacco control relative to other health issues, types of services offered, and perceptual indicators of network effectiveness.

- Send the survey by mail or e-mail, along with letters of support and a cover letter explaining the project, to all network organizations and potential respondents.

The survey can be Web based or handwritten. If it is mailed, include a postage-paid return envelope.

- One week after mailing, follow up with a telephone call to each respondent and discuss receipt of the survey and any questions about completion. Continue follow-up by telephone call and/or e-mail weekly or every other week, until further efforts seem fruitless. Aim for approximately 80%–90% response. Dillman[48] reviews effective general survey methods using both mail and telephone.

- Depending on the number of networks studied, the size of each network, and budget constraints, visit each site shortly after the survey is mailed and interview as many network members as possible, especially those who are most heavily involved. If the survey form has not been completed, go through the questionnaire during the interview to maximize the response rate and discuss in-depth perceptions and attitudes about network involvement to help provide a rich contextual understanding of the operation and evolution of the network and its goals.

- Obtain all key available secondary data relevant to the study, including contextual data such as differences in tobacco use and tobacco control funding across networks, if multiple networks are being compared. Ideally, multiple outcome indicators also would be available for comparison with network-level measures over time.

- Code, analyze, and interpret all network data. Decide whether to use symmetrical and confirmed network data, symmetrical and unconfirmed network data, or both for the analysis. Unconfirmed data are the raw survey results for network involvement, based on the reports from each organization in the network. Confirmed data, validated against parties listed in the survey responses, are considered to be far more reliable if the goal of the research is to establish the existence of links in the absence of objective data. In the absence of symmetry and confirmation, unconfirmed data can be used. These data can provide potentially valuable information on "weak tie" relationships.[49] In addition, asymmetrical ties may be desired to reflect certain types of links, such as when trying to determine reputation or network influence (i.e., who lists whom as most influential).

- Report baseline network findings within each network studied and across multiple networks to network participants and key officials involved in tobacco control policy.

- Repeat the data-collection process after about 12–18 months and/or after a significant event that might alter network activities and structure in major ways (see "when?" question). Data should be collected at least twice and preferably three times to enable thorough understanding and explanation of network evolution and progress. Code, analyze, and interpret the results from all data-collection efforts, and compare findings within and across networks over time. Compare network data with tobacco control outcomes.

As noted previously, this data-collection method is extremely thorough and will provide an in-depth understanding of network structures and processes in tobacco control. Conducting this sort of data collection is highly recommended, but budget and time constraints may limit what is possible. To accommodate these constraints, the approach can be streamlined in several ways. Several alternatives to the full-blown data-collection effort are listed below.

- Use a limited procedure for reputational sampling. Identification of most network organizations can usually be obtained from a subgroup of the members of the full network, especially those who are most heavily involved in and most knowledgeable about the network. Caution should be exercised here, however, because this approach tends to underidentify network members who are not well connected.

- Conduct a partial network analysis by focusing only on a limited set of organizations that most informants believe to be the key network members. This approach might involve collecting data from 20–25 organizations versus 50–75 or more in the full network. Connections among the subsets of network agencies can be confirmed because they would report their links to one another. Connections to the larger network could still be reported, but these links would not be confirmed, providing a somewhat less reliable picture of the full network.

- Collect data from a small number of networks. This approach limits generalizability but can still produce valuable information on network "best practices" if the networks studied are carefully selected. For example, two or three quitline networks in states with well-established programs could be compared with two or three quitline networks in other states in which the program is just getting started. Another option is to study GTRN in two or three regions, comparing network structures and patterns of involvement.

- Limit the number of types of network involvement to only the two or three most important ones (e.g., resource sharing, information sharing, and referrals).

- Collect data on network involvement only from a single key informant at each organization, rather than using multiple informants. Single informants can be asked to check with other organizational members to ensure that survey responses reflect the *organization's* network and not just the respondent's network.

- Do not conduct interviews with network members. Limit network visits to one or two before data collection and one visit later to present and discuss findings. Substitute on-site interviews of most network members with telephone interviews as part of the survey follow-up process. Use of limited interviews is especially appropriate when multiple networks are compared or when network members are scattered geographically across a wide area, as with GTRN.

- Examine network evolution across two time periods only (instead of three or more), and conduct data collection at two-year intervals.

The information collected from either of these approaches can be used to develop an exercise for mapping network assets for the development, deployment, analysis, redesign, and simulation of networks.

Case Study of Network Analysis in Tobacco Control Evaluation

As a case study of network analysis in tobacco control, a project headed by Doug Luke of Saint Louis University, Missouri, is examined here. The project, performed in 2004, shows how the technique can be used as part of the process evaluation of tobacco control programs. Evaluation of the tobacco control process typically focuses on "counting" activities. Program evaluation includes determination of factors such as the amount of funding, numbers and types of prevention activities, and the number of countermarketing advertisement spots aired. This type of evaluation of local and state tobacco control programs ignores the complexity of the systems of agencies,

organizations, and people who coordinate activities to achieve a common goal of reducing the health burden of smoking and tobacco use.

A state comprehensive tobacco control program typically consists of a lead agency directing tobacco control funds to a series of state and local contractees. The lead agency also coordinates activities with voluntary agencies such as the American Cancer Society (ACS) and the American Lung Association (ALA). State and local coalitions provide guidance and outreach. Finally, a state program may include other types of partners, including public relations firms, local law enforcement agencies, or state attorney general offices. Network analysis is an analytic tool that is particularly appropriate for evaluating state tobacco control programs by using this type of systems perspective. The purpose of this case study is to show how network analysis is being used in an ongoing multistate project to evaluate tobacco control programs.

Collection of Network Data from State Tobacco Control Programs

The network analysis data reported here came from two large-scale multistate projects to evaluate tobacco control programs. These projects were conducted by the Center for Tobacco Policy Research, Saint Louis University School of Public Health,[50] and were funded by the American Legacy Foundation and the Chronic Disease Directors Association. The primary goals of these process evaluation studies were to assess (1) the implementation of CDC guidelines for *Best Practices for Comprehensive Tobacco Control Programs*[51] by state tobacco control programs, and (2) changes in state programs in response to massive cuts in funding.

The network analysis data were collected to facilitate understanding of the

ISIS Examines Its Own Network

To bring home the concepts of network analysis for ISIS members, a short proof-of-concept exercise was performed before a summit meeting in the Washington, DC, area in January 2004.

A questionnaire was designed and distributed to the meeting participants, who represented government agencies such as NCI and CDC, tobacco control research and advocacy organizations, and academic institutions. Each stakeholder was asked eight questions. The questions included requests for identification of their greatest needs and desired future interactions and other organizations with which they had financial, professional, or networking interactions.

Network involvement was analyzed based on these responses by using the Inquiring Knowledge Networks On the Web system from the University of Illinois at Urbana-Champaign. This system is a Web-based environment for conducting network analyses. Network results were illustrated graphically by using a series of network plots reflecting which organizations were linked and the ways in which they were linked. (See network on facing page.)

Within a very small nonrepresentative sample, this exercise nonetheless provided the ISIS stakeholders with a good overview of many of the network concepts discussed in this chapter, including centrality, cliques, and referral networks. More important, it served as a catalyst for productive dialogue between experts in networks and other disciplines, with an eye toward integrating network methods as part of a broader systems approach to tobacco control.

Note. TTAC = Tobacco Technical Assistance Consortium; U of Wisc = University of Wisconsin; ACS = American Cancer Society; TTURC = Transdisciplinary Tobacco Use Research Center; RWJF = Robert Wood Johnson Foundation; CTC = Center for Tobacco Cessation; CDC = Centers for Disease Control and Prevention; CFTFK = Campaign for Tobacco-Free Kids; Legacy = American Legacy Foundation; NCI = National Cancer Institute; SDSU = San Diego State University; JHSPH = Johns Hopkins School of Public Health; IGTC = Institute for Global Tobacco Control; RTI = Research Triangle Institute International; Uni of IL Chi = University of Illinois at Chicago; ORI = Oregon Research Institute; SAMHSA = Substance Abuse and Mental Health Services Administration.

structure of these complex state tobacco control programs, to identify other state characteristics related to program structure, and to determine whether changes in program funding and political support are associated with changes in program structure. The network analysis had three phases: network delineation, network data collection, and network analysis.

As discussed here, network delineation is the process of defining and identifying the network. In this case, the manager of the state tobacco control program was asked to identify every agency partner that played a critical role in planning and implementing the state tobacco control program. A modified snowball sampling approach was used to complete the list of program partners by contacting members on the initial list and asking whether any important partners had been omitted from the list. For the states evaluated in 2002, the tobacco control networks typically ranged from 14 to 17 partners. In addition to the lead agency (usually the state health department), the other commonly observed types of program partners included regional coalitions (in all 10 states), statewide coalitions (9 of 10 states), contractees (10 states), ACS (10 states), ALA (7 states), and the American Heart Association (6 states).

Once the network for each state was defined, an expert informant from each network partner agency was asked to participate in the study. In the network analysis, four primary pieces of relational network information were collected: (1) funding relationships among partners, (2) frequency

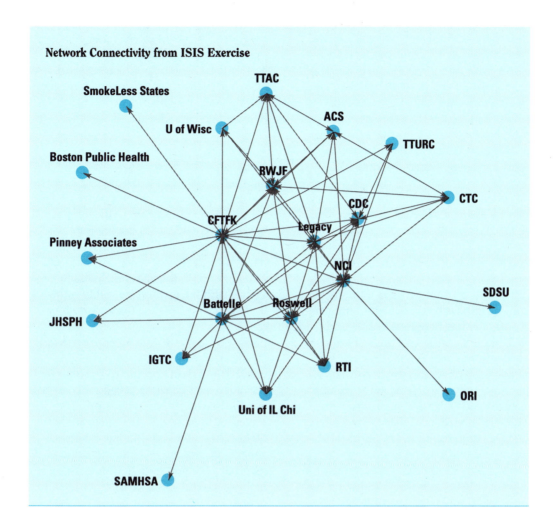

Network Connectivity from ISIS Exercise

of contact, (3) degree of cooperation, and (4) perceived importance of network partners in achieving state tobacco control goals. The next section presents results from the question on frequency of contact.

Information Learned about Tobacco Control Program Networks

A primary purpose of the evaluation of state tobacco control programs was to explore the influence of state financial and political climates on the structure and processes of tobacco control programs. Financial and political climate ratings were produced for each state according to a number of criteria. States were seen as having a positive financial climate for tobacco control if they (1) were meeting CDC recommendations for the amount of money budgeted for tobacco control, (2) had relatively high levels of per capita spending on tobacco control, (3) had set a high excise tax on cigarettes, and (4) had not securitized funding from the Master Settlement Agreement. States were rated as having a positive political climate if they had (1) multiple tobacco control "champions" in positions of authority and influence, (2) support for tobacco control from the governor, (3) support for tobacco control from the legislature, and (4) a low tobacco industry presence in the state. The ratings for political and financial climates were combined in a summary scale that could range from –9 to +9. Table 6.1 shows the ratings for the states evaluated in 2002. During this time, Indiana, Mississippi, and Hawaii had relatively positive climates for tobacco control. However, Wyoming, Michigan, Oklahoma, and Missouri had more challenging environments.

To determine whether political or financial climate was related to network structure, the contact networks for each state were examined. The contact networks for Indiana and Mississippi, two states with relatively positive climates, are shown in figure 6.1. A link connects two partners if they have contact with each other at least once per month. Contact is defined broadly and includes face-to-face meetings, telephone conversations, and e-mail. Examination of this network reveals which partners are more centrally located in the contact network and which are more peripheral. For example, the Indiana Tobacco Prevention and Cessation Agency (ITPC) is the lead agency for Indiana, and it has frequent contact with all 14 other network members. Boys and Girls Clubs (B&G Clubs), on the other hand, meets only monthly with three of the network members. Thus, ITPC plays a more central role in the communication network in the Indiana tobacco control

program. This result can be measured more formally by calculating Freeman's betweenness centrality—the measure of how often a particular network member lies "in between" any two other network members, linking members who are not directly connected.[52]

A high score for betweenness centrality indicates a node that is central in a network and can be considered to be a gatekeeper or controller of information. In the network figures here, nodes with the highest scores for betweenness are colored purple and nodes with the lowest scores are colored yellow. For both Indiana and Mississippi, the agency with the greatest centrality is the lead agency for the state tobacco program.

Finally, the centrality for an entire network can be assessed with the centralization index. This index is calculated by summing the differences between all centrality scores and the maximum centrality score. The scores for Indiana and Mississippi are both higher than 20%. This finding indicates a moderate amount of communication hierarchy—that is, both networks have a few highly central nodes and many peripheral nodes.

The contact networks for Michigan and Oklahoma, two states with much poorer

Table 6.1 Ratings of Political and Financial Climates for 10 States in 2002

State	Political support	Financial support	Total score
Indiana	Very strong	Strong	+5
Mississippi	Very strong	Strong	+4
Hawaii	Strong	Very Strong	+4
Pennsylvania	Moderate	Strong	+2
Washington	Strong	Moderate	0
New York	Moderate	Moderate	−1
Wyoming	Challenging	Strong	−3
Michigan	Challenging	Moderate	−3
Oklahoma	Challenging	Challenging	−5
Missouri	Challenging	Challenging	−9

Figure 6.1 Contact Networks for Two States with Strong Financial and Political Climates (Indiana, left; Mississippi, right)

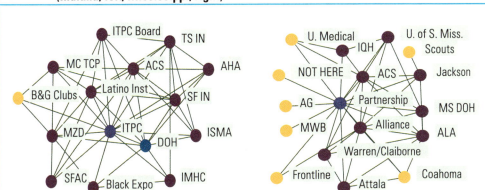

Notes. Indiana (left) had a centralization index of 22.7%, and Mississippi (right) had a centralization index of 20.5%. ITPC = Indiana Tobacco Prevention and Cessation Agency; TS IN = Tobacco Smart Indiana; MC TCP = Marion County Tobacco Control Program; ACS = American Cancer Society; AHA = American Heart Association; B&G Clubs = Indiana Alliance of Boys and Girls Clubs; Latino Inst = Indiana Latino Institute; SF IN = Smokefree Indiana; MZD = MZD Advertising; ISMA = Indiana State Medical Association; DOH = Indiana State Department of Health; SFAC = Smokefree Allen County; Black Expo = Indiana Black Expo; IMHC = Indiana Minority Health Coalition; U. Medical = University Medical Center; U. of S. Miss. = University of Southern Mississippi; IQH = Information and Quality Healthcare; Scouts = Girl Scouts of Gulf Pines; Jackson = Partnership for a Healthy Jackson County; AG = Attorney General's Office; Partnership = Partnership for a Healthy Mississippi; MS DOH = Mississippi State Department of Health; MWB = Maris, West & Baker; Alliance = Mississippi SmokeLess States Alliance; ALA = American Lung Association; Warren/Claiborne = Partnership for a Healthy Warren/Claiborne Counties; Frontline = Frontline State Board; Coahoma = Partnership for a Healthy Coahoma; Attala = Partnership for a Healthy Attala.

Figure 6.2 Contact Networks for Two States with Weak Financial and Political Climates (Michigan, left; Oklahoma, right)

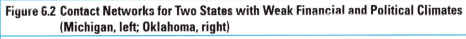

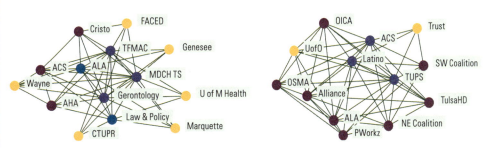

Notes. Michigan (left) had a centralization index of 10.4%, and Oklahoma (right) had a centralization index of 6.6%. FACED = Faith Access to Community Economic Development Corporation; Cristo = Cristo Rey Community Center; TFMAC = Tobacco Free Michigan Action Coalition; Genesee = Genesee County Smokefree Multi-Agency Resource Team; ACS = American Cancer Society; ALA = American Lung Association; MDCH TS = Michigan Department of Community Health, Tobacco Section; Wayne = Wayne County Smoking and Tobacco Intervention Coalition; Gerontology = Center for Social Gerontology; U of M Health = University of Michigan Health System; AHA = American Heart Association; Law & Policy = Tobacco Control Law & Policy Consulting; Marquette = Marquette County Tobacco-Free Coalition; CTUPR = Center for Tobacco Use Prevention and Research; OICA = Oklahoma Institute for Child Advocacy; Trust = Tobacco Settlement Endowment Trust; UofO = University of Oklahoma Health Sciences Center; Latino = Latino Agency; SW Coalition = Southwest Tobacco Free Oklahoma Coalition; TUPS = Oklahoma State Department of Health Tobacco Use Prevention Service; OSMA = Oklahoma State Medical Association; Alliance = Oklahoma Alliance on Health or Tobacco; TulsaHD = Tulsa City-County Health Department; NE Coalition = Northeast Tobacco Free Oklahoma Coalition; PWorkz = PreventionWorkz.

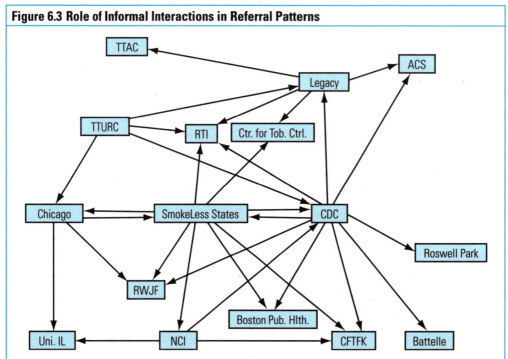

Figure 6.3 Role of Informal Interactions in Referral Patterns

Notes. TTAC = Tobacco Technical Assistance Consortium; ACS = American Cancer Society; Legacy = American Legacy Foundation; TTURC = Transdisciplinary Tobacco Use Research Center; RTI = Research Triangle Institute International; Ctr. for Tob. Ctrl. = Center for Tobacco Control; CDC = Centers for Disease Control and Prevention; RWJF = Robert Wood Johnson Foundation; Boston Pub. Hlth. = Boston Public Health; Uni. IL = University of Illinois; NCI = National Cancer Institute; CFTFK = Campaign for Tobacco-Free Kids.

climates for tobacco control, are shown in figure 6.2. One difference between these two networks is that instead of having only one highly central agency, each state has three central agencies, again indicated by purple nodes. For example, in Oklahoma, the Latino Agencies (Latino) and ACS join the lead agency, the Tobacco Use Prevention Service (TUPS), and are collectively the most central nodes in the state network. The low network centralization indices (10.4% for Michigan and 6.6% for Oklahoma) also show that these networks have a much more active communication structure than was seen for Indiana and Mississippi.

The preliminary interpretation of these patterns is the presence of a relationship between financial and political climates and structures for communication about tobacco control. The hypothesis is that lead

agencies in states with positive financial and political climates have the financial and political resources that allow them to take a strong leadership role in the tobacco control program. Conversely, in states that have poor climates, lead agencies no longer have these resources, and thus no longer are the most central agencies in the programs. In fact, a process of network adaptation may be in effect. When funds and support are scarce, tobacco control agencies may reconfigure their relationships to ensure sustainability of the program. In a sense, they may be "sharing the load" when times are tough.

This relationship is apparent for all 10 states, as evidenced by a fitted linear regression line and a smoothed local regression curve (locally weighted scatterplot smoother) (figure 6.3).[53] In addition, the relationship between the financial and political climates

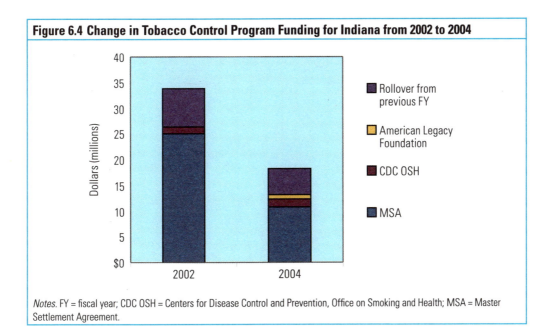

Figure 6.4 Change in Tobacco Control Program Funding for Indiana from 2002 to 2004

Legend:
- Rollover from previous FY
- American Legacy Foundation
- CDC OSH
- MSA

Notes. FY = fiscal year; CDC OSH = Centers for Disease Control and Prevention, Office on Smoking and Health; MSA = Master Settlement Agreement.

for tobacco control and the communication structure is moderately positive. The more positive the climate, the more hierarchical is the communication network ($r = .32$).

Because of the small number of states considered in the calculations, these interpretations must necessarily be tentative. However, a second phase of the state evaluation project allowed longitudinal examination of this hypothesis. In 2004, eight state tobacco control programs were evaluated, including a return visit to Indiana. Between the two evaluation periods, there was major upheaval in the Indiana program. The tobacco control program lost approximately one-half of its funding (figure 6.4). In addition, the state had a new governor who was perceived as being much less supportive of tobacco control (figure 6.5). Consequently, Indiana had a much more challenging financial and political climate for tobacco control in 2004 than it had in previous years. The communication networks for both 2002 and 2004 are shown in figure 6.6. The tobacco control network is the same size in 2004, but it has a very different structure. The centralization index

is much lower (decrease from 23% to 13%). This finding indicates a communication structure that is more active. At the same time, the density has increased from 49% to 59%. Density is the proportion of observed ties to possible ties. The higher density indicates that more of the agency partners talked to each other directly in 2004. Thus, there has been a shift in Indiana—as the climate worsened, the network apparently adapted by "flattening" the communication structure and increasing the amount of direct contact. This change over time is consistent with the hypothesis that state climates influence structures of the state tobacco control program.

Network Research Questions for Tobacco Control, Discovery, Diagnosis, and Design

The research described above provides an example of how network analysis can be conducted in a tobacco control context, but it is highly descriptive. Based on research like this, however, network leaders can use findings to help build and strengthen

Figure 6.5 Change in Perceived Political Support for Tobacco Control from Two Indiana Governors, Governor Frank O'Bannon (2002, left) and Governor Joseph Kernan (2004, right)

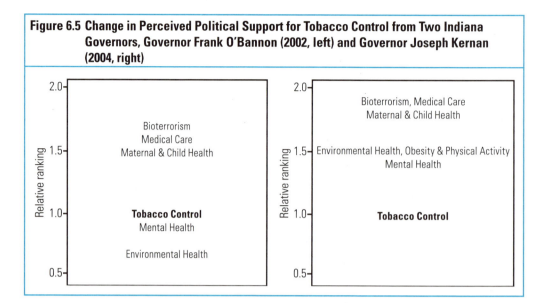

Figure 6.6 Change in Indiana's Tobacco Control Contact Network Structure from 2002 (left) to 2004 (right)

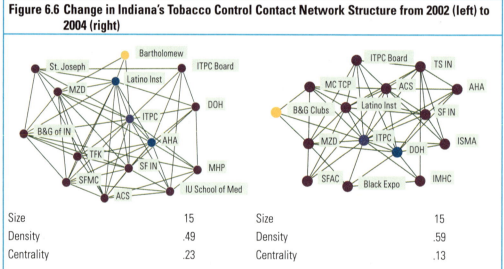

Size	15	Size	15
Density	.49	Density	.59
Centrality	.23	Centrality	.13

Notes. Bartholomew = Bartholomew County; St. Joseph = St. Joseph County; ITPC = Indiana Tobacco Prevention and Cessation; Latino Inst = Indiana Latino Institute; MZD = MZD Advertising; DOH = Indiana State Department of Health; B&G of IN = Indiana Alliance of Boys and Girls Clubs; AHA = American Heart Association; TFK = Tobacco Free Kids; SF IN = Smokefree Indiana; MHP = Madison Health Partners; SFMC = Smokefree Marion County; IU School of Med = Indiana University School of Medicine; ACS = American Cancer Society; TS IN = Tobacco Smart Indiana; MC TCP = Marion County Tobacco Control Program; ISMA = Indiana State Medical Association; SFAC = Smokefree Allen County; IMHC = Indiana Minority Health Coalition; Black Expo = Indiana Black Expo.

their network. Recent work by Provan and colleagues[39] was discussed earlier in this chapter. These researchers proposed a series of questions that might be asked by network leaders and participants to guide their efforts in translating network data into practice. In addition, Contractor and colleagues[54] at the "collaboratory" of Science of Networks in Communities at the University of Illinois at Urbana-Champaign have proposed an innovative, high-risk, high-payoff strategy for basic network research and its transfer to the practice of enabling networks within various communities. They refer to it as the "3D"—discovery, diagnosis, and design—model.

Drawing on ideas from both groups of researchers, this chapter proposes a series of questions that can guide the development of research on tobacco control networks. In addition, the questions proposed have a very practical orientation, demonstrating how network leaders and policy officials might use network analysis in tobacco control. The questions are organized around the concepts of discovery, or learning about who is connected to whom; diagnosis, or analyzing network relationships; and design, which involves application of findings to build, maintain, and strengthen the network.

Discovery

The questions listed here are designed to help a community discover existing communication and knowledge networks. (If only the tobacco control network knew what the tobacco control network knows.) These questions focus on some ways in which network data collection can contribute to a deeper understanding of the structure of a tobacco control network. An important aspect of identification is to determine the capacity of network stakeholders to know "who knows what."

1. What specific organizations and/or individuals constitute a particular tobacco control network?

2. Are individual tobacco control stakeholders able to identify which organizations are included in the network and which are not?

3. Are there large differences between self-identification of network ties and the reports of others in the tobacco control network (i.e., unconfirmed versus confirmed ties)? Does everyone really know who is connected to whom and in what ways?

4. Are individual tobacco control stakeholders able to identify others in the tobacco control community who share specific interests and areas of expertise so they might coalesce into a "community of practice"?

5. Are tobacco control stakeholders able to identify other key organizations and groups outside the tobacco control community that may have expertise and resources needed by those within the network?

6. Can tobacco control stakeholders identify organizations within the network that may have working relationships with these critical outside groups?

Diagnosis

Once the network has been discovered and identified, detailed network analysis methods, both qualitative and quantitative, are used to diagnose network structure and processes. They help the community to diagnose the "health" of the network. These questions focus on what specific attributes are normally assessed in the process of network diagnosis.

1. Which organizations are most central in the network in that they use both direct and indirect measures of centrality? Are these the organizations most essential for addressing client and program needs?

2. Are some network relationships especially strong and others weak? Is the relative strength of ties consistent with network needs for essentials such as information and resources?

3. Who are the connectors, information brokers, and boundary spanners in the network who can meet network needs in areas such as research, funding, and services? Do these important roles even exist in the network? Do the appropriate

organizations and individuals occupy these roles?

4. Is the network broadly connected, highly fragmented, or divided into subgroups and cliques? Which specific subgroups of network organizations have strong working relationships?

5. Is the flow of essentials such as information, knowledge, clients, and funding needed for tobacco control efforts being efficiently and effectively distributed throughout the network? Where are the gaps? Where are the redundancies?

6. Are critical network ties based solely on personal relationships, or have they become institutionalized so they are sustainable over time, as key individuals come and go?

7. Do network members have links to other groups and organizations outside the network that may be helpful to the full network for vital actions such as attracting needed resources and information and influencing policy?

8. How are these external ties structured? Are they primarily through core or peripheral network members? Are network members able to draw on these external ties to "explore" and/or "exploit" the outside environment in ways that might benefit tobacco control efforts?

9. How is the network governed? Are mechanisms and structures in place to facilitate and guide the coordinated actions of network members so tobacco control efforts are appropriately integrated and coordinated?

10. How has the network evolved over time, as evidenced in several waves of data collection? Specifically, has reasonable progress been made in establishing critical network ties and building effective network governance mechanisms?

11. What level of trust and cooperation exists among tobacco control agencies trying to work together? Have trust and cooperation increased or decreased over time?

12. What have been the benefits, drawbacks, and expectations of network involvement? Have these changed over time?

13. Within a particular service domain such as tobacco control, how do networks in some communities, states, or regions compare, along the dimensions described here, with other networks trying to perform similar services?

14. What is the network's *capacity for scanning*—that is, the extent to which it has human and automated "probes" that can bring new information into the network?

15. What is the network's *capability for absorption*—that is, the extent to which it can absorb relevant information scanned from outside the network?

16. What is the network's *efficiency for distribution*—that is, the extent to which it can selectively and strategically distribute the information it absorbs to the appropriate nodes that need it?

17. What is the level of *congestion* within the network due to bottlenecks—that is, the extent to which certain organizations or individuals are holding up the flow of knowledge or resources, because their "circuits are too busy with unnecessary networking"?

18. What is the network's *robustness against disruption*—that is, the extent to which built-in redundancies in the links within the network help to prevent unraveling of the network when one individual or organization departs?

19. What is the network's *vulnerability to external sources*—that is, the extent to which links among members of the network are being brokered by nodes outside the network?

Design

Discovery (identification) and diagnosis contribute to building a deep understanding of one or more tobacco control networks by using the tools and techniques of network analysis. However, once this understanding has been established, it is up to network leaders and members to work with network researchers to put the findings to use. The design phase involves efforts to modify network structures and relationships to enhance the effectiveness of the network. The focus of this phase is on helping the community collectively identify strategies to design (tune) a network to accomplish its goals more effectively. This strategy could apply to an existing network or to a latent or nascent network that needs a jump-start.

Designing a network includes identifying links or nodes that must be restructured, as well as identifying social incentives and technical infrastructures necessary for the network design to be successfully implemented. This "rewiring" of the network is frequently difficult, because it may require changes in the structure and patterns of behavior that have evolved over the life of the network.

The recommendations made here relate to changes network leaders and members may want to consider, not changes that must be addressed. Such changes would be implemented slowly and would be guided by such considerations as a thorough understanding of network context, the individuals involved, and what is politically possible. Networks can be changed to operate more efficiently and effectively, and network analysis provides a rationale for making the necessary changes on the basis of data, rather than assumptions and general observations.

The design questions presented build on the identification and diagnosis questions already discussed. Design is simply the application and use of this knowledge. The design questions are more general than the questions about identification (discovery) and diagnosis, focusing on the types of issues

---

Linking Systems and Networks: Agent-Based Models

One area that may hold promise for network methods is use of agent-based simulations of networks, a concept from system dynamics. In such simulations, autonomous agents operating under specific rules create evolutionary outcomes.[a] In a tobacco control context, for example, one might simulate the long-term consequences of including specific organizations in a network, adding links (e.g., by creating cross-functional teams), dropping links (e.g., by creating firewalls), or offering incentives for specific types of resource flows among certain members within the network. "What if" scenarios could then be based on these assumptions.

Interest in development of agent-based computational models and multiagent simulation environments has been substantial.[b] Blanche, a computer application developed by Contractor and Monge,[c] is one such computational network modeling environment especially well suited to simulate and visualize changes in a network based on multitheoretical, multilevel mechanisms. Another more distant but promising area is the potential "docking" of the aggregate system dynamics models and agent-based computational network models. Such approaches may help to improve the collective validity and usefulness of these models for practitioners interested in designing networks.

[a]Sterman J. D. 2000. *Business dynamics: Systems thinking and modeling for a complex world.* New York: McGraw-Hill/Irwin.

[b]Gilbert, N., and K. G. Troitzsch. 1999. *Simulation for the social scientist.* Berkshire, UK: Open Univ. Press.

[c]Monge, P. R., and N. Contractor. 2003. *Theories of communication networks.* New York: Oxford Univ. Press.

that might be addressed by an organizational network focused on tobacco control.

1. How can understanding of factors such as who is involved in the network, who knows what, and the location of key information and resources be enhanced? Members of the tobacco control network must have access to all network identification data so they can develop relationships with other network members as needed.

2. How can the network be redesigned to operate more efficiently? How can redundant ties be limited and weak or nonexistent ties in key areas be strengthened? Which relationships should be direct and which should be indirect, brokered by other organizations and individuals? Tobacco control organizations should collaborate to enhance effectiveness, but networks with ties that are too dense are inefficient because everyone is too busy networking to get anything else done.

3. How can the network be redesigned to operate more effectively? Which types of relationships seem to work best? How can these be expanded to other areas of the network? Networks should be redesigned so organizations with assets and skills critical for particular aspects of tobacco control (e.g., information and certain client services) have a high degree of centrality and are not peripheral in the network's structure.

4. Consistent with question 3, what overall types of network design and structure are most appropriate for accomplishing different types of network outcomes? For example, dense networks may work best for achieving collective action, and small-world networks with ties to outside groups may be best for exploring and importing new ideas. In general, however, as noted earlier in this chapter, effective networks typically display "focused integration," with an appropriate mix of weak and strong ties and some fragmentation.

5. In light of existing levels of trust, how can trust be enhanced among network members, especially if the network is to be highly collaborative and not based on hierarchy or contracts? Should trust building focus on key subgroups or cliques of organizations first and then be expanded to others? Have certain low-trust relationships been identified and thus circumvented in the building of network ties?

6. How can the benefits of network collaboration that have been identified be maintained and reinforced? How can the drawbacks be minimized?

7. How can the appropriate network governance structure be established and sustained so network activities and interactions can be encouraged, coordinated, and facilitated on an ongoing basis? What should such a governance structure look like? Who should lead it?

8. How can critical network ties be institutionalized? Tobacco control organizations should work to ensure that key network ties, especially broker ties, are not dependent on a single individual.

9. Based on comparative network analysis across multiple networks, what "best practices" can be established? How can these practices be effectively implemented?

Summary

Network analysis represents an important and currently underused approach for assisting leaders in health care services, public health practice, and development and implementation of health policy, especially in the area of tobacco control. Network analysis can be a powerful tool for strengthening tobacco control efforts at local, state and regional, national, and international levels. Network analysis can be done (1) by identifying existing networks and who is involved, (2) by diagnosing how these networks are structured and governed and how they operate, and (3) by using this knowledge to help network leaders design networks that work together more effectively to enhance a broad range of tobacco control efforts. This chapter provides an overview of how network analysis might be accomplished and why it would be beneficial for tobacco control programs. The structural data provided by network analysis must be combined with an in-depth knowledge of the nature of the problem being addressed, the services and capacities of the organizations involved, and the social and political contexts in which the network is embedded.

Conclusions

1. Solving complex future issues in tobacco control will require replacing silos of information and activity with greater linkage of tobacco stakeholders through networks.

2. Networks of tobacco control stakeholders form a foundation of the systems environment envisioned for the future of tobacco control. Many components of a systems approach are built around the presumption of stakeholder networks that span multiple levels of tobacco control activity and transcend geography and discipline. These components include building organizational capacity; participatory approaches to planning, implementation, and evaluation; optimization of resources and effort; and dissemination of knowledge and best practices.

3. Network analysis holds the potential for facilitating understanding and strategic management of linkages between stakeholder groups.

4. Numerous theories of network behavior currently coexist, and core concepts that describe networks now have broad acceptance, particularly those related to network attributes and behavior.

5. Network applications in public health are at an early stage. However, they have shown promise in recent studies, particularly in areas where disparate organizations have a common goal. Recent tobacco control applications of networks include the North American Quitline Consortium and Global Tobacco Research Network.

6. Network attributes potentially serve as a measure of the health of tobacco control efforts, as evidenced by a case study correlating network centrality with the strength of political and financial support for tobacco control.

7. In the future, tobacco control programs could consist of multiple networks with specific functional objectives, linked in turn as part of a "network of stakeholders."

References

1. Kilduff, M., and W. Tsai. 2003. *Social networks and organizations.* Thousand Oaks, CA: Sage.

2. Watts, D. J. 1999. *Small worlds: The dynamics of networks between order and randomness.* Princeton: Princeton Univ. Press.

3. Brass, D. J., J. Galaskiewicz, H. R. Greve, and W. Tsai. 2004. Taking stock of networks and organizations: A multilevel perspective. *Academy of Management Journal* 47 (6): 795–817.

4. Wasserman, S., and J. Galaskiewicz, eds. 1994. *Advances in social network analysis: Research from the social and behavioral sciences.* Thousand Oaks, CA: Sage.

5. Granovetter, M. 1985. Economic action and social structure: The problem of embeddedness. *American Journal of Sociology* 91 (3): 481–510.

6. Burkhardt, M. E., and D. J. Brass. 1990. Changing patterns or patterns of change: The

effects of a change in technology on social network structure and power. *Administrative Science Quarterly* 35 (1): 104–27.

7. Burt, R. S. 1992. *Structural holes: The social structure of competition.* Cambridge, MA: Harvard Univ. Press.

8. Uzzi, B. 1997. Social structure and competition in interfirm networks: The paradox of embeddedness. *Administrative Science Quarterly* 42 (1): 35–67.

9. Gulati, R. 1995. Social structure and alliance formation patterns: A longitudinal analysis. *Administrative Science Quarterly* 40:619–52.

10. Bickman, L. 1996. Implications of a children's mental health managed care demonstration evaluation. *Journal of Mental Health Administration* 23 (1): 107–17.

11. Morrissey, J. P., M. Calloway, W. T. Bartko, M. S. Ridgely, H. H. Goldman, and R. I. Paulson. 1994. Local mental health authorities and service system change: Evidence from the Robert Wood Johnson Program on Chronic Mental Illness. *Milbank Quarterly* 72 (1): 49–80.

12. Provan, K. G., and H. B. Milward. 2001. Do networks really work? A framework for evaluating public sector organizational networks. *Public Administration Review* 61 (4): 400–409.

13. Morrissey, J. P., M. Calloway, M. Johnson, and M. Ullman. 1997. Service system performance and integration: A baseline profile of the ACCESS demonstration sites. *Psychiatric Services* 48:374–80.

14. Provan, K. G., L. Nakama, M. A. Veazie, N. I. Teufel-Shone, and C. Huddleston. 2003. Building community capacity around chronic disease services through a collaborative interorganizational network. *Health Education and Behavior* 30 (6): 646–62.

15. Safford, S. 2004. Why the Garden Club couldn't save Youngstown: Civic infrastructure and mobilization in economic crises (MIT-IPC-04-002). Cambridge, MA: Massachusetts Institute of Technology, Industrial Performance Center.

16. Owen-Smith, J., and W. W. Powell. 2004. Knowledge networks as channels and conduits: The effects of spillovers in the Boston biotechnology community. *Organization Science* 15 (1): 5–21.

17. Contractor, N., S. Wasserman, and K. Faust. 2006. Testing multitheoretical multilevel hypotheses about organizational networks: An analytic framework and empirical example. *Academy of Management Review* 31 (3): 681–703.

18. Salancik, G. R. 1995. Wanted: A good network theory of organization. Review essay. *Administrative Science Quarterly* 40 (2): 345–49.

19. Scott, J. 2000. *Social network analysis: A handbook.* 2nd ed. Thousand Oaks, CA: Sage.

20. Monge, P. R., and N. Contractor. 2003. *Theories of communication networks.* New York: Oxford Univ. Press.

21. Provan, K. G., J. M. Beyer, and C. Kruytbosch. 1980. Environmental linkages and power in resource-dependence relations between organizations. *Administrative Science Quarterly* 25 (2): 200–225.

22. Cook, K. S. 1977. Exchange and power in networks on interorganizational relations. *Sociological Quarterly* 18 (1): 62–82.

23. Olson Jr., M. 1965. *The logic of collective action: Public goods and the theory of groups.* Cambridge, MA: Harvard Univ. Press.

24. Marwell, G., and P. Oliver. 1993. *The critical mass in collective action: Toward a micro-social theory.* Cambridge: Cambridge Univ. Press.

25. Westphal, J. D., R. Gulati, and S. M. Shortell. 1997. Customization or conformity? An institutional and network perspective on the content and consequences of TQM adoption. *Administrative Science Quarterly* 42 (2): 366–94.

26. Ibarra, H. 1992. Homophily and differential returns: Sex differences in network structure and access in an advertising firm. *Administrative Science Quarterly* 37 (3): 422–47.

27. Allen, T. J. 1970. Communication networks in R&D laboratories. *R&D Management* 1 (1): 14–21.

28. Conrath, D. W. 1973. Communication environment and its relationship to organizational structure. *Management Science* 20:586–603.

29. Wellman, B. 2001. Computer networks as social networks. *Science* 293:2031–34.

30. Baum, J. A. C. 1996. Organizational ecology. In *Handbook of organization studies,* ed. S. R. Clegg, C. Hardy, and W. R. Nord, 77–114. Thousand Oaks, CA: Sage.

31. Human, S. E., and K. G. Provan. 2000. Legitimacy building in the evolution of small-firm multilateral networks: A comparative study of success and demise. *Administrative Science Quarterly* 45 (2): 327–65.

32. O'Toole Jr., L. J. 1997. Treating networks seriously: Practical and research-based agendas in public administration. *Public Administration Review* 57 (1): 45–52.

33. Agranoff, R. 2003. *Leveraging networks: A guide for public managers working across organizations.* Arlington, VA: IBM Center for The Business of Government.

34. Alter, C., and J. Hage. 1993. *Organizations working together.* Thousand Oaks, CA: Sage.

35. Moreland, R. L., and L. Argote. 2003. Transactive memory in dynamic organizations. In *Leading and managing people in the dynamic organization,* ed. R. Peterson and E. Mannix, 135–62. Mahwah, NJ: Lawrence Erlbaum.

36. Brandenburger, A. M., and B. J. Nalebuff. 1996. *Co-opetition.* New York: Currency.

37. Eisenberg, M., and N. Swanson. 1996. Organizational network analysis as a tool for program evaluation. *Evaluation and the Health Professions* 19 (4): 488–506.

38. Provan, K. G., M. A. Veazie, N. I. Teufel-Shone, and C. Huddleston. 2004. Network analysis as a tool for assessing and building community capacity for provision of chronic disease services. *Health Promotion Practice* 5 (2): 174–81.

39. Provan, K. G., M. A. Veazie, L. K. Staten, and N. I. Teufel-Shone. 2005. The use of network analysis to strengthen community partnerships. *Public Administration Review* 65 (5): 603–13.

40. Goodman, R. M., M. A. Speers, K. McLeroy, S. Fawcett, M. Kegler, E. Parker, S. R. Smith, T. D. Sterling, and N. Wallerstein. 1998. Identifying and defining the dimensions of community capacity to provide a basis for measurement. *Health Education and Behavior* 25 (3): 258–78.

41. Chaskin, R. J., P. Brown, S. Venkatesh, and A. Vidal. 2001. *Building community capacity.* New York: Aldine de Gruyter.

42. Ring, P. S., and A. H. Van de Ven. 1994. Developmental processes of cooperative interorganizational relationships. *Academy of Management Review* 19 (1): 90–118.

43. D'Aunno, T. A., and H. S. Zuckerman. 1987. A life-cycle model of organizational federations: The case of hospitals. *Academy of Management Review* 12 (3): 534–45.

44. Gulati, R., and M. Gargiulo. 1999. Where do interorganizational networks come from? *American Journal of Sociology* 104 (5): 1439–93.

45. Provan, K. G., and H. B. Milward. 1995. A preliminary theory of interorganizational network effectiveness: A comparative study of four community mental health systems. *Administrative Science Quarterly* 40 (1): 1–33.

46. Provan, K. G., K. R. Isett, and H. B. Milward. 2004. Cooperation and compromise: A network response to conflicting institutional pressures in community mental health. *Nonprofit and Voluntary Sector Quarterly* 33 (3): 489–514.

47. Knoke, D., and J. H. Kuklinski. 1982. *Network analysis.* Thousand Oaks, CA: Sage.

48. Dillman, D. A. 1978. *Mail and telephone surveys: The total design method.* New York: John Wiley and Sons.

49. Granovetter, M. 1983. The strength of weak ties: A network theory revisited. *Sociological Theory* 1:201–33.

50. Center for Tobacco Policy Research. 2005. Best practices project. St. Louis: Saint Louis Univ. School of Public Health, Center for Tobacco Policy Research. http://ctpr.slu.edu/bp.php.

51. Centers for Disease Control and Prevention. 1999. Best practices for comprehensive tobacco control programs, August 1999. Atlanta: U.S. Department of Health and Human Services, Centers for Disease Control and Prevention, National Center for Chronic Disease Prevention and Health Promotion, Office on Smoking and Health. http://www.cdc.gov/tobacco/research_data/stat_nat_data/bestprac-dwnld.htm.

52. Freeman, L. C. 1979. Centrality in networks conceptual clarification. *Social Networks* 1 (3): 215–39.

53. Cleveland, W. S. 1979. Robust locally weighted regression and smoothing scatterplots. *Journal of the American Statistical Association* 74:829–36.

54. Contractor, N. 2006. Team Engineering Collaboratory (TECLAB)/Science Of Networks In Communities (SONIC). Program description. Urbana-Champaign: Univ. of Illinois, Team Engineering Collaboratory. http://sonic.ncsa.uiuc.edu.

7

What We Know: Managing the Knowledge Content

This chapter presents a unified framework for applying knowledge management and translation (KMT) in public health areas, such as tobacco control. The approach integrates KMT in a system that considers purpose, people, process, and product. This framework then is used to examine two current examples of KMT methodology in tobacco control:

- *Review of KMT in the tobacco control efforts of the National Cancer Institute (NCI) through a formal review of knowledge management based on data gathering and personal interviews*

- *A private-sector project that used concept mapping to help a diverse group of tobacco control stakeholders to collaboratively design a knowledge-base taxonomy for tobacco control*

Knowledge is of two kinds: we know a subject ourselves, or we know where we can find information upon it.

—Samuel Johnson (1709–84)

Introduction

This chapter examines issues in the development and maintenance of KMT infrastructure for tobacco control based on previous work applying KMT to public health, related work in other areas, and a summary of two research projects. These projects include a knowledge infrastructure review of current tobacco control efforts at NCI and the use of concept mapping to help tobacco control stakeholders develop a taxonomy for a tobacco control knowledge base.

More than two centuries ago, Samuel Johnson summarized the fundamental case for knowledge management in the quotation cited here. Today, knowing where to find knowledge and sharing the knowledge that resides within ourselves form the linchpin of the ability to link the efforts of tobacco control stakeholders in a systems environment. Formal KMT methodologies represent a process by which access to this knowledge can be designed and developed both locally and globally.

To disseminate new knowledge, tobacco control researchers, like researchers in virtually every scientific field, rely on publication in peer-reviewed journals. This dissemination tactic is necessary for two reasons: (1) it ensures that the research methods and results have been reviewed by knowledgeable experts, providing some safeguard that the information is credible; and (2) publishing in refereed journals still is an integral part of the academic promotion and tenure process and so is an important part of the culture of most academic organizations. Unfortunately, journals represent an ineffective dissemination strategy at best, because in virtually every scientific field, it often is impractical to keep abreast of a growing mass of published information.

In tobacco control, because researchers come to the field from the perspectives of so many different disciplines, the literature is particularly fragmented. For example, a search for recent tobacco control citations in *New Citations*[1] yields articles in publications specializing in medicine, pharmacology, cancer, psychology, addiction, and public health, as well as a growing number of journals devoted to tobacco control. *Current Citations* is a citation resource of the Centers for Disease Control and Prevention (CDC). Resources such as this are helpful for identifying the available literature because the citations are written in the language of the discipline in which they reside. However, accessibility of these resources to all frontline practitioners is limited. Similarly, resources that are excellent first steps in translating and synthesizing evidence from the extensive literature on KMT include the Tobacco Technical Assistance Consortium;[2] CDC's *Guide to Community Preventive Services*;[3] and NCI's Cancer Control Plan, Link, Act, Network with Evidence-based Tools (PLANET).[4]

However, practitioners often need knowledge refinement, tailored programmatic tools, and information, which are not necessarily available in "prepackaged" databases. There is a need for enhancement of these existing services and of mechanisms that reward researchers for publishing in refereed journals and for disseminating research output and other knowledge to sources more available to practitioners. Similar mechanisms must be made available for researchers to tap into the experiential knowledge of frontline practitioners and the tacit knowledge of experts in other disciplines.

Today, organizations grapple with the ever-increasing and complex web of health knowledge that influences many facets of life. The first step in this effort is to differentiate between knowledge and information. Information is data such as the pattern of adult smokers in the United States. Knowledge involves interpretation of information within some context. Knowledge also includes experiences, expertise, and routines that sometimes can be expressed only through action. Therefore, understanding the significance of the pattern of adult smokers in the United States in terms of its economic and societal impacts constitutes a source of knowledge about tobacco control that can have a profound influence on the health of the nation. Knowledge is a fundamental component of how organizations function. Increasingly, organizations in pursuit of success are looking for effective ways to manage what they know.

Knowledge Management and Translation

Definition

Knowledge management has been formally defined as "the organization, creation, sharing and flow of knowledge within organizations."[5] Knowledge translation refers to the process by which knowledge is rendered usable by its end users. The first of these two definitions is quoted from *Wikipedia,* an Internet-based encyclopedia that, in and of itself, represents a good example of the evolution of knowledge management in a systems environment. In first-generation KMT solutions, people would attempt, often unsuccessfully, to create all-encompassing proprietary knowledge "systems" through means such as intranets and databases. Second-generation solutions frequently follow the core systems concepts of chaos and complexity theory. Namely, these include the adoption of simple rules that ultimately gather, maintain, and translate knowledge in forms that can be best used by those who need it. *Wikipedia* itself uses such simple rules, built around interlinked components known as "wikis"

that users can update. A stakeholder-based mechanism for review and acceptance preserves accuracy and integrity. Unlike a traditional top-down effort to create a new encyclopedia, *Wikipedia* harnesses the power of its own readers to create a knowledge base that is truly encyclopedic, but often updated within minutes after new events happen.

Within such a systems environment, knowledge management forms an integral part of a new approach to tobacco control and public health. Previous chapters in this monograph discuss the use of systems models—networks of stakeholders and adaptive organizations—to address increasingly complex issues in this field. KMT forms the "glue" that holds these components together by providing the knowledge needed for these components to function and interact.

At a practical level, KMT involves both the methodologies and infrastructure needed to use knowledge effectively. It comprises strategies, processes, and technologies for identifying, capturing, and leveraging knowledge to advance a field of study. In concert with other integrated systems approaches in tobacco control, KMT strategies can manage and disseminate knowledge ranging from evidence-based tobacco control practices to the needs and experiences of the practitioner community.

Within the cycle of planning, implementation, and evaluation (see chapter 4), KMT is central to implementation strategies as a resource for maintaining explicit knowledge that, in turn, forms an evidence base. In addition, such strategies also are intimately connected to the development of both systems and networks for tobacco control, by drawing on the large body of tacit knowledge in the form of the needs and expertise of tobacco control stakeholders. As has been demonstrated in other fields, such tacit knowledge is critical to optimizing the efforts of a widely diverse range of stakeholders.

Dimensions

Nonaka and colleagues[6] differentiate the raw data that drive the organizational knowledge infrastructure in terms of *explicit* and *tacit knowledge.* Both kinds of knowledge are created by individuals and amplified as part of the knowledge system in an organization. *Explicit knowledge* constitutes factual information that generally is contained within data. It often is precise and can be formally articulated in organizations. *Tacit knowledge* is formally defined as "knowledge that enters into the production of behaviors and/or the constitution of mental states but is not ordinarily accessible to consciousness."[7] Tacit knowledge generally is present in individuals. It is the subjective know-how in individuals and often is more difficult to express than explicit knowledge, except through action and experience.

These two kinds of knowledge frequently converge, as when both the facts of a study and the knowledge of its principal investigator are important to changing outcomes. Leveraging this knowledge is perhaps the most critical issue facing effective implementation of a KMT infrastructure to link research and practice in tobacco control so researchers and practitioners can share needs, experiences, and best practices in support of improved outcomes for tobacco control.

As a formal science, KMT methodologies have become the cornerstone of a revolution in knowledge-intensive organizational behavior. In the context of public health and specifically tobacco control, development of formal knowledge infrastructures holds the potential to integrate systems approaches such as system dynamics and network analysis as part of a broader knowledge-based framework for the linkage between research and practice. The four common types of knowledge management projects are to build knowledge repositories, improve knowledge access and use, enhance the underlying knowledge

environment, and manage knowledge as an asset. In a review of corporate knowledge-management projects across 24 companies, Davenport and colleagues[8] summarize eight key success factors behind these systems:

1. Linkage to economic performance and industry value

2. Existing technical and organizational infrastructure

3. Standard but flexible form of knowledge structure

4. Knowledge-friendly culture

5. Clear purpose and language among staff

6. Change in motivational practices

7. Multiple channels of knowledge transfer

8. Senior management support

Replicating these success factors from the private sector to public health involves numerous challenges. These include coordination of KMT efforts across multiple organizations with different cultures, the need to develop a consistent and universally accepted knowledge infrastructure, and budgetary constraints. At the same time, such a knowledge infrastructure has the promise to form a cornerstone for evidence-based decision making in public health and for linking research to practice and practice to research. Moreover, the current state of tobacco control, with its multiple stakeholder organizations operating in an environment of declining financial resources, can particularly benefit from a consistent and successful knowledge infrastructure.

As part of research on the application of managing knowledge content from multiple stakeholders in the public health system, a metalevel framework is envisioned that applies knowledge management and knowledge translation concepts and strategies to the health policy, evidence, experience, and contact base in the field (figure 7.1).

Knowledge Management Concepts

Lau[9] outlines a conceptual framework for knowledge management that comprises a set of knowledge management concepts for the health setting, revolving around the production, use, and refinement of both explicit and tacit knowledge in an underlying social context. The types of knowledge addressed include clinical and administrative policy, research evidence, practice experience, and resource contact that are considered critical and relevant to specific settings. An overview of this framework, as shown in figure 7.2,

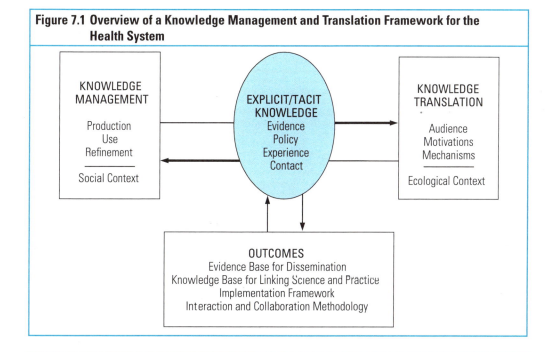

Figure 7.1 Overview of a Knowledge Management and Translation Framework for the Health System

---

Benefits of Knowledge Infrastructure for Tobacco Control

For tobacco control, potential outcomes of a consistent knowledge infrastructure include

- *Evidence base for effective dissemination,* which serves as a repository for evidence-based practices in tobacco control, potentially in much the same way the Cochrane Collaboration[a] provides the medical profession with an accessible meta-analysis of evidence-based medical research
- *Knowledge base for linking science and practice* so stakeholders in both communities can share needs and approaches
- *Implementation framework* for policy changes and consensus practices in tobacco control
- *Interaction and collaboration methodology,* which links large, geographically and politically diverse groups of tobacco control stakeholders in a cycle of planning, implementation, and evaluation for ongoing tobacco control efforts

[a]Cochrane Library. 2003. http://www.cochrane.org.

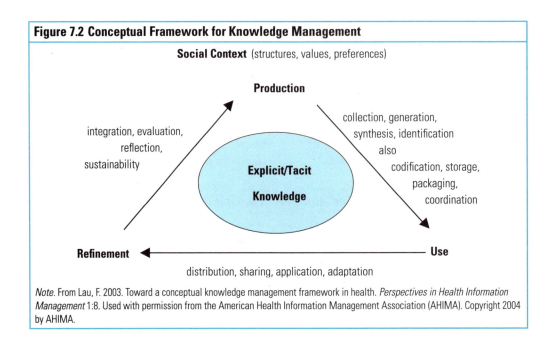

Figure 7.2 Conceptual Framework for Knowledge Management

Social Context (structures, values, preferences)

Production

integration, evaluation, reflection, sustainability

collection, generation, synthesis, identification also codification, storage, packaging, coordination

Explicit/Tacit Knowledge

Refinement ← Use

distribution, sharing, application, adaptation

Note. From Lau, F. 2003. Toward a conceptual knowledge management framework in health. *Perspectives in Health Information Management* 1:8. Used with permission from the American Health Information Management Association (AHIMA). Copyright 2004 by AHIMA.

involves three key components: knowledge production, use, and refinement.

Knowledge production is the process of creating and organizing policy, evidence, experience, and contacts. In a health care context, sources of this knowledge include policy syntheses, research findings, local practices, and resource contacts. The phase of knowledge production includes collection of local experience, such as organizational practice norms and values, generation of new knowledge from primary research (e.g., randomized trial or case study), synthesis of research findings, policy advice and local experience through a critical review process, and identification of individual or organizational resource contacts willing to share their knowledge.

As knowledge is created, a formal process is needed to organize this knowledge as artifacts or intellectual resources. This process involves codification of knowledge by using the appropriate nomenclature; computer-based storage for later retrieval and maintenance; packaging with appropriate content details and delivery

modalities; and coordination of intellectual resource contacts on such details as expertise, experience, locations, and availability.

Knowledge use refers to the manner in which stakeholders use explicit and tacit knowledge in a local setting. In a tobacco control environment, these stakeholders can span a broad range of roles, including researchers, advocates, practitioners, leaders, and legislators. The types of knowledge they use can range from specific research results to linkage with other stakeholders and their expertise. Factors in knowledge use include distribution to targeted audiences through channels such as print and online media; sharing through interpersonal communication; application in a local setting in policy or practice; and adaptation to the values, cultures, and norms of the local environment.

Knowledge refinement refers to ways knowledge sources are institutionalized within organizations over time as part of routine, accepted practices. Knowledge refinement is an ongoing process of managing the information that is extant in the knowledge base. Factors in knowledge refinement include integration with existing work processes and practice norms; evaluation by using measures (e.g., quality, use, and impact); reflection on the knowledge source through subjective interpretations by stakeholders; and ongoing sustainability of the knowledge management approach.

All three of these factors exist within a larger *social context* affecting how the overall stakeholder group—including policy makers, practitioners, researchers, and the public—interacts with knowledge. This social context encompasses the social structures (e.g., organizations, rules, and processes) in which these stakeholders operate; values guiding beliefs and actions; and preferences on a wide range of health issues, based on belief systems and needs. This context creates a unique environment for knowledge management that is difficult to replicate outside of it.

Knowledge Translation Concepts

Knowledge management focuses on the systematic process of producing, using, and refining explicit and tacit knowledge in and across organizations. Knowledge translation is concerned with the dynamics necessary to convert explicit knowledge to tacit knowledge and vice versa across individual, group, organizational, and societal levels. The proposed framework for translation comprises members of the audience, their motivations, and the different mechanisms for the ongoing conversion of tacit and explicit knowledge within an underlying ecological context. An overview of this framework, as shown in figure 7.3, involves three key components: an audience, motivations, and mechanisms.

The audience consists of stakeholders, such as policy makers who make legal, financial, or administrative decisions; practitioners

who assist in clinical decisions for clients and families; researchers involved in scientific inquiries to generate new health knowledge; and others ranging from advocates, activists, and legislators to the general public. An important dynamic that determines the success of any effort at knowledge translation is the ability to distinguish among the types of audiences involved. Different audiences have different knowledge needs that must be recognized when translating the policy, evidence, experience, or contact to address a particular issue.

Motivations for knowledge translation depend on the specific audience. Motivations may include decision making for clinical, administrative, or legislative issues; education to improve knowledge and performance; innovation to generate new knowledge; or advocacy to influence the actions of others.

Mechanisms that translate explicit and tacit knowledge into usable forms of health policy, evidence, experience, and/or personal contact include a combination of different forms of explicit knowledge to add value, articulation of tacit knowledge in print or electronic form, internalization of explicit knowledge as intellectual capability, and sharing of tacit knowledge with others through socialization.

This environment for knowledge translation exists in an *ecological context* that views the health system as an ecosystem with interrelated components interacting with each other at different levels over time, in a complex and unpredictable manner.[10] The quality and effect of these interactions are contingent on different situational contexts. These include the organizational context in the health care environment; the cultural context that encompasses values, beliefs, and norms; the political–legal context such as legislation, mandates, and privacy issues; and the surrounding media environment for communication and interaction.

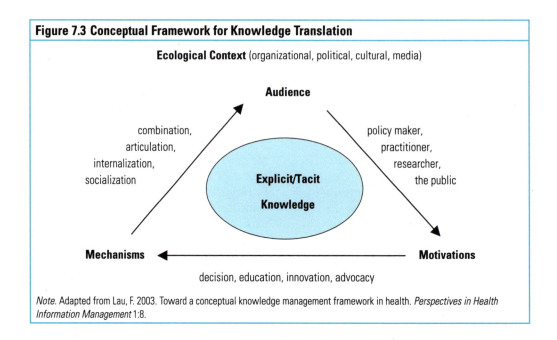

Figure 7.3 Conceptual Framework for Knowledge Translation

Ecological Context (organizational, political, cultural, media)

Audience

combination,
articulation,
internalization,
socialization

Explicit/Tacit Knowledge

policy maker,
practitioner,
researcher,
the public

Mechanisms

Motivations

decision, education, innovation, advocacy

Note. Adapted from Lau, F. 2003. Toward a conceptual knowledge management framework in health. *Perspectives in Health Information Management* 1:8.

Integration of Knowledge Management and Translation

Effective management of the content of explicit and tacit knowledge requires consideration of all of the concepts described in the frameworks for knowledge management and knowledge translation. Although the two frameworks address different aspects of managing and translating knowledge, they are complementary in nature and should be considered in synchrony for maximal effects. Therefore, in producing, using, and refining tobacco control knowledge such as policy, evidence, experience, and contact in and across organizations, one should also take into account members of the intended audience, their respective motivations, and the mechanisms available for translating such knowledge, within the underlying social and ecological contexts. Table 7.1 summarizes specific considerations for each aspect of the integrated KMT concepts.

As table 7.1 implies, the integration of knowledge management and knowledge

translation has specific ramifications for the processes of knowledge production, use, and refinement to address specific audiences and their motivations. *Knowledge production* requires consideration of factors related to generating knowledge for effective translation. These factors include the following:

- Collection of local experience in such a way that stakeholders articulate it from a tacit to explicit form

- Generation of new knowledge by articulating tacit knowledge from research findings into published form

- Synthesis of this knowledge in forms such as systematic reviews

- Identification of intellectual resources as sources of tacit knowledge

Once generated, the knowledge should be organized by methods that facilitate effective translation. This process encompasses the codification of collected experience, evidence, and other resources into explicit knowledge in the following steps:

Table 7.1 Integrated Concepts of Knowledge Management and Translation

Concept	Audience	Motivations	Mechanisms
Production	Who generates and/or organizes the knowledge and whom is it for?	What are the motivations for creating and organizing the knowledge?	What translation mechanisms should be included when creating and organizing the knowledge?
Use	Who uses the knowledge?	What are the motivations for using the knowledge?	What translation mechanisms should be included when using the knowledge?
Refinement	Who refines the knowledge and whom is it for?	What are the motivations for refining the knowledge?	What translation mechanisms should be included when refining the knowledge?

- Use accepted vocabularies such as that of the *International Classification of Diseases* (10th revision)[11] and Health Level 7[12] (an exchange standard for clinical data)

- Code this knowledge into online repositories

- Package it in a variety of content, media, and delivery formats

- Coordinate intellectual resource contacts within this knowledge base to enhance their availability as sources of tacit knowledge

Knowledge use through translation should take place in contexts that are relevant to different audiences and their motivations. This context must influence factors such as the distribution of explicit knowledge in appropriate forms and the sharing of tacit knowledge through socialization. The presentation should be tailored to different audiences. The application and/or adaptation of explicit or tacit knowledge must be oriented to local settings.

Knowledge refinement involves formulating a presentation of concepts that is geared to specific audiences and their motivations. This process requires integration of new knowledge with existing knowledge by socializing new knowledge in tacit form; internalizing new explicit knowledge into tacit knowledge; and conversely, articulating new knowledge from tacit to explicit form. The process also entails evaluation of the impact of this knowledge by articulating tacit experience into a quantifiable explicit form, reflection of the experience of using this knowledge, and assessment of the sustainability of the KMT effort.

The common thread running through each of these issues is the need to develop a consistent approach for KMT that encompasses the unique needs and motivations of each of the stakeholder audiences, such as policy makers, practitioners, and researchers. Moreover, as discussed later in this chapter, these issues point to the need to integrate knowledge management strategies for health care environments within the broader area of systems thinking—for example, the use of systems approaches involving adaptive behavior and feedback to address complex issues. Accomplishment of this integration requires the following procedures:

- Infusing the collection of explicit knowledge into research and practice experience

- Leveraging the use and maintenance of networks as a source of tacit knowledge

- Using this knowledge in a framework of systems-level planning, implementation, and outcomes evaluation

- Creating an integrated framework for leveraging knowledge within the broader public health system

Framework for Strategy of Knowledge Management and Translation

The concepts described under the knowledge management and knowledge translation frameworks provide a rich taxonomy and models of understanding that can be used to devise specific strategies and actions for implementation. Three broad strategies are envisioned to manage the complex knowledge content that spans multiple stakeholder organizations, as is the case for tobacco control: (1) the 4Ps (purpose, people, process, and product) of KMT; (2) the underlying KMT infrastructures; and (3) the KMT strategy maps. Figure 7.4 shows this KMT strategy framework.

Four Ps of Knowledge Management and Translation

The 4Ps of KMT refer to the four aspects of KMT that should be leveraged as an essential part of an integrated KMT strategy—purpose, people, process, and product. These 4Ps provide the necessary focus and means to implement an effective knowledge infrastructure in and across organizations.

Purpose

Management of complex knowledge content, such as tobacco control policy, practice, and experience that span multiple stakeholder organizations or audiences, requires a shared understanding of the overall mandate, vision, goals, and objectives, even though they are high level, abstract, and evolving. Such a mental model can serve as

a road map from which concrete plans can be developed and implemented. This purpose encompasses four key actionable items:

- *Agendas* are needed that are specific to individual audiences, such as the research agenda, the political agenda, and the public's agenda, in the case of tobacco control. The intent is to ensure that *everyone knows who should do what*.

- *Relevance* ensures that the coordinated agendas fit the mandate, goals, and activities of the stakeholder organizations. The intent is to ensure that *everyone knows that who should do what is relevant*.

- *Timelines* provide an overall schedule to implement coordinated agendas for stakeholder organizations according to priority, need, and the availability of resources. The intent is to ensure that *everyone knows that who should do what is relevant when*.

- *A business case* with well-articulated justifications for proceeding is essential for successful implementation of KMT. The intent is to ensure that *everyone knows that who should do what is relevant and justified when*.

People

Even with the best-coordinated agendas, nothing will happen unless the appropriate human resources are in place to implement these plans. Within the complex public health system, an effective KMT infrastructure that spans different stakeholder organizations requires the ongoing engagement of specific types of people, including the following:

- Knowledge champions are leaders who are respected in the field or have positional power to lead, lobby, or advocate for specific causes, expecting others to follow or comply with their actions. Their presence and actions are

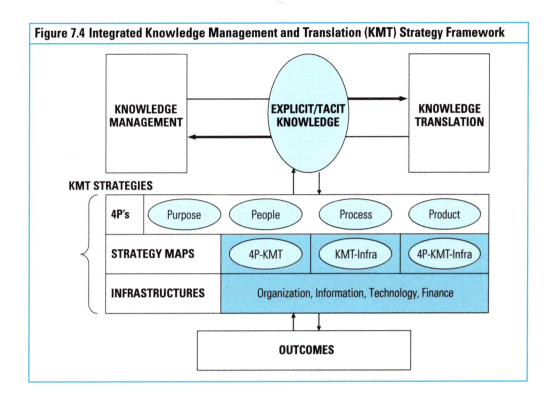

Figure 7.4 Integrated Knowledge Management and Translation (KMT) Strategy Framework

crucial in introducing change in and across organizations because of their stature and conviction.

- *Knowledge brokers/managers* work as intermediaries to translate the knowledge required by different audiences according to their specific motivations. They are knowledgeable in KMT methodologies and are responsible for translating knowledge such as health policy, evidence, experience, and contact into tailored content, media, and formats that are relevant to local practice.

- *Knowledge architects* are responsible for the planning, design, implementation, and support of KMT systems in organizations or groups. Knowledge architects usually are trained in KMT and are responsible for the strategic, financial, technical, and organizational aspects of the knowledge infrastructures.

- Communities of practice are individuals and groups in and across organizations

that share common agendas and work practices. They provide the critical mass needed to collectively produce, use, and refine health policy, evidence, experience, and contact in ways that fit the specific motivations of different audiences.

Process

Process is made up of the activities that enable people in and across stakeholder organizations to work collectively on the coordinated KMT agendas. Key processes that form part of the KMT strategy and infrastructure include the following:

- *Consensus building* enables stakeholders to identify and negotiate a diverse set of issues or options to reach agreement on key issues or solutions.

- *Capacity building* enables stakeholders to develop local and practical expertise to address a specific health area or issue.

- *Knowledge development* enables stakeholders to engage in specific KMT activities related to health issues.

- *Network development* enables stakeholders across organizations to collectively engage in KMT activities.

Products

Products serve as the tools that enable people to work collectively on coordinated agendas through specific KMT processes. Representative tools that form part of the KMT strategy and infrastructure include groupware, knowledge repositories, tools for knowledge development, and tools for knowledge access, as follows:

- *Groupware* includes software tools for communication, coordination, and collaboration, which allow individuals, groups, and organizations to work together electronically and virtually on specific KMT activities.

- *Knowledge repositories* usually are interactive knowledge bases accessible through the Internet that contain a wide range of health knowledge content in various media and delivery formats.

- *Knowledge development tools* are software tools for generation and organization of knowledge content.

- *Knowledge navigation/access tools* are software tools used by audiences to retrieve specific knowledge content from knowledge repositories according to specific motivations.

The 4Ps provide a framework for implementation of a KMT strategy. Moreover, their components form an important part of the planning checklist for such an implementation. In a public health setting such as tobacco control, these factors also ensure that the unique needs of individual stakeholder groups are addressed as an integral part of the design and implementation effort.

Underlying Infrastructures

The 4Ps provide the focus and means to implement KMT in and across organizations. However, the underlying KMT infrastructures provide the necessary foundations on which the 4P-KMT strategy can be deployed. Key aspects of the KMT infrastructures include the following:

- *Organization infrastructure* refers to the structures, procedures, and norms by which organizations can work collectively to manage and translate knowledge. The components include the sites of explicit and tacit knowledge resources in and across organizations; the procedures behind knowledge-related tasks; and the cultural norms and customs of stakeholder organizations.

- *Technology infrastructure* refers to the information technology capacity and tools with which organizations deploy the knowledge infrastructure, including software applications, computer networks, telecommunications, and Internet connectivity.

- *Information infrastructure* refers to the underlying electronic databases, library resources, and data definitions and taxonomies available in and across organizations as input into the knowledge infrastructure.

- *Financial infrastructure* encompasses the mechanisms used to define and measure the value of knowledge infrastructures. These mechanisms include the investment portfolios that finance the human and physical resources required, intellectual assets representing the value of knowledge resources, and the return-on-investment measures of this value relative to the original investment.

These components serve to illustrate the larger point that a KMT infrastructure encompasses an integration between computer and database technology and the surrounding organizational environment. This point underscores the concept that the KMT infrastructure cannot be purely approached as a computing issue. Instead, it should be seen in the context of the larger goals of affected stakeholder organizations.

4P-Knowledge Management and Translation Strategy Maps

KMT strategy maps provide detailed mapping of the actionable items under the 4P and infrastructure strategies to achieve the desirable outcomes. These strategy maps are intended to offer guidance in planning and implementing a knowledge infrastructure. Three KMT strategy maps are described here: 4P-KMT, KMT infrastructures, and 4P-KMT infrastructures.

4P-Knowledge Management and Translation Strategy Map

The 4P-KMT map is focused on the actionable items under the 4P strategy for KMT in and across organizations. For example, with respect to purpose, one needs to define the relevant agendas, the timelines, and the business case with regard to who should produce, use, and refine the knowledge, based on members of the audience, their motivations, and translation mechanisms. At the same time, the local social and ecological contexts must be considered. Table 7.2 shows the 4P-KMT strategy map.

Strategy Map for Knowledge Management and Translation Infrastructure

The strategy map for KMT infrastructures focuses on the actionable items under the KMT infrastructure strategy in and across organizations. For example, with respect to organization infrastructure, one needs to establish the appropriate structure, procedures, and norms for the production, use, and refinement of knowledge. This process must take into account members of the audience, their motivations, and different translation mechanisms, as well as the local social and ecological contexts, such as affected stakeholder groups and their interaction with the broader health care system. Table 7.3 shows this strategy map.

Strategy and Outcome Map for 4P-Knowledge Management and Translation Infrastructures

The strategy and outcome maps for 4P-KMT infrastructures focus on the actionable items under the 4P strategy, taking into account issues related to the underlying KMT infrastructure and the desired outcomes. The purpose is to establish a comprehensive infrastructure for KMT. This strategy map (figure 7.5) can be used as a framework to expand its actionable items into a more detailed strategy map for each type of knowledge involved, which in turn can be expanded into detailed checklists for final planning and implementation. (For more details on 4P-KMT infrastructures, see appendix 7A.)

Case Study: Knowledge Management in Tobacco Control

An illustrative case study of the current role of KMT in tobacco control efforts is presented here. A series of discussion meetings with key informants were conducted in June and July 2004 to examine KMT in the domain of tobacco control, as part of a substantive study of large-scale

Table 7.2   4P-Knowledge Management and Translation Strategy Map

	Production	Use	Refinement
Purpose	Define relevant agendas, timelines, and business case; and decide who should produce what knowledge	Define relevant agendas, timelines, and business case, and decide who should use what knowledge	Define relevant agendas, timelines, and business case, and decide who should refine what knowledge
People	Identify champions, brokers, managers, and communities of practice to produce knowledge	Identify champions, brokers, managers, and communities of practice to use knowledge	Identify champions, brokers, managers, and communities of practice to refine knowledge
Process	Incorporate consensus building and knowledge-development process to produce knowledge	Incorporate consensus building and knowledge-development process to use knowledge	Incorporate consensus building and knowledge-development process to refine knowledge
Products	Produce knowledge through groupware, knowledge development, and repository and access tools	Use knowledge through groupware, knowledge development, and repository and access tools	Refine knowledge through groupware, knowledge development, and repository and access tools

Note. Each 4P-knowledge management and translation strategy is specifically based on the audience, motivations, and different translations in social and ecological contexts.

Table 7.3   Strategy Map for Knowledge Management and Translation Infrastructure

	Production	Use	Refinement
Organization	Establish structures, procedures, and norms for producing knowledge	Establish structures, procedures, and norms for using knowledge	Establish structures, procedures, and norms for refining knowledge
Technology	Establish applications, networks, and connectivity for producing knowledge	Establish applications, networks, and connectivity for using knowledge	Establish applications, networks, and connectivity for refining knowledge
Information	Develop internal and external databases and information resources needed for producing knowledge	Develop internal and external databases and information resources needed for using knowledge	Develop internal and external databases and information resources needed for refining knowledge
Finance	Establish investment portfolios, intellectual assets, and return on investment for producing knowledge	Establish investment portfolios, intellectual assets, and return on investment for using knowledge	Establish investment portfolios, intellectual assets, and return on investment for refining knowledge

Note. Each 4P-knowledge management and translation strategy is specifically based on the audience, motivations, and different translations in social and ecological contexts.

change in health systems. The scope of these discussions was focused mainly on the recent Cancer Control PLANET[4] initiative and several related Web-based knowledge resources outlined here, including the Cancer Biomedical Informatics Grid (caBIG)[13] and the Cancer Intervention and Surveillance Modeling Network (CISNET).[14] These efforts provide real-life case illustrations of the current state of the KMT infrastructure that is emerging within the field and the challenges involved.

Key informants identified by the study team were invited to discussion meetings in person or by telephone to share their thoughts about KMT by using tobacco control or related areas as the domain. (See appendix 7B for discussion questions.) These key informants were researchers, policy makers, information-

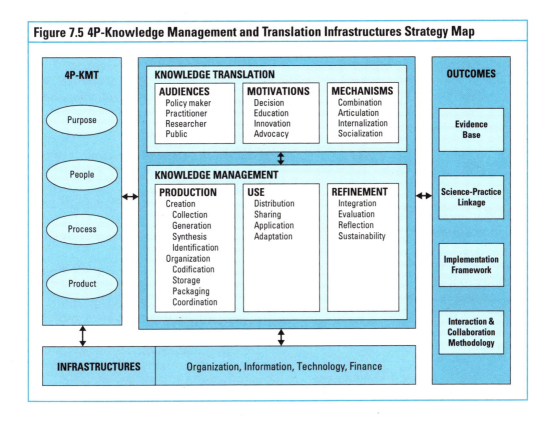

Figure 7.5 4P-Knowledge Management and Translation Infrastructures Strategy Map

management professionals, community-based practitioners, and advocates involved with tobacco control and/or cancer control from NCI and selected partner organizations such as CDC and the Campaign for Tobacco-Free Kids. NCI was chosen as a focus organization because of its central role in funding and developing an infrastructure for tobacco control efforts and its key support for the Initiative on the Study and Implementation of Systems (ISIS). Definitions related to KMT (appendix 7A) were provided before the meetings to familiarize informants with KMT terms. The team also reviewed information on these initiatives that NCI published on its Web site. The purpose of this review was to facilitate an understanding of the nature of the KMT efforts, especially in the area of tobacco control.

Chapter findings are organized around the types of tobacco control and related knowledge needed and those currently managed, how such KMT efforts can be viewed as part of an emerging KMT infrastructure, and suggested ways to advance this infrastructure to better meet the ongoing challenges in tobacco control.

Tobacco Control and Related Knowledge

At the discussion meetings, different types of tobacco and cancer control knowledge resources were reviewed with key informants from NCI and partner organizations. These resources included Cancer Control PLANET[4] as an example of an evolving Web-based knowledge repository, as well as the Surveillance, Epidemiology, and End Results (SEER)[15] registry program, CISNET,[14] and audience segmentation tools such as the Consumer Health Profiles (CHP),[16] as related knowledge resources that can be leveraged in tobacco control as part of the KMT efforts. Key aspects of the newly established caBIG were presented to illustrate an evolving collaborative knowledge network that may be considered for the tobacco control domain. In addition, information was presented on the problem of missing, incomplete, or conflicting knowledge for some aspects of tobacco control, especially at the systems level. Related KMT efforts and needs are described here.

Cancer Control PLANET and Tobacco Control

Cancer Control PLANET[4] is a Web portal for cancer control launched in April 2003 and developed over two years as a collaborative effort among key government and nongovernment agencies, including the following:

- *National Cancer Institute:* An agency of the U.S. Department of Health and Human Services (DHHS) that serves as the federal government's principal agency devoting resources to scientific research on cancer; also the coordinating agency for PLANET.

- *Centers for Disease Control and Prevention:* A DHHS agency focused on control and prevention of disease, injury, and disability. The Division of Cancer Prevention and Control of the National Center for Chronic Disease Prevention and Health Promotion is the lead CDC agency in the area of tobacco control.

- *American Cancer Society:* A nationwide nongovernmental organization dedicated to cancer prevention and treatment.

- *Substance Abuse and Mental Health Services Administration:* A federal agency involved with issues of substance abuse and mental health that provided the review of tobacco control programs for PLANET.

- *Agency for Healthcare Research and Quality:* A DHHS agency dedicated to

improvement of the quality of health care. This agency supports the U.S. Preventive Services Task Force, which develops recommendations on effective clinical preventive interventions such as screening, counseling, and medication regimens.

- *American College of Surgeons Commission on Cancer:* A professional organization that joined as a PLANET partner in 2006 to help promote evidence-based comprehensive cancer control through its state-based liaison physician program.

PLANET's Web portal provides profile data on cancer nationally and by county and state, risk factor data by state, and resource information to assist program planners, educators, and researchers in the design, implementation, and evaluation of evidence-based cancer control programs. Users of the portal are assisted in "assessing the profile and risks of cancer within a state, identifying potential partner organizations already working with high-risk populations, understanding current research findings and recommendations, accessing evidence-based programs and products, and finding guidelines for planning and evaluation."[4] As part of this Web portal, PLANET provides detailed step-by-step instructions for its audience to establish a comprehensive cancer control program in the local setting.

The portal also covers a wide range of cancer-related topics, including information on specific cancers (e.g., breast cancer), diet, nutrition, physical activity, tobacco control, and sun exposure safety. In the tobacco control domain, the same five-step approach to cancer control planning is used. The user audience can assess local program priorities based on state cancer profiles and risks for current smokers; identify local program and research partners involved in work related to cancer and tobacco control; determine the effectiveness of different tobacco control interventions; access research-tested tobacco control programs and products; and plan and/or evaluate a local tobacco control program. Key aspects of this tobacco control portal that illustrate the KMT efforts are highlighted here.

- *State cancer profiles and risk factor data on current smokers* are available from sources such as the SEER registry program, the National Program of Cancer Registries, the Behavioral Risk Factor Surveillance System, and the Current Population Survey Tobacco Use Supplement. The types of information that can be obtained cover such areas as the prevalence of cancer for specific sites, incidence, mortality, and survival statistics, as well as smoking patterns and targets for smoking cessation in different population segments at the national and state levels and sometimes at the regional level. Coupled with additional statistics on local tobacco control policies and experiences, such knowledge resources can be used in planning specific tobacco control initiatives and evaluating their effectiveness based on local priorities and needs.

- *Potential partners* can be identified through up-to-date directories listing regional tobacco control programs and information on contacting researchers. The organizations listed in the program directory include the American Cancer Society, the CDC Tobacco Control Network, and NCI's Cancer Information Service, which makes available regional representatives to provide coordination and support in local tobacco control initiatives. The researchers are potential partners who already are involved with tobacco control research in academic institutions, research foundations, or medical centers in different regions of the United States. These contacts provide the expertise and resources

needed to plan, implement, and evaluate specific tobacco control initiatives at the local level.

- *Effective research-based tobacco control intervention strategies* include current systematic reviews and recommendations, available electronically via the Web from such sources as the *Guide to Community Preventive Services,* the *Clinical Guide to Tobacco Use Counseling,* and the *Clinical Practice Guideline on Tobacco Cessation.* These evidence-based knowledge resources are distributed by reputable groups including the Community Preventive Services Task Force, the U.S. Preventive Service Task Force, the Public Health Service, the Agency for Healthcare Research and Quality, CDC, and NCI.

- *Research-tested tobacco control programs and products* are appraised for quality and made available to the audience according to their specific needs. NCI and the Substance Abuse and Mental Health Services Administration conduct ongoing peer reviews of scientifically tested tobacco control programs and products published by researchers for adoption by others. These knowledge resources can be downloaded at no cost and modified for local implementation by following specific guidelines for program adaptation. The adaptation includes determining the needs of the audience, working with expert advisors to maintain the integrity of the original program, pilot testing the modified program, and evaluating the implemented program for its effectiveness.

- *Planning and evaluation of local tobacco control programs* can be accomplished by using the comprehensive cancer control planning framework from CDC. This planning framework outlines a specific set of objectives, planning activities, and outcomes that should be addressed to successfully implement a cancer control initiative such as a local tobacco control program. The processes outlined in the framework are based on actual experiences from several states that undertook comprehensive cancer control planning in recent years.

The design and implementation of PLANET as a dynamic knowledge repository have been an ongoing iterative process, with a great deal of effort spent on ensuring that it provides up-to-date knowledge resources, translated in ways that are usable to a wide range of audiences. An online "train-the-trainer" course also is available on PLANET, based on a 3.5-hour course delivered around the country through Comprehensive Cancer Control Leadership Institutes, to increase the uptake of PLANET in the field. When the site is accessed, limited information automatically is collected. The information includes the name of the domain and the Internet address of the provider, the Web site, and the computer used; the date and time of the visit; and the pages visited. Because of privacy concerns, it is not feasible to monitor how the audience actually uses the knowledge resources through the site, such as which products were downloaded from the Research-Tested Intervention Programs. A more formal evaluation on the effectiveness of PLANET will be conducted through a follow-up survey of those who have completed the 3.5-hour in-person training. Other issues on enhancing the adoption and use of PLANET in tobacco control include the following:

- Finding ways to encourage successful champions to take the evidence on what works in tobacco control and make it theirs as part of the knowledge transfer process

- Developing a version of PLANET for clinicians, with additional features such as real-time delivery of evidence at the point of patient contact, with concise

one-page fact sheets by topic area, to help them incorporate the available evidence as their choice of interventions in practice

- Translating the instruments used by researchers to simple program evaluation tools and sharing their experiences with the appropriate audience to encourage the adoption of evidence as part of practice norms

Surveillance, Epidemiology, and End Results Registry

The SEER program of cancer registries[15] is a broad information source on cancer incidence and survival in the United States. When used in conjunction with its companion suite of analytic tools, SEER can be a valuable knowledge resource for statistics on cancer. Available statistics include the following:

- Cancer survival based on follow-up of cancer cases over time, measured in a number of different ways depending on intended purpose

- Probabilities of developing or dying from cancer

- Statistics that pool data from different sources to analyze cancer patterns and trends in particular segments of the population

The SEER program is an important knowledge resource for tobacco control, with its extensive repository of statistical evidence indicating that smoking is a major cause of many cancers.

Cancer Intervention Surveillance Network

CISNET[14] is a community of NCI-sponsored researchers who use modeling to improve understanding of the impact of cancer control interventions (i.e., prevention, screening, treatment) on population trends in incidence and mortality. These models are also used to project future trends and to help determine optimal cancer control strategies. When possible, comparative modeling projects are undertaken to answer important cancer control questions using an agreed upon set of common model inputs and outputs. CISNET's interactive, Web-based software for profiling models enables researchers to document components of their models in predefined templates. The synthesis of these disparate models into a common format enables comparison of model structures, tracking of model versions, searching of model components, and replication of the model and results by others. The design of CISNET has been an iterative process, ensuring that the tools developed are meaningful and useful to the research community. CISNET can be a valuable knowledge resource for tobacco control in terms of access to modeling expertise in predicting the effects of tobacco control interventions in cancer. One example is Levy's recent simulation study[17] of the effects of tobacco policy on lung cancer in the population. The findings provide insights on (1) the effects of tobacco policies on the number of deaths attributed to smoking, (2) whether new tobacco products and related products may reduce risk of cancer, and (3) finding ways to coordinate tobacco control policies with improved detection and treatment of lung cancer.

Consumer Health Profiles

Being able to narrow audiences based on more than demographic characteristics is a critical component of social marketing approaches. Audience segmentation systems rely on a combination of demographic and lifestyle data to define lifestyle groups and provide insights into how to market to them. Systems such as these are used extensively in consumer marketing and have been applied to social marketing campaigns since the mid-1990s.

NCI has developed CHP,[16] a tool to support the use of audience segmentation information by health education program planners and implementers. The profiles in CHP are summaries of the demographics, health care attitudes, behaviors, media habits, and lifestyle characteristics of consumers in selected "lifestyle clusters." These profiles also outline suggested strategies for reaching these audiences with health information and behavioral interventions. Organizations can use these profiles along with maps and reports as a planning aid to identify and target underserved or at-risk populations most in need of cancer education and outreach programs. Used in conjunction with other resources such as the State Cancer Legislative Database,[18] NCI's *Making Health Communications Programs Work: A Planner's Guide* (also known as the Pink Book),[19] CDCynergy,[20] and PLANET, CHP can be a valuable resource for knowledge about tobacco control. These resources can be helpful in developing intervention programs for tobacco control by using approaches such as social marketing to increase reach and efficacy in specific population segments (e.g., female teenage smokers).

The knowledge resources described here are illustrations of KMT efforts that NCI has undertaken over the last few years in cancer and tobacco control to produce, use, and refine explicit and tacit knowledge for a specific audience. Resources such as PLANET, SEER, and CHP can help stakeholders understand the patterns and effects of smoking and can reveal which tobacco control interventions are effective. In addition, the CISNET initiative can foster interactions and collaboration across different groups of stakeholders, encouraging them to work collectively toward a common set of agendas for tobacco control.

Cancer Biomedical Informatics Grid: Evolving Knowledge Network

Launched by NCI in February 2004, caBIG[13] is a collaborative initiative to build an integrated biomedical informatics infrastructure for sharing data, tools, and expertise. Nearly 900 individuals from more than 50 cancer centers and 30 other organizations across the United States were participating by the end of 2006. The overall aim of caBIG is to create a virtual community of researchers to expedite cancer research through the development of a set of common vocabularies and data elements, with standards-based software applications and technology platforms. It is expected that the researchers and organizations that make up this community will be able to easily share the resulting data, tools, and infrastructures. In addition, caBIG tools and infrastructure are freely available to all and are widely applicable beyond cancer.

Members of this virtual community have been working to define the agenda, projects, and priorities for this initiative. Activities of caBIG are organized into "workspaces," each addressing a specific area of need identified by the community. The two types of workspaces are domain specific and crosscutting. Overall strategic planning and management and two types of working groups have been established to coordinate specific pilot projects within the workspaces. An online knowledge repository has been created as an inventory to store the data, application, and infrastructure artifacts and documentation generated to support various caBIG projects. NCI provides financial support for members to take part in these working groups and to work on specific projects. Current projects under the two workspaces are briefly described here.

Clinical trial management systems deploy existing and develop new information, applications, processes, services, and infrastructures used to support the design, implementation, and administration of clinical trials. Examples include (1) the caBIG clinical protocols portal, a Web-based application that enables researchers to share protocols; and (2) the C3D, a remote application that captures data for conducting clinical trials by using standardized vocabularies and common data elements.

In vivo imaging focuses on identifying the ways in which the wealth of information provided by such imaging, performed at academic and other research centers across the country, can be shared, optimized, and most effectively integrated. The in vivo imaging technologies and modalities addressed include systems for research and clinical imaging of live patients and animals (including single-cell organisms) used as model systems for human disease.

Integrative cancer research tools are being developed and deployed to enable integration and sharing of basic and clinical cancer research data among researchers at different centers. These include tools used to support research on pathway mapping, proteomics, microarrays, and gene expression. In addition, raw data can be shared across platforms and organizations.

Tissue banks and pathology tools are being developed and deployed to enable the integration and sharing of information from repositories of cancer specimens from cancer research centers. These include tools that can enhance identification of tissue banks and access to research samples. They can also leverage existing sample-tracking systems and management systems for pathology information, providing additional support for decision making and analytic capabilities.

Vocabularies and common data elements refer to the development of cancer ontology content and standardization of clinical terms used in cancer research. Examples include the NCI National Cancer Data Standards Repository and the Common Data Elements development and harmonization program. Because these activities and resources are part of the crosscutting workspace, it is expected that the outputs will be shared among other working groups and their projects under the domain workspace.

The architecture workspace is involved in developing architectural policies and standards based on the open-source environment principles. Its purpose is to ensure consistent application of these principles across groups in the caBIG community and to achieve seamless integration and sharing of the knowledge resources in cancer research.

In 2006, caBIG added a new special interest group focusing on population science. Its work includes analyzing key opportunities for and barriers to using informatics to strengthen population science, including data sharing and intellectual property issues, interoperability issues, and specific tools to enable population research (such as tools for generating standardized questionnaires).

An evolving informatics infrastructure, caBIG connects researchers and organizations in cancer and biomedical research to accelerate the pace at which their activities can be conducted in a coordinated and collaborative manner. Although its current emphasis is on the cancer and biomedical research community, the philosophy, objectives, framework, and process of caBIG can be readily applied to bringing stakeholder groups together to advance the field of tobacco use prevention and control. More important, the tobacco control field can build directly on caBIG's interoperable infrastructure and tools to avoid both duplicating efforts and creating new "silos" that do not permit researchers to integrate data from multiple sources.

Systems-Level Tobacco Control Knowledge: Missing Pieces

Over the years, the tobacco control community has made great strides in the prevention and control of tobacco use by conducting research on smoking and implementing tobacco control policies and intervention programs. A vast amount of knowledge about tobacco control has been accumulated during this time, as is illustrated through the various KMT efforts in tobacco and related cancer control initiatives at NCI. However, for some aspects of tobacco control, knowledge is missing, incomplete, or conflicting, especially at the systems level. Such deficiencies are seen as major obstacles to effective prevention and control of tobacco use in society.

During the discussion meetings on KMT, the key informants offered their views on the major types of tobacco control knowledge that they perceived to be missing, incomplete, or conflicting. These obstacles include the following and are described below:

- Lack of current data on the tobacco industry

- Need for knowledge about current activities in tobacco control

- Need for knowledge of current needs in tobacco control efforts and who should address these needs

- Lack of "receptor capacity" in local settings, in terms of the ability of some local program staff with insufficient expertise and experience to absorb new ideas

- Need to make research findings more relevant

Lack of intelligence about the tobacco industry is problematic because the industry constantly adapts to counter tobacco control efforts and maintain profits.[21,22] Without such intelligence it is difficult to know where attention should be focused and where the scarce resources should be deployed to anticipate and counteract the actions of the industry.

Knowing who is doing what in tobacco control is difficult. Many stakeholders are committed to tobacco control, and new initiatives, such as research findings, policy initiatives, and intervention programs, are continually being introduced. Even though these diverse initiatives are worthy in their own right, they tend to put tobacco control in a constant state of flux, making it difficult to keep abreast of all the happenings in the field.

Knowing who should do what in tobacco control also is difficult, because stakeholders, such as policy makers, researchers, practitioners, and the public, may have their own agendas, priorities, and so they engage in tobacco control in different ways. Such diverse motivations have led to duplication of efforts, competition for resources, and even conflicting results. Some efforts have been made to improve communication among stakeholders, but better coordination and collaboration still are needed.

Lack of receptor capacity in tobacco control in local settings is another obstacle to efficacious tobacco control. The concept of "receptor capacity" refers to the ability to absorb new ideas and paradigms. It has become an increasingly key issue as stakeholder organizations restructure their public health programs and combine multiple initiatives (e.g., obesity, smoking, and physical activity), often with reduced funding and human resources. Consequently, some local program staff have insufficient expertise and experience in tobacco control and thus do not know what knowledge is needed, where to find this knowledge, or how to apply it in the local setting.

Research should be more relevant to practitioners so it can be more applicable

in the field setting. The current funding mechanisms are largely research driven, and less attention is given to the needs of stakeholders. This situation has led to gaps between the results of research and the knowledge required in the field to develop effective tobacco control programs. There also is a perception that tobacco control researchers conduct their studies, publish their findings, and move on to the next project without translating their knowledge into meaningful instruments that can be used by tobacco control policy makers and practitioners.

National Cancer Institute's Emerging Knowledge Management and Translation Infrastructure

The knowledge resources and initiatives described thus far represent selected KMT efforts that NCI has undertaken over the past years. These efforts have evolved both as part of an overall organizational strategy and from the practical day-to-day need to move the cancer and tobacco control agendas forward. Here, these KMT efforts are examined under the lens of the proposed framework for KMT strategy. Thus, how the field of public health can move toward a systems view of establishing a coherent KMT strategy, leading to the intended KMT outcomes, can be demonstrated. The components of the strategy maps for 4P-KMT infrastructure are briefly described by using tobacco control as the focus. The illustrations include both existing KMT efforts in tobacco control through NCI and suggested efforts drawing on those from cancer control.

Tobacco Control and Related Knowledge Resources

Based on the types of tobacco control and related knowledge resources described earlier in this chapter, an example of a high-level map of tobacco control knowledge can be produced according to explicit and tacit knowledge. The knowledge resource examples included are PLANET, SEER, CISNET, CHP, and caBIG. All of these resources are considered explicit knowledge in that they capture specific knowledge related to tobacco and/or cancer control as tangible objects. In addition, some of these resources, notably caBIG, focus more on the interaction of tacit knowledge with explicit knowledge by nurturing the formation of face-to-face and virtual knowledge networks within and between organizations.

This knowledge map also identifies systems-level knowledge sources for tobacco control that are perceived to be missing, incomplete, or conflicting. Examples include public data on tobacco industry strategies and products; a coordinated agenda for tobacco control research and practice; existing tobacco control policy, research, and practice initiatives; knowledge brokers at the local, state, and national levels; and improved mechanisms for knowledge translation, especially by researchers. Table 7.4 shows this high-level example of a tobacco control knowledge map.

4P-Knowledge Management and Translation Strategy for Tobacco Control

Again, the strategic components of the 4P-KMT strategy for tobacco control at NCI are purpose, people, process, and products. For each strategic action, the actionable items that should be considered to achieve effective tobacco control can be defined. Related resources for knowledge of cancer control (e.g., CISNET and caBIG) should be expanded, adapted, and adopted for the tobacco control domain. The 4P strategic actions and the corresponding actionable items are described here.

Purpose

The relevant agenda, timelines, and business case for the production, use, and refinement of the resources for tobacco control knowledge at NCI need to be defined based on the specific audiences, their motivations, and translation mechanisms. The knowledge should include (1) resources for the explicit and tacit knowledge of tobacco control currently managed at NCI and other stakeholder organizations, and (2) the systems-level tobacco control knowledge viewed as missing or incomplete.

Table 7.4   High-Level Map of Tobacco Control Knowledge

Type of knowledge	Explicit knowledge	Tacit knowledge
Policy	PLANET, caBIG, tobacco industry data, TC agenda, existing TC initiatives, knowledge translation	caBIG, tobacco industry data, TC agenda, existing TC initiatives, knowledge translation
Evidence	PLANET, SEER, CISNET, caBIG, existing TC initiatives, knowledge translation	caBIG, existing TC initiatives, knowledge translation
Experience	PLANET, CISNET, CHP, tobacco intelligence, existing TC initiatives, knowledge translation	tobacco intelligence, existing TC initiatives, knowledge translation
Contact	PLANET, CHP, existing TC initiatives, knowledge brokers, knowledge translation	caBIG, existing TC initiatives, knowledge brokers, knowledge translation

Notes. PLANET = Plan, Link, Act, Network with Evidence-based Tools; caBIG = Cancer Biomedical Informatics Grid; TC = tobacco control; SEER = Surveillance, Epidemiology, and End Results; CISNET = Cancer Intervention and Surveillance Modeling Network; CHP = Consumer Health Profiles.

People

There is a need to identify the champions of tobacco control knowledge, brokers and managers, architects, and communities of practice within and outside NCI who can help to define and implement the resources for tobacco control knowledge needed as part of the emerging KMT strategy. This is especially true for tobacco control knowledge at the systems level in ways that can benefit the entire tobacco control community.

Process

Rigorous yet adaptable methods and approaches must be used to encourage interaction and collaboration among stakeholder organizations using the knowledge infrastructure at NCI. The tobacco control community needs methods for consensus building and capacity building, development of tobacco control knowledge resources, and a network in which tobacco control knowledge converges. These methods should be sufficiently generic to incorporate different knowledge domains, including tobacco control and other areas as needed.

Products

Appropriate groupware that can facilitate the various communication, coordination, and collaboration tasks needed by the tobacco control community needs to be incorporated in knowledge resources. This groupware includes technologies such as real-time Web conferencing, asynchronous discussion forums, and brainstorming and concept-mapping tools. Also needed are robust knowledge repositories with the appropriate navigation and access tools that can be used to manage and translate the resources for tobacco control knowledge available through and needed by the tobacco control community.

Knowledge Management and Translation Infrastructure: Strategy for Tobacco Control

Application of the principles of KMT infrastructure outlined in this chapter as a strategy for tobacco control at NCI can be examined in terms of the underlying organization, technology, information, and finance infrastructures needed. For each strategic infrastructure, parameters for corresponding infrastructure that could help achieve a more effective knowledge framework for tobacco control can be proposed. Strategic components and corresponding parameters for infrastructure are described here.

Organization

There is a need to define the organizational structures, procedures, and norms appropriate for the production, use, and refinement of resources for tobacco control knowledge aimed at specific audiences based on their motivations and through tailored translation mechanisms. Because of the large number of stakeholders involved in tobacco control, the organizational infrastructures being used must be sufficiently flexible and adaptable to accommodate the different bureaucracies that are in place.

Technology

Appropriate computer applications, networks, and connectivity components must be incorporated to ensure that the technology infrastructure can support the deployment of the proposed KMT framework for tobacco control. This infrastructure needs to support the ongoing interactions of the tobacco control community, as well as the day-to-day management and use of robust online repositories of knowledge and tools for knowledge development and navigation and access by different tobacco control stakeholders within and outside individual organizations.

Information

Electronic databases, library resources, and data dictionaries relevant to tobacco control need to be established. In particular, there is a need (1) to synthesize the vast amount of information on tobacco control and related issues, including all relevant tobacco control policies, practices, and experiences; and (2) to coordinate contact information for use by the tobacco control community.

Finance

There is a need to establish a balanced investment portfolio so that the resources for tobacco control knowledge can be used effectively. A means of evaluating these resources as intellectual assets must be established. Where feasible, the return on investment for the production, use, and refinement of specific resources for tobacco control knowledge for selected audiences should be estimated.

Knowledge Management and Translation Strategy and Outcome Maps for Tobacco Control

The strategies for 4P-KMT and KMT infrastructures for tobacco control can be expanded by creating the corresponding detailed strategy and outcome maps. The intent of these maps is to provide a set of checklists that can be helpful for planning and implementing the KMT infrastructure for tobacco control. Figure 7.6 and tables 7.5 and 7.6 show examples of these maps.

KMT efforts, which often have their roots in addressing specific needs, must move toward a greater level of synthesis to serve the future global needs of tobacco control. Initial efforts in this area have tended to be largely centered on databases. The 4P-KMT framework outlined here provides a valuable mechanism for extending these efforts to a more integrated environment encompassing the needs of its stakeholders for both explicit and tacit knowledge. This environment has the potential to move in some important directions:

- From contact directories to repositories of tacit knowledge

- From data sources to an integrated KMT environment

- From silos of information and knowledge created for specific needs to an infrastructure for the global knowledge needs of tobacco control, driven by the 4P-KMT framework

Moreover, these needs point to the importance of integrating the KMT environment for tobacco control with other systems efforts. Examples include using network analysis as a factor in managing tacit knowledge, integrating KMT with data that drive systems models, and leveraging a systems management environment in the ongoing planning and oversight process inherent to the 4Ps. Seen as part of an integrated systems environment, the efforts in process in tobacco control research and programs form the beginnings of a valuable knowledge infrastructure for tobacco control, with the aid of a more global view of their future evolution.

Case Study: Concept Mapping of Knowledge Base for Tobacco Control

One case study illustrates several key components of the KMT framework. It involves use of concept mapping to help create a knowledge base for tobacco control. (See chapter 4 for a more detailed description of methodology for concept mapping.) In this case study, planners from stakeholder organizations in the public and private sectors were identified and brought together through a coordinated effort to generate new tobacco control knowledge in a way that could be codified, stored, and packaged. In doing so, these planners engaged in a process of knowledge translation. They socialized through the planning session and articulated their tacit knowledge on tobacco control as ideas that eventually were turned into formal explicit knowledge. As the audience

Figure 7.6 4P-Knowledge Management and Translation (KMT) Strategy Maps: Templates for Knowledge Resources Needed in Tobacco Control

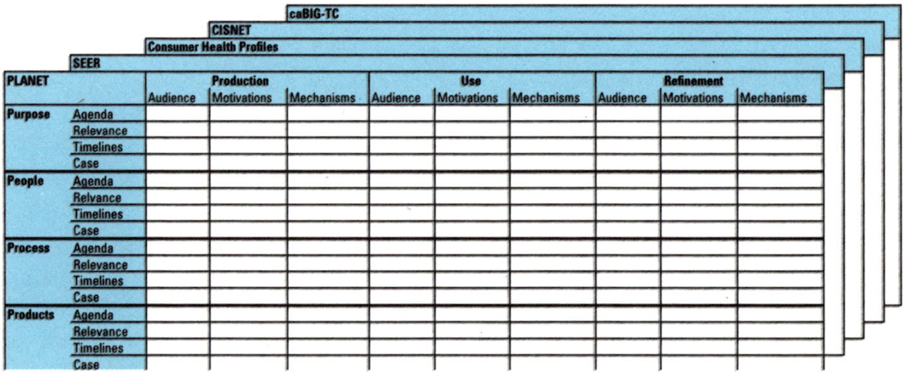

Notes. caBIG-TC = Cancer Biomedical Informatics Grid; CISNET = Cancer Intervention and Surveillance Modeling Network; SEER = Surveillance, Epidemiology, and End Results; PLANET = Plan, Link, Act, Network with Evidence-based Tools.

Table 7.5 Example of Detailed Knowledge Management and Translation (KMT) Strategy Checklist for Cancer Control PLANET: One Knowledge Resource Being Deployed in Tobacco Control

	PLANET-RTIPs	Production		
		Audience	**Motivations**	**Mechanisms**
Purpose	Agenda	Encourage researchers, policy makers, practitioners, and the public to participate in RTIPs; increase total number of RTIPs available	Identify specific motivations for researchers, policy makers, practitioners, and the public that can increase their participation in RTIPs	Increase socialization, articulation, and internalization opportunities for researchers, policy makers, practitioners, and the public to promote RTIP participation
	Relevance	Determine relevance of RTIPs for specific audiences to increase participation	Determine relevance of RTIPs based on audience motivations for decision, education, innovation, or advocacy to increase participation	Translate relevant RTIPs with timelines to specific audiences through articulation, internalization, or socialization to increase participation
	Timelines	Establish timelines to implement RTIPs for audiences that can increase their participation	Establish timelines to implement RTIPs based on specific audience motivations for decision, education, innovation, or advocacy	Translate relevant RTIPs with timelines to specific audiences through articulation, internalization, or socialization to increase participation
	Case	Develop business case to justify the value of RTIPs to specific audiences to increase participation	Develop business case to justify RTIPs with timelines based on specific audience motivations for decision, education, innovation, and advocacy to increase participation	Translate business case with justified relevant RTIPs and timelines to specific audiences through articulation, internalization, or socialization to increase participation

Notes. PLANET = Plan, Link, Act, Network with Evidence-based Tools; RTIPs = Research-Tested Intervention Programs.

Table 7.6 Example of Knowledge Management and Translation (KMT) Strategy and Outcome Map for Tobacco Control, Based on Resources for Tobacco Control Knowledge and Potential Linkage to Desired Outcomes

Type of knowledge	Evidence base	Science–practice linkage	Implementation framework	Interaction and collaboration methodology
PLANET	▪ State cancer profiles relevant to TC ▪ RTIPs ▪ Community guides on TC	▪ RTIPs for TC ▪ Feedback on local TC programs	▪ Five-steps planning approach for TC ▪ CDC cancer control planning framework adapted for TC	Contact list of regional TC programs and researchers
SEER	Cancer epidemiology and statistics relevant to TC	People/population statistics for TC	Companion suite of tools for data collection, analysis, and reporting on TC	Sharing of experience with people and of population statistics for TC
CISNET	▪ Modeling of TC impacts ▪ Metadata-level description of models	Replication of model and results with local data on TC	Iterative design process to share metadata-level description of models	Modelers to understand and share models through metadata-level description
CHP	Lifestyle clusters on tobacco use	Feedback on lifestyle clusters and link to TC	Combined use with other resources such as CDC Pink Book and State Legislations Database on TC	
caBIG		▪ Relevance of TC research ▪ Feedback on TC programs	TC agendas, policies, and infrastructures and projects for TC community	Workspaces and working groups for different focuses of TC (e.g., more smoking prevention, cessation, and environment)

Notes. PLANET = Plan, Link, Act, Network with Evidence-based Tools; TC = tobacco control; RTIPs = Research-Tested Intervention Programs; CDC = Centers for Disease Control and Prevention; SEER = Surveillance, Epidemiology, and End Results; CISNET = Cancer Intervention and Surveillance Modeling Network; CHP = Consumer Health Profiles; caBIG = Cancer Biomedical Informatics Grid.

of this process of knowledge translation, the planners assumed the roles of researchers, policy makers, practitioners, and the public. They were motivated by the innovation in creating a tobacco control knowledge base. They used the mechanisms of concept mapping to articulate their ideas from tacit to explicit knowledge.

Two support companies conducted this project on behalf of CDC to create a conceptual framework to guide the development of a knowledge base for use in tobacco control programs and research. The project engaged members of a diverse stakeholder group in a process

that mapped their ideas and defined a taxonomy for the subsequent knowledge base. A planning group identified an initial group of 36 participants, including stakeholders in the private and public sectors at federal, state, and local levels. They were asked to brainstorm ideas by completing the following focus prompt: "Specific information I would need to plan, implement, and evaluate a tobacco prevention and control program or to conduct tobacco control research is..."

The participant group generated 184 ideas, which the planning group synthesized into a set of 97 unique ideas used in subsequent analyses. Each participant was asked to sort these statements into categories that made sense and to rate each statement for importance on a scale of 1 to 5 (1 = relatively unimportant; 5 = extremely important).[23-25]

A concept mapping analysis[26] was then performed on these statements to organize and display this information in a series of easily readable concept maps and displays for pattern matching.[27-29] These maps show the relationships among the 97 ideas, the clustering of the ideas into themes or issues, and the relative importance of the ideas as rated by the participants (figure 7.7).

The multivariate analysis generated maps and other statistical results that participants then interpreted in a structured, facilitated session. Using the concept map analysis, the participants identified 12 clusters of issues relevant to knowledge management in tobacco control: (1) data on knowledge, attitude, and behavior; (2) evaluation; (3) tools to assess

capacity; (4) collaboration for sustainability; (5) models and methods; (6) planning; (7) smoking cessation; (8) tobacco industry; (9) background; (10) legislation; (11) impact of policy; and (12) influencing policy.

Participant ratings then were displayed graphically on a concept map, with clusters that represent groupings of ideas mapped according to their relationship(s). Rating values are shown as the height of individual clusters, with higher clusters relatively more important. For instance, the clusters for "evaluation, knowledge, attitude, and behavior data," and "tobacco industry" were seen as relatively important; and the cluster for "smoking cessation" was ranked lowest in importance. Figure 7.7 shows this cluster rating map. The planning group used these clusters and their ratings to create the taxonomy shown in table 7.7 for the planned knowledge base for tobacco control.

The taxonomy categories and the 97 statements within categories provide a

Figure 7.7 Cluster Rating Map for Tobacco Knowledge Base

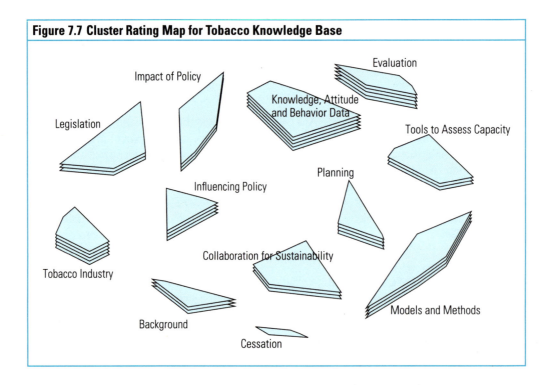

comprehensive and detailed list of issues that should be considered in developing a tobacco control knowledge base. The concept map clusters and the ultimate taxonomy categories are closely correlated. Moreover, the statements in each cluster provide details on specific information the stakeholders wanted to see in the knowledge database. For example, statements in the highest rated cluster, "evaluation," included both evaluation methods and measures for tobacco control, as well as their relationship to outcomes. Typical statements included the following:

- "Examples of evaluation designs and evaluation tools that could be adapted"

- "Identification of key indicators for evaluation—what to measure and monitor"

- "Measures for evaluation of health outcomes such as decrease in tobacco-attributable morbidity and mortality"

Similarly, statements within the cluster for "tobacco industry" ranged from marketing initiatives and policy positions to specific tactics to counter tobacco control efforts. Participants in the highly rated cluster for "knowledge, attitude, and behavior data" proposed data sources ranging from public attitudes to hard data (e.g., population surveillance data). Some of statements for this cluster, such as "Indicators and data sources for each major goal area," also pointed to sublevels of taxonomy to be considered within the design of the knowledge base.

The process the planning group followed in defining this taxonomy from the concept maps serves as a good example of how stakeholder input can evolve into a pragmatic, deliverable outcome. It was informed by both the participant statements and the clusters resulting from an analysis of these statements, as well as participant ratings of these cluster categories. The end result was a knowledge base taxonomy that was isomorphic and in many cases identical to the categories derived from participant data.

Table 7.7   Categories for Knowledge Base Taxonomy and Related Clusters from Concept Mapping

Concept map clusters	Taxonomy category
Legislation Influencing policy	Policy
Influencing policy	Influencing policy
Impact of policy	Impact of policy
Planning Background Models and methods	Policy and program planning
Evaluation	Policy and program evaluation
Knowledge, attitude, and behavior data	Sources of data
Tools to assess capacity	Assessment tools
Models and methods	Models and methods
Collaboration for sustainability	Working with communities
Tobacco industry	Tobacco industry
Background	History of tobacco control
Smoking cessation	Smoking cessation
Models and methods	Harm reduction

In addition to analyzing participant input to help define the knowledge base categories, the process provided valuable input on how subgroups of participants differ about what is important. Using a technique known as pattern matching,[27–29] the project compared relative importance ratings of several subgroups, including federal versus state and local levels of government and participants from the public sector versus those not from the public sector. Private-sector participants include stakeholders such as private industry and nongovernmental organizations.

Figure 7.8 shows results of two pattern matches. The correlation between cluster importance ratings for the federal government versus those in state or local government was extremely high ($r = .94$). This finding indicates strong agreement on the relative importance of these ideas for inclusion in a database for tobacco knowledge management. However, the correlation between cluster importance

ratings in the public sector and those not in the public sector was relatively lower ($r = .55$). This finding indicates that the two groups have different opinions about what should be included in the database for tobacco knowledge management. Representatives from public agencies thought that the importance of including ideas related to evaluation was high. Representatives from nonpublic agencies ranked ideas related to "knowledge, attitude and behavior data" as more important.

This concept-mapping study had several immediate products. First, it created the potential categories for a knowledge management database for tobacco prevention and control. The detailed statements in each category provide more specific information to guide knowledge management. In addition, the process enabled prioritization of categories, indicating which should be emphasized in the database. Perhaps most important, the process provided a summary of the

---

Concept Mapping and the 4P-Knowledge Management and Translation (KMT) Approach

The case study outlined here not only serves as a practical example of designing a knowledge base taxonomy from stakeholder input, but it also aligns in several key ways with the 4P approach outlined earlier for designing KMT strategy and infrastructure. As discussed at the beginning of this case study, this project served above all as a structured process that acquired tacit knowledge and translated it to explicit knowledge. Other parallels include the following:

- The tobacco prevention and control knowledge concepts derived from concept mapping serve as an innovative method of knowledge generation, as part of the knowledge production process.

- By including a wide range of stakeholders and analyzing their responses, this process highlights the generation of new knowledge by a specific audience on the basis of their motivations, by using the mechanism of articulation to translate tacit knowledge into an explicit form.

- Use of a visual map for linking knowledge to the evidence base and the science–practice linkage is similar to the broader process described earlier of creating a 4P-KMT infrastructures strategy map in designing a knowledge infrastructure.

The end product of this process is highly relevant tobacco knowledge that can be applied as explicit knowledge resources by using the KMT infrastructures mentioned earlier. Moreover, this knowledge can be expanded by using 4P-KMT strategy maps to detail the purpose, people, process, and products, as part of an integrated KMT effort.

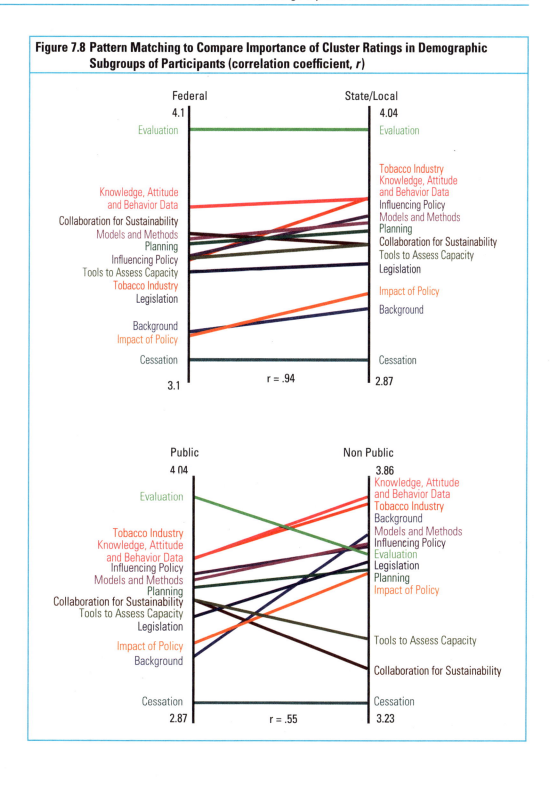

Figure 7.8 Pattern Matching to Compare Importance of Cluster Ratings in Demographic Subgroups of Participants (correlation coefficient, _r_)

Integrating Knowledge Management and Translation (KMT) with a Systems Approach to Tobacco Control

Beyond serving as a technology infrastructure for sharing information, KMT strategies have the potential to share a base of knowledge that helps the tobacco control environment evolve and, as such, form an important part of the systems strategies discussed in other chapters of this monograph.

A key example is in the interface between KMT and tobacco control networks. Overcoming turf issues and developing more effective collaboration are critical to advancing the tobacco control community as a whole. Other relevant objectives include better coordination of initiatives from different stakeholder organizations; improved translation mechanisms to enable sharing of tobacco control knowledge in ways that are relevant and meaningful to the stakeholder organizations; and translating tobacco control knowledge into action that can be implemented by practitioner communities. Ongoing dialogue that results from bringing researchers, practitioners, policy makers, and the public together to engage in such activities as joint planning, sharing lessons, role playing, and thinking outside the box can help the tobacco control community become a network of tobacco control knowledge.

Another challenge is to keep abreast of the strategies and actions of the tobacco industry. As discussed in chapter 2, this approach is analogous to the concept of disease in epidemiology. The host (human) has an illness (cancer) caused by an agent (tobacco) through a vector (tobacco industry). The vector and the agent, in this case the tobacco industry and tobacco products, respectively, are in a constant state of flux and disguise, leading to manifestations of the illness in varying forms and severity in unsuspecting or maimed hosts. The tobacco control community needs knowledge to be able to anticipate and counter tobacco industry actions.

perspectives of key stakeholders in the tobacco control field with regard to crucial elements and priorities for inclusion in this database. Through this process, a consensus framework based on the ideas of the participants was created.

Summary

An integrated KMT strategy for tobacco control is outlined here. This strategy, in turn, addresses a larger goal—the broad sharing of knowledge in a systems environment and the sustainability of this knowledge as this system evolves. As the tobacco control community moves toward this goal, it increases its ability to address more complex issues and improve public health outcomes.

The tobacco control domain is complex and dynamic, and many stakeholders are involved. Stakeholders in this domain need to address parts of a puzzle. However, no one has all the current requisite knowledge to understand or address the entire system. The kinds of knowledge needed range from very specific information, such as how many schools have effective smoke-free policies or ongoing statistics on use of hotlines for help in stopping smoking (quitlines), to the broad base of tacit information required for sharing of best practices or network building. Where can one find this knowledge, and how valid is it? How will this knowledge be updated over time? A system must be developed to collect and synthesize such knowledge for distribution and sharing, without causing information overload for the tobacco control community.

The fundamentals of a KMT infrastructure for the tobacco control domain are outlined here as a step toward the systematic production, use, and refinement of explicit and tacit tobacco control knowledge for specific audiences, based on their motivations, through different translation mechanisms. A strategic approach to KMT can advance such efforts from a project-by-project basis to becoming a coherent knowledge infrastructure, in which tobacco control and other initiatives can converge as a comprehensive set of knowledge resources. By addressing the respective components of the KMT framework, at the level of detail that makes sense for the organization based on its expertise and resources, the tobacco control community can advance to work collaboratively as a network of tobacco control knowledge enabled by technology.

Conclusions

1. Effective knowledge management is based on a social context revolving around knowledge production, use, and refinement, as well as an ecological context based on audience, motivations, and mechanisms.

2. A formal strategy for knowledge management is essential to the creation of a consistent knowledge environment. One framework defines knowledge capabilities in terms of purpose, people, process, and products, together with a knowledge management and translation infrastructure defined in terms of its underlying organization, technology, information, and finance infrastructures.

3. A review of resources for tobacco control knowledge at the National Cancer Institute confirmed the existence of extensive resources for tobacco control, combined with growth areas for the future, such as integration, visibility among stakeholders, and knowledge gaps.

4. A concept-mapping project that engaged stakeholders to examine specific information needed for tobacco prevention, control, or research yielded clusters of knowledge categories that helped form the taxonomy for a planned knowledge base for tobacco control.

Appendix 7A.   4P-Knowledge Management and Translation Infrastructures: Strategy and Outcome Maps

The infrastructures map is focused on the actionable items under the strategy of four Ps (purpose, people, process, and product). The map takes into account the underlying issues of the infrastructure for knowledge management and translation (KMT) and the desired outcomes, to establish a comprehensive KMT infrastructure. Figure 7A.1 shows this strategy map.

Depending on need, the components of this 4P-KMT infrastructures strategy map can be expanded to provide further details. The actionable items in the 4P-KMT and the KMT infrastructures strategies can be elaborated into detailed strategy maps for each type of knowledge involved. In addition, each of the actionable items can be further elaborated into detailed checklists that can be used in final implementation planning and execution. The KMT strategy also can be mapped to outcomes to ensure that they are being achieved. Figures 7A.2 and 7A.3 and table 7A.1 provide examples of detailed KMT strategy maps.

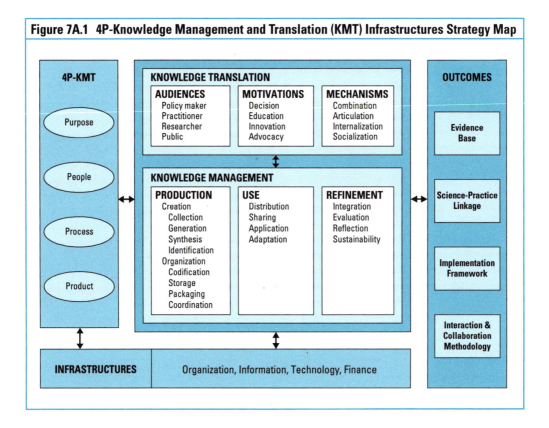

Figure 7A.1   4P-Knowledge Management and Translation (KMT) Infrastructures Strategy Map

4P-KMT	KNOWLEDGE TRANSLATION			OUTCOMES
Purpose	**AUDIENCES** Policy maker Practitioner Researcher Public	**MOTIVATIONS** Decision Education Innovation Advocacy	**MECHANISMS** Combination Articulation Internalization Socialization	**Evidence Base**
People	**KNOWLEDGE MANAGEMENT**			**Science-Practice Linkage**
Process	**PRODUCTION** Creation Collection Generation Synthesis Identification Organization Codification Storage Packaging Coordination	**USE** Distribution Sharing Application Adaptation	**REFINEMENT** Integration Evaluation Reflection Sustainability	**Implementation Framework**
Product				**Interaction & Collaboration Methodology**
INFRASTRUCTURES	Organization, Information, Technology, Finance			

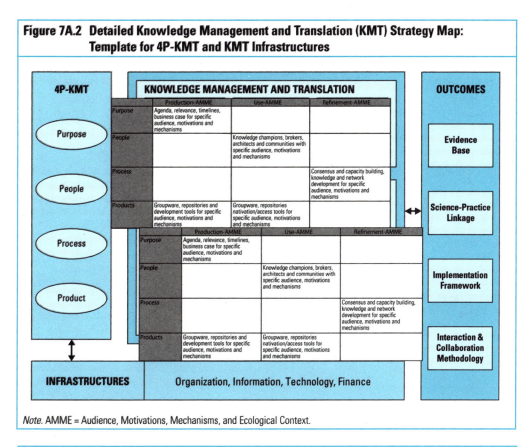

Figure 7A.2 Detailed Knowledge Management and Translation (KMT) Strategy Map: Template for 4P-KMT and KMT Infrastructures

Note. AMME = Audience, Motivations, Mechanisms, and Ecological Context.

Figure 7A.3 Example of Template for Detailed 4P-Knowledge Management and Translation Strategy Map for Production, Use, and Refinement of Particular Type of Knowledge

Type of Knowledge		Production			Use			Refinement		
		Audience	Motivations	Mechanisms	Audience	Motivations	Mechanisms	Audience	Motivations	Mechanisms
Purpose	Agenda									
	Relevance									
	Timelines									
	Case									
People	Agenda									
	Relevance									
	Timelines									
	Case									
Process	Agenda									
	Relevance									
	Timelines									
	Case									
Products	Agenda									
	Relevance									
	Timelines									
	Case									

Note. Each cell can contain a detailed checklist of actionable items for implementation.

Another important knowledge map links the knowledge resources to the corresponding outcomes. The rationale for this knowledge-outcome map is to ensure that the KMT strategy for each type of knowledge resource being deployed is able to accomplish the intended

Table 7A.1   Example of Detailed 4P-Knowledge Management and Translation (KMT) Strategy Checklist for Production of Particular Type of Knowledge

| Type of knowledge | | Production | | |
		Audience	Motivations	Mechanisms
Purpose	Agenda	Define agendas for researchers, policy makers, practitioners, and the public	Define agendas based on the audience motivations for decision, education, innovation, or advocacy	Translate agendas for audience through combination, articulation, internalization, or socialization
	Relevance	Determine relevance of agendas for researchers, policy makers, practitioners, and the public	Determine relevance of agendas based on the audience motivations for decision, education, innovation, or advocacy	Translate relevant agendas with timelines to audience through combination, articulation, internalization, or socialization
	Timelines	Establish timelines to implement agendas for researchers, policy makers, practitioners, and the public	Establish timelines to implement agendas based on the audience motivations for decision, education, innovation, or advocacy	Translate relevant agendas with timelines to audience through combination, articulation, internalization, or socialization
	Case	Develop business case to justify agendas with timelines for researchers, policy makers, practitioners, and the public	Develop business case to justify agendas with timelines based on the audience motivations for decision, education, innovation, and advocacy	Translate business case with justified relevant agendas and timelines to audience through combination, articulation, internalization, or socialization

Note. Checklist outlines how the purpose of particular knowledge resource can be defined in terms of agenda, relevance, timelines, and business case, for specific audiences and their motivations, through different translation mechanisms.

outcomes. In the study presented here, the proposed outcomes are the establishment of an evidence base for dissemination, a knowledge base for linking science and practice, an implementation framework for change, and an interaction and collaboration methodology. By performing mapping using the specific types of explicit and tacit knowledge resources being deployed, the salient aspect of each knowledge that can contribute to the respective outcome can be determined. Table 7A.2 shows an example of this knowledge-outcome map.

Table 7A.2   Example of Knowledge-Outcome Map

Type of knowledge	Evidence base	Science–practice linkage	Implementation framework	Interaction and collaboration methodology
Knowledge A	Web knowledge repository			
Knowledge B		Coordinated contacts Translated knowledge		
Knowledge C			4P-KMT infrastructure strategy maps	
Knowledge D				4P-KMT strategy framework

Note. 4P-KMT = 4P-knowledge management and translation.

Appendix 7B.   Discussion Questions Used in National Cancer Institute Review of Knowledge Management and Translation

Discussion Questions

1. Types of knowledge being managed

   (a) What do you think are the important types of knowledge needed to advance tobacco control in the United States? Why do you think these types of knowledge are important?

   (b) How much of this tobacco control knowledge do you think is being managed through your organization and others? Is it being managed effectively? If so, how? If not, why not?

2. Challenges and suggestions for knowledge management and translation (KMT)

   (a) What do you think are the key challenges in managing tobacco control knowledge across these networks of organizations? What are the barriers and incentives?

   (b) What suggestions do you have to improve the ways this tobacco control knowledge is managed within and across the networks of tobacco control organizations? Which is the highest priority action item?

3. Experience of KMT in practice

   (a) What should local/state communities do to share their questions, viewpoints, findings, and lessons regarding specific local tobacco control programs and interventions through your organization?

   (b) What other experiences and lessons would you like to share with the study team, in terms of managing tobacco control knowledge within and across the networks of tobacco control organizations?

Definition of Knowledge Management and Translation Terms

- **Knowledge**—A fluid mix of framed experience, practice routines, contextual information, and expert insight that provides a mental framework for evaluating and incorporating new experiences and information in domains such as tobacco control.
- **Explicit and tacit knowledge**—Explicit knowledge often is precise and can be formally articulated in organizations such as a tobacco control policy or program. Tacit knowledge is the know-how or expertise in tobacco control that resides within individuals.
- **Knowledge management**—A set of formal and informal structures, processes, and measures used to manipulate explicit and tacit knowledge within and across organizations such as those in tobacco control.
- **Knowledge conversion**—Ongoing processes to translate between explicit and tacit knowledge, such as in tobacco control through combination, internalization, articulation, and socialization.

- **Knowledge networks**—A collection of individuals, groups, and organizations with the requisite explicit and tacit knowledge that work collaboratively to generate ideas, products, and services, such as specific tobacco control policies and intervention programs within and across these networks of organizations.
- **KMT framework in health**—The production, use, and refinement of explicit and tacit knowledge within a particular social context of the health system such as in tobacco control.

Figure 7B.1 provides the KMT framework in health and illustrates linkages within knowledge conversion.

Figure 7B.1 Knowledge Management and Translation Framework in Health

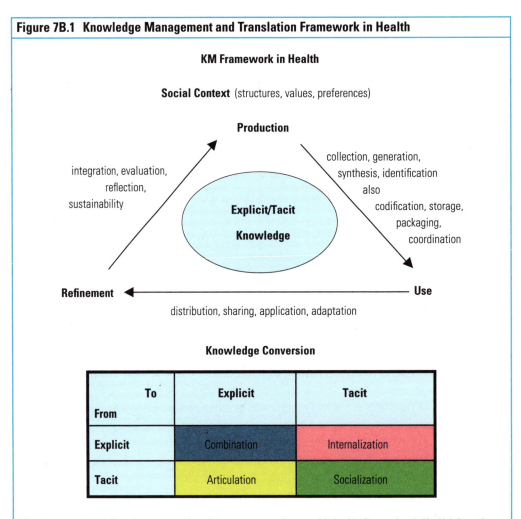

Note. From Lau, F. 2003. Toward a conceptual knowledge management framework in health. *Perspectives in Health Information Management* 1:8. Used with permission from the American Health Information Management Association (AHIMA). Copyright 2004 by AHIMA. KM = Knowledge Management.

References

1. Centers for Disease Control and Prevention. 2005. New citations. Atlanta: U.S. Department of Health and Human Services, Centers for Disease Control and Prevention, National Center for Chronic Disease Prevention and Health Promotion, Tobacco Information and Prevention Source. http://apps.nccd.cdc.gov/shrl/newcitationssearch.aspx (for November 11, 2005, through December 29, 2005).

2. Tobacco Technical Assistance Consortium. 2005. Web site. http://www.ttac.org.

3. Centers for Disease Control and Prevention. 2005. *Guide to community preventive services.* Atlanta: Department of Health and Human Services, Centers for Disease Control and Prevention, National Center for Health Marketing, Community Guide Branch. http://thecommunityguide.org.

4. National Cancer Institute. 2005. Cancer Control PLANET: Plan, Link, Act, Network with Evidence-based Tools. http://cancercontrolplanet.cancer.gov.

5. Wikipedia. 2005. Knowledge management. http://en.wikipedia.org/wiki/knowledge_management.

6. Nonaka, I., H. Takeuchi, and K. Umemoto. 1996. A theory of organizational knowledge creation. *International Journal of Technology Management = Journal International de la Gestion Technologique* 11 (7–8): 833–45.

7. Eliasmith, C., ed. 2005. *Dictionary of philosophy of mind.* Waterloo, ON: Univ. of Waterloo, Philosophy Department. http://philosophy.uwaterloo.ca/minddict.

8. Davenport, T. H., D. W. De Long, and M. C. Beers. 1998. Successful knowledge management projects. *Sloan Management Review* 39 (2): 43–57.

9. Lau, F. 2003. Toward a conceptual knowledge management framework in health. *Perspectives in Health Information Management* 1:8.

10. Street Jr., R. L. 2003. Communication in medical encounters: An ecological perspective. In *Handbook of health communication,* ed. T. L. Thompson, A. M. Dorsey, K. I. Miller, and R. Parrott, 63–89. Mahwah, NJ: Lawrence Erlbaum.

11. World Health Organization. 2003. International classification of diseases, 10th revision (ICD-10). http://www.who.int/classifications/apps/icd/icd10online/.

12. Health Level 7. 2006. What is HL7? http://www.hl7.org.

13. Cancer Biomedical Informatics Grid. 2006. Welcome to the caBIG community Website. https://cabig.nci.nih.gov.

14. Cancer Intervention and Surveillance Modeling Network. 2006. http://cisnet.cancer.gov.

15. Surveillance, Epidemiology, and End Results. 2006. http://seer.cancer.gov.

16. National Cancer Institute. n.d. Consumer Health Profiles. National Cancer Institute, Office of Communications, Cancer Information Service Research Program. http://cis.nci.nih.gov/research/CHP_FACT_SHEET.pdf.

17. Levy, D. T. 2005. A simulation of tobacco policy, smoking and lung cancer. Calverton, MD: Pacific Institute for Research and Evaluation. http://cisnet.cancer.gov/grants/lung/levy.html.

18. State Cancer Legislative Database. 2006. http://www.scld-nci.net.

19. National Cancer Institute. 2002. Making health communication programs work: A planner's guide. Bethesda, MD: National Cancer Institute. http://www.cancer.gov/pinkbook.

20. Centers for Disease Control and Prevention. 2006. CDCynergy. CD-ROM. http://www.cdc.gov/healthmarketing/cdcynergy/index.htm.

21. National Cancer Institute. 2005. *ASSIST: Shaping the future of tobacco prevention and control* (Tobacco control monograph no. 16, NIH publication no. 05-5645). Bethesda, MD: National Cancer Institute. http://cancercontrol.cancer.gov/tcrb/monographs/16/index.html.

22. National Cancer Institute. 2006. *Evaluating ASSIST: A blueprint for understanding state-level tobacco control* (Tobacco control monograph no. 17, NIH publication no. 06-6058). Bethesda, MD: National Cancer Institute. http://cancercontrol.cancer.gov/tcrb/monographs/17/index.html.

23. Rosenberg, S., and M. P. Kim. 1975. The method of sorting as a data-gathering procedure in multivariate research. *Multivariate Behavioral Research* 10 (4): 489–502.

24. Coxon, A. P. M. 1999. *Sorting data: Collection and analysis.* Quantitative Applications in the Social Sciences series 127. Thousand Oaks, CA: Sage.

25. Weller, S. C., and A. K. Romney. 1988. *Systematic data collection*. Qualitative Research Methods series 10. Thousand Oaks, CA: Sage.

26. Trochim, W. M. K. 1989. An introduction to concept mapping for planning and evaluation. *Evaluation and Program Planning* 12 (1): 1–16.

27. Trochim, W. M. K. 1989. Outcome pattern matching and program theory. *Evaluation and Program Planning* 12 (4): 355–66.

28. Trochim, W. M. K. 1985. Pattern matching, validity, and conceptualization in program evaluation. *Evaluation Review* 9 (5): 575–604.

29. Trochim, W. M. K., and J. A. Cook. 1992. Pattern matching in theory-driven evaluation: A field example from psychiatric rehabilitation. In *Using theory to improve program and policy evaluations,* ed. H. Chen and P. Rossi, 49–69. Westport, CT: Greenwood.

ISIS: Synthesis and Conclusions

This chapter examines common themes and potential areas of synthesis from a systems thinking perspective across the areas studied in the Initiative on the Study and Implementation of Systems (ISIS). It then presents conclusions based on the findings of its core group of researchers. These conclusions are based on the four core research areas of ISIS—systems organization, system dynamics and modeling, system network methods, and systems knowledge management and translation, as well as a set of crosscutting conclusions. The conclusions are used jointly to form a potential action plan for the future of systems thinking in tobacco control.

The whole is greater than the sum of its parts.

—Fritz Perls (1893–1970)

Introduction

The ultimate aim of ISIS is better health. The basic premise of this project is that the next major round of advances in health resulting from tobacco control will evolve through the adoption of systems thinking. Tobacco control and public health in general stand at a crossroads where further large-scale gains will come through the ability to understand and solve increasingly complex, evolving issues. Systems thinking may provide the means to accomplish these gains by transforming the fragmented ad hoc system that currently characterizes tobacco control to one that is more effectively self-organized, integrated, connected, and adaptive.

This chapter examines the areas studied within this project from a synergistic systems thinking viewpoint and presents the current conclusions of the ISIS team. These conclusions have the potential to move the tobacco control community toward a more integrated environment of systems thinking. The underlying unifying conclusion is that systems thinking is an ecological process, rather than just the implementation of an assortment of techniques or methods. Systems thinking is not about using a specific tool, but as Checkland states, it "is a way of looking at the world."[1] It is an inevitable evolution toward an environment that equips the tobacco control community to solve challenging, complex issues in tobacco control and public health, based on a clear set of fundamentals:

1. Simple rules by which to navigate complex adaptive systems and participatory processes that engage stakeholders at all levels

2. Feedback and evaluation mechanisms that allow adaptive, evolutionary change

3. Tools and infrastructure needed to enable functioning as a system of networked stakeholders

4. Methods for organizing and transforming the knowledge in the system to achieve more effective systemic change

Tobacco control already is heading in this direction, and this project equally reflects and factors in the evolution. Consequently, the purpose here is to encourage and channel a trend that already is in process—one in which the choice is between doing it well and sooner or doing it poorly over a longer period. With the conclusions in this chapter, this challenge is framed around guidelines that could enable the next steps in implementing real-world systems approaches to tobacco control issues.

A systems environment is dynamic. The general conclusions of this project complement the recommendations of individual chapters and are not independent of them. The systems approaches on which this project was based are among the most important of a broad array of approaches that can contribute substantially to the overall future of the systems environment in tobacco control. The four key research approaches explored in this project and the major conclusions relevant to them are presented here.

Systems Organizing

Systems organizing is about an evolution from traditional management theory to a "learning organization"[2] or an adaptive systems perspective within a systems environment. Its major message is the evolution of current concepts of managing and organizing by transforming traditional top-down, command-and-control structures to encompass participatory approaches, community-based methods, organizational change and dynamics, and effective evaluation of such efforts. Methods of organization are envisioned as a continuum from formal organization in the traditional management sense to self-organizing, community-level groups, partnerships, or collaborations.

System Dynamics

System dynamics involve methods that facilitate a more constructive examination of complex adaptive systems by modeling the behavior of actions and their consequences, both intended and unintended. These methods are particularly well suited to tobacco control, which encompasses an ongoing struggle with countervailing factors that change over time and can be strengthened. There is considerable promise in a range of systems approaches, including formal system dynamics modeling techniques, group processes that harness the problem-solving capabilities of multiple stakeholders, and ancillary methods such as simultaneous equations modeling. These approaches constitute tools that help address problems that are increasingly dynamic and complex.

System Networks

Networks represent the backbone of a system by harnessing the power of linking diverse stakeholder groups. Networks offer the means to have the greatest influence on the largest number of people in the shortest time, even more than do system dynamics models and knowledge management. Moreover, research findings suggest that countervailing forces against tobacco control often function within a network environment.[3] Understanding the formation and management of networks and using the knowledge to foster healthy networks in tobacco control are critical components of a systems environment in tobacco control.

Systems Knowledge

The management and transfer of shared knowledge form the basis of interaction between stakeholders in a systems environment. This monograph outlines a comprehensive, sophisticated infrastructure for knowledge management and transfer that is based on integrating existing silos of information and manages both explicit knowledge (what we know we know) and tacit knowledge (what we do not know

we know; unconscious lessons from experience). This knowledge environment must be collaborative, in keeping with the needs of the stakeholders it supports, and evolving to meet the changing needs and methods underlying a systems approach to tobacco control.

This project serves the dual purposes of performing original research, as a way of demonstrating the potential for systems thinking approaches in tobacco control, and of exploring the future of a systems environment for tobacco control and public health. ISIS work was accomplished through the efforts of a diverse, transdisciplinary team, which itself served as an example of a successfully functioning system. This chapter examines the implications of this effort within the broader context of recent tobacco control efforts, together with their potential trends toward an integrated systems environment for tobacco control. It then presents the conclusions reached at the two-year point of this ongoing endeavor.

Synthesis: Looking Back and Looking Over the Horizon

The systems thinking approaches studied in this project were selected for reasons beyond their future applicability to tobacco control. In a very real sense, they were seen by the principals of the project as self-evident trends that already are starting to evolve in tobacco control and public health. Moreover, they are not simply islands of automation taking place in isolation. They are part of a consistent trend that tracks throughout the recent history of tobacco control efforts.

Starting with the release of the 1964 Surgeon General's report on smoking and health,[4] efforts to improve public health by controlling tobacco use evolved from interventions aimed at the individual[5] to community-based interventions such as the Community Intervention Trial for Smoking Cessation (COMMIT) and the American Stop Smoking Intervention Study for Cancer Prevention (ASSIST), both funded by the National Cancer Institute (NCI). COMMIT focused on resources for education, health care, and smoking cessation,[6–9] and ASSIST focused on policy-level interventions such as taxes and legislation.[10,11] Interventions that address elements of the tobacco control problem as an interrelated system are a logical next step in the process, supported by recent successes in applying systems approaches to other areas such as business and defense.[2,12] Figure 8.1 tracks this evolution in tobacco control strategy and its correlation with evolution toward increasing use of systems methods in tobacco control methodology.

These trends lead to a core argument for the future of systems thinking in tobacco control. It is clear that tobacco control is using systems methodologies at increasing levels over time, but much greater benefits would be derived from *using them in a consistent, self-conscious, and methodologically integrated manner.* The most efficacious direction would be promotion of greater integration of systems approaches applied to the complex problems of tobacco control and public health.

Even in the absence of efforts such as this project, these trends toward application of systems methods to tobacco control would continue to boost use and importance. Focusing the work of stakeholders on collaborative use of these systems approaches would create an environment that drives further integration of these methods. Table 8.1 shows examples of recent efforts to apply systems methods to tobacco control. (For more information about any of the programs or references in table 8.1, see chapters 2 and 3.)

Figure 8.1 Trends over Time in Tobacco Control Strategy and Methodology

Tobacco Control Strategy	The Past	Tobacco Control Methodology
Emphasis on individual behavior change • Biobehavioral research • Smoking cessation • School-based programs		• Individual controlled trials • Separate organizational focus • Publication of results limited to peer-reviewed journals
Emphasis on population-level/environmental change • Policy/media advocacy • Coalition model • Explicit knowledge sources		• Collaborative population-based studies • Logic models (cause and effect) • Broader dissemination strategies • Web access to knowledge and data
Emphasis on system-level change • Person-environment interaction • Networks • Tacit and explicit knowledge resources • Research to practice to research		• System models (evolving models with feedback) • Participatory stakeholder-based methodologies • Networks and knowledge bases

The Future

Table 8.1   Examples of Recent Systems Efforts in Tobacco Control

Systems methodology	Tobacco control efforts
Systems organizing Managing and leading as a system	■ Mapping Integration of Research and Practice Project ■ State and local SoTC mapping project ■ Projects on CDC's Environmental Public Health Indicators
System dynamics Modeling and understanding dynamic change	■ SimSmoke simulation model of prevalence and consumption[a] ■ Prototype simulation modeling effect of tobacco control on health outcomes in morbidity and mortality due to lung cancer[b] ■ Tracking evolution of SoTC versus strength of tobacco industry counterefforts over time
System networks Understanding and managing stakeholder networks	■ Global Tobacco Research Network ■ Tobacco Harm Reduction Network ■ Tobacco Surveillance Epidemiology and Evaluation Network ■ Transdisciplinary Tobacco Use Research Centers ■ Cancer Intervention and Surveillance Modeling Network ■ Prevention Research Centers
Systems knowledge and its management Managing content and infrastructure for explicit and tacit knowledge	■ Community Guide project ■ Cancer Control PLANET dissemination effort ■ CDC TIPS Smoking and Health databases ■ Tobacco Technical Assistance Consortium

Notes. SoTC = Strength of Tobacco Control; CDC = Centers for Disease Control and Prevention; PLANET = Plan, Link, Act, Network with Evidence-based Tools; TIPS = Tobacco Information and Prevention Source.

[a] Levy, D. T., F. J. Chaloupka, J. Gitchell, D. Mendez, and K. E. Warner. 2002. The use of simulation models for the surveillance, justification and understanding of tobacco control policies. *Health Care Management Science* 5 (2): 113–20.

[b] Karash, R. 2003. Applying systems thinking to tobacco control. Minutes of the 1st ISIS Systems Thinking Summit, Washington, DC.

The tobacco control community increasingly faces the limits of using systems approaches such as these piecemeal as individual components of a tobacco control strategy. Each of these approaches addresses a need, and their implementation in tobacco control borrows to some extent from the existing processes. For example, members of the ASSIST evaluation team participated in creating a logic model for systems evaluation as part of the strength of tobacco control (SoTC) measure of state-level tobacco control efforts.[13] In addition, NCI's Plan, Link, Act, Network with Evidence-based Tools (Cancer Control PLANET) project for cancer control encompasses elements of both knowledge management and networks in providing tools for implementing evidence-based tobacco control.[14] Also, the project on Environmental Public Health Indicators of the Centers for Disease Control and Prevention (CDC) uses participatory methods and development of logic models.[15]

An integrated systems environment, encompassing these elements and more, would extend the reach of all these efforts by providing access to broader stakeholder groups, knowledge, simulation models, and other systems constructs. Promoting an integrated systems environment can lead to a "critical mass" and precipitate action to address and solve even more complex issues and to optimize improvement in outcomes.

A key finding of this investigation is that methodological features can cut across systems approaches. This finding suggests that integration of approaches is feasible and would result in better performance, improved use, and greater efficiency. For example, many systems approaches use structured brainstorming, conceptual mapping, and network analysis techniques that share quantitative methods, such as multidimensional scaling and cluster analysis. In addition, many of these approaches involve creating and maintaining data in what could become common data environments. These commonalities fall into three areas:

- *Process:* Logistical processes behind the use of a methodology

- *Technology:* Hardware and software infrastructure on which the methodology is implemented

- *Analysis:* Algorithms and analysis techniques that underlie a methodology

Some of the common methodologies across the systems approaches studied in the ISIS project are listed here by the three dimensions of process, technology, and analysis, with an eye toward how they might work together in the future (table 8.2).

Table 8.2 demonstrates a considerable overlap in methodology that, with proper planning and oversight, could form the basis for a more consistent, integrated approach across these and other areas. There has been little recognition of these methodological similarities among the different systems

traditions that tend to operate independently of one another. Examples of overlapping methodologies are as follows:

- Concept mapping and some network analysis methods share a common core of quantitative multivariate analyses, such as multidimensional scaling and cluster analysis, and could, in turn, share a common software architecture and computing environment as tools.[16,17]

- Similarly, there is a great deal of procedural overlap between the brainstorming and data-gathering processes in nearly all of these systems approaches. This overlap can pave the way for more integrated use of group processes in tobacco control projects.

- Knowledge management and translation and systems methods share the need to mine and visualize data, as well as similar front-end processes of data gathering.

At a broader level, all these approaches represent mixed methods that share common elements, such as collaboration,

Table 8.2 Common Methodological Elements across ISIS Systems Approaches

Approach	Process	Technology	Analysis
Systems organizing	Concept mapping Structured brainstorming Group processes Data gathering Participant feedback	Data mining Internet use Database management Graphic visualization	Multivariate analysis methods (e.g., multi-dimensional scaling) Clustering methods
System dynamics	Structured brainstorming Group processes Data gathering	Programmable modeling languages Data mining Database management Graphic visualization	Solution of differential equations Fuzzy logic
Network analysis	Data gathering Participant feedback	Data mining Internet use Database management Graphic visualization	Multivariate analysis methods (e.g., multi-dimensional scaling) Clustering methods Data optimization Fuzzy logic
Knowledge management	Data gathering Participant feedback	Data mining Database management Graphic visualization	Data optimization Clustering methods Fuzzy logic

structured processes, algorithms, and data representations. They have both quantitative and qualitative aspects in common, and all approach problems from a systems perspective. As part of an historical trend, they hold the potential for further systems integration around a larger concept that brings all these approaches together. Some examples of this potential integration include the following.

First, combining system dynamics modeling with network analysis may help in understanding tobacco control as an evolutionary process in which some system parts develop more productively than others. Depending on the overall strategy, this understanding can be used to set priorities and allocate resources. System dynamics modeling can indicate where networks might best be strengthened or developed, adapt more effectively, and encourage innovation in the system. Conversely, if strategy dictates, lower priority activities can be redirected or phased out.

Second, combining systems organizing with system dynamics modeling in a new structured form of system modeling with participation of multiple stakeholders can lead to other benefits. Currently in system dynamics modeling, it is typical to begin with brainstorming for potential elements of the system ("stocks" and "flows"). (See chapter 5 for definitions.) These elements usually are grouped or categorized, either by the analyst or by the group as a whole. Structured methods could be used, as in concept mapping, to enable each participant to organize the system dynamic model components individually. Subsequently, these components could be algorithmically or statistically combined into a group model that would enable exploration of stakeholder perspectives.

Third, system dynamics modeling can be combined with knowledge management to access existing knowledge in a particular

area or for horizon scanning to understand emerging developments in areas of interest. These techniques also can assist in exploring topics not previously integrated with understanding or practice. For all stakeholders, this combination helps in understanding the options that are so important in developing strategy.

Fourth, combining network analysis and knowledge management has the potential to lead to a better understanding of unknown areas by confirming gaps in knowledge where no one has ventured. This understanding can be used to develop research agendas relevant to multiple stakeholders or to advance strategy development. Work in this area may uncover useful knowledge from networks that cross into other disciplines less directly related to tobacco control, such as public health factors that are concomitant with tobacco use. Importantly, this is an approach for eliciting and processing tacit knowledge from diverse sources for broader access by many tobacco control stakeholders.

Finally, combining all four approaches would promote a shared strategy that recognizes tobacco control as an adaptive system. The strategy should help to guide new ideas toward acceptance and implementation, rather than waiting for natural evolution driven by external processes or trying to impose such concepts through brute force. This project serves as one example of providing explicit, accessible, and transparent processes to engage stakeholders at all levels in "big picture" thinking. The challenge from here will be to develop a vision that is coherent across the entire tobacco control system while promoting locally relevant and tailored missions and actions.

General Conclusions

The confluence of trends suggests that systems thinking as an organizing paradigm in public health is increasing. The signs are everywhere: the Institute of Medicine's report, *Crossing the Quality Chasm: A New Health System for the 21st Century*[18] in the field of medicine; the evolution of the Santa Fe Institute and the study of complexity;[19,20] the move to systems approaches in the management of large public[12] and private[2] organizations; and the popularization of the idea of chaos and the possibility of unexpected effects of small changes in initial conditions.[19,21] Systems approaches help in grappling with complexity, interconnectedness, rapid change, and uncertainty. The intent of this monograph is to break similar ground for tobacco control and, by extension, to demonstrate the value of systems approaches for the entire public health profession.

Tobacco control constitutes an ideal public health test laboratory for systems approaches. By its very nature, tobacco control needs to be adaptive and ecological and involves complex relationships among a profit-making industry marketing an attractive, addictive, and harmful product; the public health profession; and the population. The details of this complex relationship are constantly developing and are not always fully understood. Systems approaches can elucidate these relationships at a level that guides policy and practice and, more significantly, their evolution.

Perhaps most important, systems thinking contributes to a better understanding of an environment in which the results of single interventions frequently have unforeseen and unintended negative consequences. For example, bans on tobacco advertising may have helped to create a climate in which tobacco firms have taken a lead in sophisticated and highly effective cutting-edge marketing techniques that embed their products in movies, magazine articles, and television programs. Such techniques are much more difficult to regulate and now

are used throughout the private sector.[22,23] As another example, dependence on tobacco settlement funds may have influenced the passage of state laws that, in the eyes of some people, defend the competitive interests of major tobacco companies.[24] Systems methods hold the promise of an environment in which effects and countereffects could be more accurately modeled over time, across all affected stakeholders.

Chapter 3 presents the fundamental argument for applying systems methods to the complex issues that stand between stakeholders and improved health outcomes. Here, a roadmap for putting these ideas into practice is presented. The first two years of the ISIS endeavor and reflection on both the outcomes and future directions of systems thinking efforts lead to some initial conclusions about desirable directions for systems thinking in tobacco control specifically and public health more generally. These conclusions, developed as part of a group process in the ISIS innovation team, revolve around the four broad approaches under study in ISIS—systems organizing, system dynamics, system networks, and knowledge management—along with a complementary set of crosscutting recommendations intended as short-term action items. Table 8.3 outlines these conclusions.

The conclusions can be viewed, in the spirit of complex adaptive systems, as "relatively simple rules [that] can lead to complex innovative systems behavior,"[18(p64)] if followed by the tobacco control community in the framework of the four core approaches under study in ISIS. These conclusions are not intended to be an exhaustive list of potential systems efforts but to link synergistically to form an interdependent, systems-based environment for future tobacco control efforts. These system efforts mirror current philosophy in systems thinking on three fronts:

Table 8.3   Initial Conclusions about Directions for Systems Thinking

Approach	Directions
Systems organizing Encouraging transformation to systems culture	▪ Encourage ongoing evolution of vision and paradigms ▪ Foster a systems thinking learning environment ▪ Nurture discussion about shared purpose ▪ Remove barriers to adopting systems thinking ▪ Engender systems leadership
System dynamics Developing and applying systems methods and processes	▪ Encourage and reinforce systems thinking theory and research development ▪ Foster mixed-methods systems thinking ▪ Conduct participatory assessments of systems needs ▪ Encourage ecological perspective on implementation ▪ Foster systems evaluation
System networks Building and maintaining stakeholder relationships	▪ Create multijurisdictional and multilevel networks of stakeholders for systems thinking and action ▪ Study networks of stakeholders to determine their dynamics and effects ▪ Encourage a transdisciplinary approach by fundamentally linking specific disciplines ▪ Prepare for the impact of demographic change
Systems knowledge management and translation Building system and knowledge capacity	▪ Build capacity for systems thinking ▪ Expand public health data to enable systems analyses ▪ Integrate information silos through development of cyberinfrastructure ▪ Foster skills and culture to affect processes and outcomes ▪ Create knowledge-translation networks.
Crosscutting conclusions	▪ Create networks of excellence for systems thinking in public health ▪ Develop a Web presence for systems methods in tobacco control ▪ Foster development of systems organizing ▪ Link with systems knowledge in other fields ▪ Develop a systems curriculum in academia ▪ Create a leadership program ▪ Organize a national association and a regular national conference on systems thinking in public health ▪ Remove organizational barriers and build capacity ▪ Link with local efforts

1. They represent the key areas seen as current "gaps" in successful implementation of the kind of systems thinking environment that will lead to substantive improvements in health outcomes in tobacco control.

2. They work in concert to produce improvements in outcomes and are much less effective alone.

3. They provide the needed infrastructure and practice guidelines that underlie an ecological environment for adaptively solving complex issues in tobacco control.

In addition, these areas represent a logical evolution in perspective on the broader field of tobacco control (as outlined in chapter 2). From the 1980s, when NCI's COMMIT represented an aggressive community-level intervention effort with modest results, to the late 1990s, when projects such as ASSIST focused on population-level policy interventions, there is a clear trend toward intervening at the system level. This trend could be seen in terms of an epidemiological model, as described in chapter 2. The original ASSIST conceptual framework for tobacco control interventions (see chapter 2, figure 2.1) was published in NCI's Smoking and Tobacco Control Monograph 1—*Strategies to Control Tobacco Use in the United States: A Blueprint for Public Health Action in the 1990's*.[5] This "blueprint" proposed application of policy and other interventions across multiple channels to affect outcomes across the target populations.

This framework, which borrows conceptually from earlier representations by epidemiologists such as Sackett and associates,[25] now is nearly 15 years old. Nevertheless, it foresaw an environment in which tobacco control interventions needed to be considered in an interdependent context, pulling together the efforts of multiple stakeholder groups. In subsequent years, such an environment found its way into a broad range of tobacco control and public health efforts, to the point that it is becoming the norm for major initiatives. Examples include the following initiatives:

- The PRECEDE/PROCEED framework for the systematic development and evaluation of health education programs[26]

- Participatory tobacco control research and planning efforts with multiple stakeholders at the state and federal levels[27,28]

- The Transdisciplinary Tobacco Use Research Centers (TTURCs) initiative that established transdisciplinary tobacco control research centers at several major universities through a partnership of public and nonprofit entities[29]

Today, the efforts embodied in ISIS point toward a similar multichannel approach at multiple levels, combined with the growing realization of the need for linkage among researchers, practitioners, community-based resources, and other stakeholders, in all phases of tobacco control and public health. ISIS extends the ASSIST framework from a "push" model for interventions, for example, one that is applied to targeted channels from a central source to a systems-level model engaging all stakeholders throughout the entire research–practice continuum of tobacco control.

Specific Conclusions

ISIS is among a growing group of innovative efforts that address complexities in improving public health. Realizing the promise of improved public health outcomes in a more complex, adaptive environment requires a fresh look at how future efforts in tobacco control are conceived, funded, and executed and at the fundamentals of learning and organization. This section presents conclusions from each of the four core areas of the ISIS project, as well as a set of crosscutting conclusions. Within each of these areas, a discussion of the topic area is followed by the formal conclusion listed in italics.

Systems Organizing: Encouraging Transformation to Systems Culture

The shift to systems thinking involves a new look at what it means to "manage" tobacco control or public health efforts. If the public health system is a type of complex, self-organizing endeavor that requires different individuals, groups, and organizations to agree to coordinate efforts in some contexts and work independently in others, then traditional management models that were designed for top-down hierarchical organizations will not be appropriate for all circumstances. The move from the traditional notion of management to one of systems organizing is not a rejection of top-down management, but rather an envelopment of it. Such a change requires an understanding of the kinds of management challenges that can be organized centrally and the kinds that require facilitation of participatory and collaborative organizing. This section describes some of the major implications of this shift from managing to organizing.

Encourage Ongoing Evolution of Vision and Paradigms

Systems thinking about tobacco control, and especially the goal of achieving better integration of research and practice, represents not only the application of new areas of research but also a new way of thinking about the process of research itself. This type of shift in thinking already is taking place in other areas such as defense, business, and technology.[2,12,30,31]

A key facet of this shift involves moving past a view of systems thinking as an assortment of methodologies toward a bolder vision and more robust approach for changing the conduct of research and practice. Reaching this new vision will take foresight and a willingness to change the status quo, ranging from the activities of individual tobacco control stakeholder groups to fundamental assumptions in areas such as infrastructure, funding mechanisms, and collaboration. In a system that does not have centralized, top-down control, it is important to develop and continually evolve a common vision. This vision will never be static and will continually be pressured from all sides to adapt to the interests of some of the participants. Nevertheless, this vision development is an essential forum for communication throughout the system and for system learning.

Support for ongoing examination of systems thinking and its implications for the entire paradigm for tobacco control and public health is required to adapt a new vision for the future.

Foster a Systems Thinking Learning Environment

The systems learning environment has been described as "continually expanding its capacity to create its future."[2(p14)] The art of learning itself has evolved as society has moved in a systems direction. To take full advantage of this evolution, the learning paradigm itself must continue to change. Over time, this paradigm has moved away from the simple model of transferring static knowledge from teachers to learners and toward a more ecological approach in which teams of people adaptively pursue and discover knowledge in an atmosphere of experimentation and feedback. Similarly, an environment can be foreseen in which tobacco control stakeholders can explore and model issues in an interactive way that will lead to a broader knowledge base, better solutions, and improved health outcomes.

Today, the seeds of this type of systems learning environment in public health can be seen in efforts such as the Roadmap for Medical Research initiative of the National Institutes of Health,[32] which fosters a transdisciplinary learning approach to biomedical research, and CDC's applied research training programs for public

Creating "What If" Laboratories

There is a strong analogy between a systems learning environment and the way innovation has accelerated over time in the private sector. For example, companies built and tested products linearly in the past. Today, however, design teams can use computer-aided design and manufacturing tools as virtual laboratories in which countless "what if" questions can be explored long before hands are put on a manufacturing tool. The result is an acceleration in the pace of product design. This ability to learn iteratively, with feedback, is the hallmark of both systems thinking and contemporary process innovation.

health professionals. At a deeper level, this direction is taking shape in areas such as increased cross-agency research teams and even a proposed integration of transdisciplinary academic programs for research.[33] Such steps point to a larger trend toward leveraging a system, rather than individual expertise, in the processes of learning and discovery.

Systems learning environments must be encouraged at several levels: within the universities that train future public health professionals, within whole-of-life education, and in the course of daily life within existing research and practice environments in tobacco control. This process will involve engaging stakeholders within academia, government, professional practice, community, and the private for-profit and not-for-profit sectors. The further methodological development of systems learning environments themselves also is required. The outcome of such environments will change the process of learning and will be part of a process that facilitates the carrying capacity to tackle increasingly large and complex issues.

Nurture Discussion about Shared Purpose

Ultimately, the measure of ISIS's success will be an increased mass of stakeholders sharing this new perspective of systems thinking. How could this process be accelerated to reach the "tipping point"[34] of a new paradigm? One could envision a process, for example, in which nodes of practitioners, scientists, and policy analysts who use systems thinking create knowledge-translation networks (KTNs) around specific topics, work together through better networking techniques, adopt emerging software technologies to manage shared knowledge, and use system modeling techniques to define priorities and scope of work. Will such an ecological approach become the new landscape of tobacco control? In some sense it already is. Research efforts like the TTURCs and

an increased emphasis on community-based participatory research are pioneering many of the systems thinking approaches emphasized here. A key in such efforts is to work toward developing a strong shared purpose, marrying the promise of systems approaches with the passion of those who toil for tobacco control.

Nurturing discussion about shared purpose is the beginning of building the foundation for all other strategic discussions.

Remove Barriers to Adopting Systems Thinking

Among the most difficult aspects of moving toward a systems model are the functional and structural barriers in today's tobacco control environment. These include a lack of coordination across stakeholders, a lack of infrastructure for using participatory approaches to problem solving, silos of information, and cultural barriers ranging from how research is funded to expectations for gaining tenure in academia. Removing these barriers will require a broad, collaborative effort, and in some cases, a greater openness to transformative change.

Some of the precursors of such a collaborative systems thinking environment already exist in the form of databases linking stakeholders and public and proprietary tools such as the "Web of Science"—a commercial database linking transdisciplinary research citations across major journals.[35] Precursors also exist in the growth of online communities and information resources and in the growing use of multiple stakeholders in planning and evaluation. Much as tools such as these were forged in response to past barriers, the systems environment of the future will continue to evolve. Understanding existing roadblocks will help guide this evolution in a more productive manner.

An open, honest examination of the practical barriers to systems thinking will be a key and necessary component of implementing a systems thinking environment.

Engender Systems Leadership

Traditional management theory is evolving over time to encompass a more ecological, participatory approach both within and between organizations. This trend is examined in greater depth in chapter 4. The skill set of the systems leaders must evolve from the emphasis on managing to one of facilitating and empowering, from organizing to self-organizing, from delegation to participation, and from discrete evaluation to continuous evaluation.

The public health field should actively develop and implement education and training that encourage this evolving view of leadership and should investigate how to provide career incentives and rewards for such leadership.

System Dynamics: Developing and Applying Systems Methods and Processes

Many of the systems approaches and traditions that evolved over the past half-century show great promise in specific applications. However, it has been only in the past 10–15 years that the potential for a broader view of systems that encompasses and integrates these varied approaches has been seen—both computationally and methodologically. Component technologies such as dynamic models and simulations, stakeholder networks, knowledge bases and information infrastructures, and participatory and systems organizing methods have begun to emerge. Nevertheless, their integration into common methodologies for practice remains at an early stage. ISIS represents an important marker in what promises to be an ongoing development process for systems methods and processes. Specific conclusions reached in this area are presented here.

Encourage and Reinforce Systems Thinking Theory and Research Development

The research efforts funded by ISIS are early steps in an important direction for tobacco control and for public health in general. To see these efforts to fruition, further development in the theoretical basis and research methodology behind systems methods is required, together with the resources and infrastructure, strategic planning, and decision making needed to achieve this goal. Today, individual components of a systems approach are having an impact on tobacco control and public health. These efforts include the following:

- Early simulation of model outcomes such as reduced prevalence of tobacco use and consumption of tobacco products

- Involvement of stakeholder networks such as the Global Links program for sharing surplus surgical materials[36] and the Global Tobacco Research Network

- Harnessing the input of stakeholders for planning purposes through approaches such as concept mapping and creation of integrated tobacco control knowledge bases

Moreover, integrative efforts such as NCI's Cancer Control PLANET show the value in linking knowledge and stakeholders together with tools and methodologies. At the same time, consensus has not been reached regarding what an integrated systems environment for the future might look like.

Expanded development of systems thinking theory and research methods in tobacco control and public health is critical to achieving a consensus and, thus, substantially improved public health outcomes.

Foster Mixed-Methods Systems Thinking

Throughout the ISIS project, polarities in systems thinking were discovered: between reductionist and holistic theories, between qualitative and quantitative approaches, and between views on "soft" systems and "hard" systems. For example, examination of systems approaches ranged from quantitative (simulation-based) techniques such as system dynamics modeling and network analysis to participatory and ecological approaches such as concept mapping, community-based participatory research, and "soft" systems methods.

An important conclusion from these efforts is renewed appreciation of the broad range of systems approaches and their role in the mosaic of solving complex issues in the future. A numerical simulation may provide answers that were previously hidden, and so might a self-adaptive process involving multiple levels of stakeholders. Different systems traditions have advantages in different situations, and many might be usefully integrated or used in concert.

Stakeholders at all levels can leverage formal network concepts to understand and manage their own strategic alliances, referral patterns, growth prospects, and even succession planning to replace and continue their efforts. They can use systems concepts to move from the cynical motto that "Today's solution is tomorrow's problem" to a more strategic understanding of complex environments. Stakeholders can harness their tacit knowledge in an environment in which subjective influences, such as perception and intention, shape behavior as much as objective influences. Above all, they can use mixed methods for a deeper understanding of cause and effect as well as barriers and facilitators, helping them to analyze leverage points and priorities for action.

A mixed-methods systems approach should be encouraged and developed to more effectively address the multiple facets of complex problems.

Conduct Participatory Assessments of Systems Needs
Research and practice have evolved away from a top-down process of proposed solutions to problems toward a more dynamic process of understanding needs and working collaboratively to fill them. Many systems approaches, such as concept mapping or community-based participatory research, have the roots of their philosophy and methodology in a process that engages stakeholders to establish needs and evolve solutions.

Formalized and structured assessment of systems needs must be a cornerstone of future systems efforts and of the public health endeavor as a whole.

Encourage Ecological Perspectives on Implementation
An ecological perspective recognizes the interrelatedness of the components in the environment. In systems implementation, one example of such a perspective is "environmental scanning." This phrase, popularized in the private sector, refers to the ongoing process of observing the macroenvironment and making strategic changes based on these observations. In a tobacco control context, it constitutes a more active, interdependent, and less procedural approach to observing and reacting to factors in the environment.

The ecological approach lies at the heart of systems thinking in that it encompasses the ability to evolve according to observation and feedback. This cybernetic view of the world already has shown results in areas such as the concept of "shared situational awareness" in national defense, in which a networked force that shares information in a self-synchronizing manner has demonstrably led to greater effectiveness with smaller fighting forces.[31] In public health, it serves as a logical next step in a field that has progressed from disease control, to prevention, to cause-and-effect intervention, and now toward working systemically to affect health outcomes. Such an approach does not reject a reductionist (single-discipline) approach to

Dynamic Program Development and Evaluation Databases

The past 50 years have seen the rise of the computer and the accompanying development of databases that store critical information. In evaluation, those asked to provide data often complain that evaluation is a task they are required to do and that they get little in return for such efforts. Funders and decision makers wonder why their grantees resist evaluation and do not make use of its results. Systems thinking and approaches are beginning to change these dynamics. This can be seen, for example, in the data system used at Amazon.com, the online bookstore. Regular users of that Web site discover that when they browse for a particular book, they are given suggestions about other books that were purchased by people who also purchased the book of interest. When the user makes a purchase, this information is stored and other purchases are linked to it in a type of information network. This type of dynamic database principle adds value for all the users and enables linkages that previously were not possible.

These principles can be applied to evaluation databases. For example, imagine a Web site for designing a local tobacco control program. Users would enter descriptions of the programs they are thinking about, and its activities, outputs, and outcomes. The program could print a logic model based on the input. That is a static database application. It might be used, but it does not add much value, and it does not provide users with much incentive. However, imagine if the Web site was designed so that information from others could be provided to users as they enter their own program ideas. If users enter in a few keywords such as "local clean indoor air regulations," the program might show them what others who previously designed such programs had done, how they had managed their campaigns, and how they evaluated results. Researchers who visit the site would be able to learn about what ideas local tobacco control people are searching for, could link in relevant evidence, and could identify potential practice sites for collaboration. Funders could see how interests are evolving and could provide funding as an incentive in real time. By the time users are finished designing their programs, they would be informed by other practitioners' experience, would know the relevant evidence base, could have some potential evaluative tools and measures, and might have a lead on potential research and funding collaborations.

Many of these systems thinking principles are emerging in sites like Amazon.com, as well as wiki applications like wikipedia.com. Such dynamic planning and evaluation databases would provide greater incentives for all parties to contribute, thereby dramatically increasing the value of the database itself over time.

science. Instead, it takes advantage of the interrelationships of those theoretical and methodological approaches to address more effectively some of the most difficult public health challenges today.

An ecological approach, including systematic environmental scanning, will become a fundamental paradigm for tobacco control and public health.

Foster Systems Evaluation

Any new direction that may require substantive change in both practice and culture requires a clear appraisal of its

effectiveness. The practice of evaluation itself must evolve.

At a deeper level, the increasing connectivity across society is making research in behavioral and social sciences increasingly difficult, because control of one or more variables cannot be ensured. Behavioral and population-specific factors either cause or contribute to the diseases causing most premature mortality, so it behooves the scientific community to ensure that methods to study these factors and intervene appropriately are developed and adapted. This is fundamentally a systems process, and it further underscores the need to develop evaluation methods for assessing system behavior, such as (1) indirect measures of outcomes and (2) participatory evaluation criteria driven by stakeholders.

A move toward systems approaches requires the further development of evaluation methods that accurately reflect progress toward outcomes, while preserving the energy and innovation of interventions. In the process, it is possible to add a further degree of rigor to the practice of public health, while helping the concept of evidence continue to evolve.

Build and Maintain Network Relationships

Today's tobacco control environment is characterized by a diverse and expansive group of stakeholders at all levels of the process, including researchers, funding agencies, public health authorities, elected officials, community-level organizations, advocacy groups, and the population groups affected by tobacco control interventions. When these groups create their own agendas, the result is not only inefficiency and duplication of effort but also a lack of shared information that in turn could change outcomes. Thus, there is a need to build the important structural connections and collaborations among tobacco control stakeholders and strategies to encourage support for improved health outcomes.

Create Multijurisdictional and Multilevel Networks of Stakeholders for Systems Thinking and Action

The formation of networks that cross levels of action and jurisdiction is one of the most promising and challenging avenues for changing outcomes in tobacco control and public health. Structured collaborations of multiple stakeholders can fundamentally change the direction of efforts and outcomes. Strategies such as face-to-face

meetings of researchers, policy makers, practitioners, and clients and collaborative interaction through group processes such as concept mapping are essential for addressing the significant gaps between research and practice.[16] Such approaches also have relevance to public health more generally. For example, the disconnect between research and practice is considered to be a root cause of the slow diffusion of successful cancer treatments.[37]

Creation of multijurisdictional, multilevel stakeholder networks holds the potential for enhancing the ability of tobacco control stakeholders to work effectively and achieve breakthrough results. Creation of such networks will lead to new research priorities and reexamination of the funding and career issues that drive current tobacco control research. Moreover, such a network environment represents a new infrastructure for future tobacco control practice, giving voice to a system of participants that, in turn, will continue to evolve with changes in tobacco control and public health.

Study Networks of Stakeholders to Determine Their Dynamics and Effects

The promise of having tobacco control stakeholders operate more effectively in a network environment brings with it a concomitant need to explore the dynamics of these networks and evaluate their effects, ranging from formative evaluation such as exploratory research and concept testing to ongoing process evaluation. Some of these areas will involve new approaches to evaluation. In addition, ancillary outcomes such as cost-effectiveness, time-effectiveness, and dissemination of results may be important areas for further study.

The evolving networks of stakeholders should be actively encouraged, and evaluation of networks should be an integral part of planning for a network environment within tobacco control.

Encourage a Transdisciplinary Approach by Fundamentally Linking Specific Disciplines

The evolution of public health over the past century has increasingly engaged multiple disciplines. Therefore, today's tobacco control environment includes a broad range of experts such as clinicians, psychologists, epidemiologists, and mathematicians. The complexity of future tobacco control issues will likely require insight and expertise from multiple disciplines. These disciplines must work collaboratively to build a common base of understanding and knowledge. Moreover, the systems environment of the future will move from collaboration to integration. Disciplines such as these have become part of the overall mosaic of fields including tobacco control and public health.

Transdisciplinary approaches are a key component of a systems approach to tobacco control. The systems, networks, and knowledge infrastructures that evolve within this field should explicitly encourage integration of multiple fields of knowledge.

Prepare for the Impact of Demographic Change

Demographers make dire predictions about future shortages of human resources. There is a scarcity of skilled personnel in many areas of tobacco control. As in the good old days, key informants describe hard-to-fill vacancies and staff turnover affecting programs throughout the United States. From a systems perspective, retaining organizational memory and sharing tacit knowledge can help to protect tobacco control agencies in future demographic transitions.

Systems thinking can help to mitigate the impact of demographic change by generating feedback about performance, developing workforce skills, improving teamwork, and ensuring that services are coordinated with other agencies.

Knowledge Management and Translation: Building System and Knowledge Capacity

If a systems environment were adopted within tobacco control tomorrow, what tools would people use? How would they collaborate? What mechanisms exist for linking stakeholder efforts? How would their knowledge be disseminated? These questions all touch on the area of building capacity: creating tools and procedures that underlie the adoption of systems methods across stakeholder groups within tobacco control.

Build Capacity for Systems Thinking

A clear analogy exists between the systems environment envisioned today and the computer and Internet environment envisioned more than a decade ago. In the 1980s and 1990s, a diverse range of tools and research efforts across the public and private sectors ultimately coalesced into the integrated computer and network environment that is taken for granted in the twenty-first century. Systems thinking requires the same coalescence. This capacity development must itself be a systems-oriented effort by multiple stakeholders. Moreover, to gain public acceptance, this effort will need to engage the private sector to develop systems tools that have ongoing commercial potential in broad areas beyond tobacco control and public health.

Efforts to develop tools for systems and knowledge capacity must move forward together and proceed with an eye toward stronger standards and improved tools as systems methods are more widely adopted across many of society's areas of endeavor.

Expand Public Health Data to Enable Systems Analyses

Methods for systems thinking involve a move away from linear, top-down modes of action toward models that assess, interpret, react to, and incorporate feedback at multiple levels. Bringing such an environment to reality requires access to timely accurate data to support decisions at multiple levels. Examples of expansion of public health data include measures of the impact of social and political interventions, such as the Strength of Tobacco Control and the Initial Outcomes Index used in the recent evaluation of the ASSIST program.[13] In addition, health outcome data have been expanded in areas such as prevalence of tobacco use, consumption of tobacco products, and morbidity and mortality at the population and community levels.

The analysis and delivery mechanisms for public health data need to be evaluated in the light of a growing systems thinking environment and implemented in a way that supports this environment.

Integrate Information Silos Through Development of the Cyberinfrastructure

The current environment of multiple stake-holders in tobacco control involves multiple silos of explicit and tacit knowledge. Creditable efforts are under way to provide integrated knowledge resources in tobacco control. These efforts include CDC's Tobacco Information and Prevention Source, a central online clearinghouse for published documents on tobacco control research; CDC's State Tobacco Activities Tracking and Evaluation System; and NCI's Cancer Control PLANET, which supports evidence-based tobacco control practice with links to data, tools, and resources.

The trend toward increased knowledge translation and transfer must continue as an important part of the infrastructure for systems thinking efforts in tobacco control. Further integration of stakeholder resources and information is clearly indicated in the future.

Foster Skills and Culture to Affect Processes and Outcomes

Capacity building for systems approaches to tobacco control involves much more

than tools and data. Beyond this narrow slice of "capacity" is a multidimensional environment. This environment ranges from an organizational infrastructure that fosters collaboration and change to a culture that supports working as a system, for example, examining the processes for tenure and for research grants to encourage bridging multiple disciplines and stakeholder groups.

The human side of knowledge capacity must be addressed as organizations critically examine how to build the skills and learning culture needed to affect both the processes and outcomes of tobacco control.

Create Knowledge-Translation Networks

Participative approaches and involvement of colleagues are essential for building capacity. A knowledge-translation network could formalize and focus other networks so they can benefit from planned development. It would become the vital third leg of a three-legged stool, balancing the evidence base and progressive practice. Knowledge-translation network activities could include "better practice" colloquia, focus groups to share tacit and explicit knowledge, and collaboration on specific issues. In the long run, theory-driven exploration of better

---

Beyond Islands of Knowledge: ISIS Knowledge Review at NCI

The review of knowledge management undertaken as part of ISIS at NCI underscored the strategic importance of knowledge and a growing trend to make this knowledge accessible to a broader range of stakeholders. More important, the review provided a framework for understanding the gaps in current knowledge capabilities by exploring the scope of explicit and tacit knowledge in key areas, such as policy, evidence, experience, and contact, and by outlining the start of an action plan to fill these gaps through an integrated and planned knowledge environment.

practice also can benefit from the evolving KTN, which provides an environment for practitioners to "drive the evidence."

Knowledge-translation networks need to be developed to encourage greater integration of practice and research.

Crosscutting Conclusions

The conclusions presented here represent broad areas of effort and activity designed to accelerate an evolutionary process that already is beginning to take place in tobacco control and in public health more generally. The implementation of systems-level concepts in practice remains an area for future study. However, a number of crosscutting steps would provide a basic foundation for future systems activity. Below are near-term actions that flow from these conclusions.

Create Networks of Excellence for Systems Thinking in Public Health

The tobacco control community would benefit from development of several multidisciplinary, cross-institutional networks designed to promote systems thinking. These networks could be based on the notion of "centers of excellence." However, they would differ in that the efforts would be explicitly collaborative, that is, not based in a single institution (e.g., a specific university or organization). The networks should be dedicated to the study of systems thinking in tobacco control specifically and in public health generally. Multiple networks of this type are needed to encourage more rapid evolution and to foster a healthy sense of competitiveness. These networks should promote accelerated implementation of systems thinking theory and research development in areas such as the following:

- Encouraging development of new methods

- Exploring integration of existing methods

- Performing research on research methodology itself in areas such as systems methods, applications, and evaluation

- Researching better practices for participatory action research and systems leadership

Develop a Web Presence for Systems Methods in Tobacco Control

Systems methods are fundamentally participatory in nature. The Internet has emerged as a core medium for interaction, participation, and transfer of knowledge. The intention of this effort is to not end only as a report or monograph such as this one but to continue as a living, evolving process with one or more homes on the Internet.

Foster Development of Systems Organizing

There is a critical need for processes that bring in the diverse range of stakeholders in tobacco control, public health, and related areas and create a framework for their collaborative effort. Existing partner networks and collaborations stand to gain considerably by pursuing such joint efforts within an appropriate infrastructure. Through closer collaboration among stakeholders, the tobacco control stakeholder community will help create the conditions for emergence of more complex and effective systems in tobacco control.

Link with Systems Knowledge in Other Fields

Systems thinking is evolving rapidly, but much of that knowledge is diffused across a broad spectrum of disciplines in everything from physics to ecology. Within these disciplines, a great part of the systems discussion is buried in local technical language and conventions, making it less accessible to other disciplines. Strategies must be developed to tap into and understand the emerging systems thinking in other disciplines. One promising and relatively inexpensive option would be to seek approaches for tobacco control and public health to become structurally engaged with existing groups and organizations that explicitly encourage cross-disciplinary translation and understanding. Networks or collaborations in tobacco control are likely to be more effective than individuals in the field in eliciting an entré into established transdisciplinary endeavors.

Develop a Systems Curriculum in Academia

Much as the computer revolution was fueled by a fresh generation of newly educated technology and software experts, the systems environment of the future will be strongly aided by upcoming graduates of public health and related areas. With input from deans and administrators in public health programs, particularly at the graduate level, a curriculum addressing both component areas of systems approaches and their integration can help make this environment part of the reality of public health. An exciting recent development along these lines is a proposal of the Australian National University and the Australian Commonwealth Scientific and Research Organization for a joint institute for research integration[33] to serve as a prototype for future programs on integrative theory and methods in public health and other areas.

Create a Leadership Program

Encouraging the development of a new generation of leaders who can function in a collaborative systems environment is one of the most important short-term tasks for the adoption of systems approaches. Individuals must possess an unusual set of talents, together with a wealth of new skills and tools, to be effective systems leaders. An early priority should be to identify potential leaders and to nurture them through a broad program of education and experience. Stakeholders need to include recognized leaders in the field defining the characteristics, designing the program, and mentoring prospects.

Organize a National Association and a Regular National Conference on Systems Thinking in Public Health

A regular forum encompassing a broad range of stakeholders can become an important part of the collaborative process and transfer of knowledge that underlie a systems approach in public health. Possible benefits of such a conference include the following:

- Creating a collaboration for systems thinking in public health that integrates existing groups such as the Syndemics Network and ISIS and provides a broader venue in tobacco control to engage people

- Increasing the linkages between systems thinking groups and stakeholders in tobacco control and public health

- Encouraging systems thinking in public health communities and vice versa

- Establishing areas of common ground

- Forming special interest groups

Remove Organizational Barriers and Build Capacity

Perhaps the most challenging but potentially fruitful near-term activity is to examine the future roles of major current stakeholders in tobacco control, with an eye toward an enhanced systems environment. The most important roadblocks to a truly collaborative, systems-based approach to tobacco control, such as funding issues, incentives for academic tenure, and organizational and information silos, can be resolved only through collaboration and engagement, as a true systems effort unto itself.

Link with Local Efforts

A core theme of many of the participatory approaches with multiple stakeholders that were studied within ISIS is the importance of community-level participation in tobacco control in all phases of planning, implementation, and evaluation. Local involvement is much more than a lofty ideal. The disconnection between research and community-based practice has been identified by other researchers as a roadblock to fundamental progress in areas such as cancer and public health.[37–39] Conversely, initiatives such as the recent Community–Campus Partnerships for Health,[40] a formal effort based at the University of Washington in Seattle to link campus research and community public health stakeholders in a participatory environment, represent an important direction for the future. Specific action items in this area include establishment of local pilot projects for future tobacco control initiatives, involvement of community-level stakeholders in planning and evaluation processes, and further linkages of local groups with a broader spectrum of tobacco control stakeholders.

Near-term action items such as these represent tangible next steps that will help translate research into action in creating a systems environment for tobacco control. Taken as a group, these action items are part of an evolution toward larger objectives such as widespread adoption of systems approaches, creation and use of networks, and development of an underlying knowledge infrastructure. More important, they will help the tobacco control profession itself move toward the kinds of stakeholder collaboration and interaction that, in turn, will form a basis for working together more effectively as a system.

Summary

What would people like the world to look like 5 to 10 years from now? If this question is posed to a group of top experts in most fields, a deterministic vision usually emerges: do X, Y, and Z, and a specific outcome will happen. In comparison, the ISIS effort yielded a very different and much more important answer to this question. The vision is of a new and more ecological

environment that could potentially allow innovation to flourish as never before. The specific steps leading to improved tobacco control and public health outcomes are not yet known. However, there is a strong consensus on the basics of a process that, if allowed to naturally evolve, could create these steps and in turn dramatically change these outcomes.

Simply stated, with more inputs, more stakeholders, and better evaluation and adaptation, the infrastructure of knowledge, networks, and analysis methods needed for the support of this adaptive environment will be the key to transforming the state of public health in the future. The rubric of "systems thinking" that underlies the ISIS effort is not simply an assemblage of component technologies, such as system dynamics models, network analyses, or knowledge bases. It is instead a philosophy that reflects the basic engine of change in life, whether it is in the form of biology, economic competition, democracy, or nature itself. This rubric has a strong theoretical base and a growing level of implementation in many fields. More important, it is a fundamental shift from much of current research and practice in tobacco control and public health.

Tobacco control provides a case study for exploring the complex interplay of collaborative (e.g., differing tobacco control programs and policies) and competing (e.g., tobacco companies and supporters of tobacco companies) factors, as demonstrated in the system dynamics analysis "shard" presented in this monograph. For example, NCI Tobacco Control Monographs 16[11] (on the American Stop Smoking Intervention Study for Cancer Prevention—ASSIST) and 17[13] (on the evaluation of ASSIST) qualitatively and quantitatively characterize the complex factors that influenced tobacco control efforts within and between states. The analysis presented in Monograph 17 includes a measure called Strength of Tobacco Control (SoTC), which begins to take this complexity into account. This modeling effort starts to quantify the relationship between tobacco control efforts in the ASSIST states and countervailing influences by the tobacco companies, including their efforts to undermine ASSIST by influencing policy makers at the state and federal levels.

By understanding the interplay of these and other complex factors relative to policy and program implementation—that is, to more fully characterize the complex "system" of tobacco control—the tobacco control community increases its ability to improve public health efforts by anticipating and tracking countervailing influences. This approach could serve as a model for addressing other public health threats such as overweight and obesity and communicable disease.

In conclusion, this monograph demonstrates that the ability to maximize knowledge of and change in such complex systems depends on the ability to (1) improve information tracking and exchange (knowledge management), (2) analyze and implement complex networks, (3) analyze relationships among complex and sometimes competing variables, and (4) understand and implement organizational structures and functions that will improve health practices. There are, of course, additional challenges, but these steps provide the essential foundation of any effective public health effort.

Against this backdrop, systems approaches clearly are a major hope for substantial improvement in health outcomes in the future. Moreover, this trend mirrors fundamental changes in how problems are solved within society as a whole. Much as efficient hierarchical organizations became a fundamental concept in the twentieth century, systems thinking may become a central concept for the twenty-first century. It could fundamentally change the nature of tobacco control and public health and

play a key role in addressing a leading cause of preventable death. The conclusions offered here hold the promise of further evolution toward such a systems thinking environment that, in turn, holds the potential to substantially change the state of the nation's health.

References

1. Checkland, P. B. 1999. *Systems thinking, system practice: Includes a 30-year retrospective.* Chichester, UK: John Wiley and Sons.

2. Senge, P. M. 1990. *The fifth discipline: The art and practice of the learning organization.* New York: Currency Doubleday.

3. Trochim, W. M., F. A. Stillman, P. I. Clark, and C. L. Schmitt. 2003. Development of a model of the tobacco industry's interference with tobacco control programmes. *Tobacco Control* 12 (2): 140–47.

4. U.S. Department of Health, Education, and Welfare. 1964. *Smoking and health: Report of the Advisory Committee to the Surgeon General of the Public Health Service* (PHS publication no. 1103). Washington, DC: U.S. Department of Health, Education, and Welfare, Public Health Service, Center for Disease Control.

5. National Cancer Institute. 1991. *Strategies to control tobacco use in the United States: A blueprint for public health action in the 1990's* (Smoking and tobacco control monograph no. 1, NIH publication no. 92-3316). Bethesda, MD: National Cancer Institute. http://cancercontrol.cancer.gov/tcrb/monographs/1/index.html.

6. *American Journal of Public Health.* 1995. Community Intervention Trial for Smoking Cessation (COMMIT): 1. Cohort results from a four-year community intervention. *American Journal of Public Health* 85 (2): 183–92.

7. *American Journal of Public Health.* 1995. Community Intervention Trial for Smoking Cessation (COMMIT): 2. Changes in adult cigarette smoking prevalence. *American Journal of Public Health* 85 (2): 193–200.

8. National Cancer Institute. 1995. *Community-based interventions for smokers: The COMMIT field experience*

(Smoking and tobacco control monograph no. 6, NIH publication no. 95-4028). Bethesda, MD: National Cancer Institute. http://cancercontrol.cancer.gov/tcrb/monographs/6/index.html.

9. *Journal of the National Cancer Institute.* 1991. Community Intervention Trial for Smoking Cessation (COMMIT): Summary of design and intervention. COMMIT Research Group. *Journal of the National Cancer Institute* 83 (22): 1620–28.

10. Shopland, D. R. 1993. Smoking control in the 1990s: A National Cancer Institute model for change. *American Journal of Public Health* 83 (9): 1208–10.

11. National Cancer Institute. 2005. *ASSIST: Shaping the future of tobacco prevention and control* (Tobacco control monograph no. 16, NIH publication no. 05-5645). Bethesda, MD: National Cancer Institute. http://cancercontrol.cancer.gov/tcrb/monographs/16/index.html.

12. Krygiel, A. J. 1999. *Behind the wizard's curtain: An integration environment for a system of systems.* Washington, DC: Institute for National Strategic Studies.

13. National Cancer Institute. 2006. *Evaluating ASSIST: A blueprint for understanding state-level tobacco control* (Tobacco control monograph no. 17, NIH publication no. 06-6058). Bethesda, MD: National Cancer Institute. http://cancercontrol.cancer.gov/tcrb/monographs/17/index.html.

14. National Cancer Institute. 2005. Cancer Control PLANET: Plan, Link, Act, Network with Evidence-based Tools. http://cancercontrolplanet.cancer.gov.

15. Centers for Disease Control and Prevention. 2005. *Environmental Public Health Indicators Project.* Atlanta: U.S. Department of Health and Human Services, Centers for Disease Control and Prevention, National Center for Environmental Health. http://www.cdc.gov/nceh/indicators.

16. Trochim, W. M. K. 1989. An introduction to concept mapping for planning and evaluation. *Evaluation and Program Planning* 12 (1): 1–16.

17. Monge, P. R., and N. Contractor. 2003. *Theories of communication networks.* New York: Oxford Univ. Press.

18. Institute of Medicine. 2001. *Crossing the quality chasm: A new health system for the 21st century.* Washington, DC: National Academies Press.

19. Phelan, S. E. 1999. A note on the correspondence between complexity and systems theory. *Systems Practice and Action Research* 12 (3): 237–46.

20. Olson, E. E., and G. H. Eoyang. 2001. *Facilitating organization change: Lessons from complexity science.* San Francisco: Pfeiffer.

21. Gladwell, M. 2002. *The tipping point: How little things can make a big difference.* New York: Little, Brown and Company.

22. Beirne, M. Brandweek. Relationship marketing: Doral's direct line. 10 Aug 1998. Philip Morris. Bates No. 2071275337A/5338. http://legacy.library.ucsf.edu/tid/dwr08d00.

23. Wells, M. *USA Today.* Marlboro saddles up dude ranch promotion. 1998. Philip Morris. Bates No. 2070910462. http://legacy.library.ucsf.edu/tid/hus37d00.

24. Olson, W. 2004. Mavericks eroding settlement tobacco share. http://www.overlawyered.com/archives/000724.html.

25. Sackett, D. L., S. E. Straus, W. S. Richardson, W. Rosenberg, and R. B. Haynes. 2000. *Evidence-based medicine: How to practice and teach EBM.* 2nd ed. Edinburgh: Churchill Livingstone.

26. Green, L. W., and M. W. Kreuter. 1999. *Health promotion planning: An educational and ecological approach.* 3rd ed. Mountain View, CA: Mayfield. http://www.thcu.ca/infoandresources/planning_resources.htm.

27. Stillman, F. A., A. M. Hartman, B. I. Graubard, E. A. Gilpin, D. M. Murray, and J. T. Gibson. 2003. Evaluation of the American Stop Smoking Intervention Study (ASSIST): A report of outcomes. *Journal of the National Cancer Institute* 95 (22): 1681–91.

28. Trochim, W. M., B. Milstein, B. J. Wood, S. Jackson, and V. Pressler. 2004. Setting objectives for community and systems change: An application of concept mapping for planning a statewide health improvement initiative. *Health Promotion Practice* 5 (1): 8–19.

29. Stokols, D., J. Fuqua, J. Gress, R. Harvey, K. Phillips, L. Baezconde-Garbanati, J. Unger, et al. 2003. Evaluating transdisciplinary science. *Nicotine & Tobacco Research* 5 Suppl. 1: S21–S39.

30. Skinner, C. S., and M. W. Kreuter. 1997. Using theories in planning interactive computer programs. In *Health promotion and interactive technology: Theoretical applications and future directions,* ed.

R. L. Street Jr., W. R. Gold, and T. Manning, 39–66. Mahwah, NJ: Lawrence Erlbaum.

31. Alberts, D. S., and R. E. Hayes. 1942. *Power to the edge: Command and control in the information age.* CCRP Publication Series. Washington, DC: U.S. Department of Defense. http://www.dodccrp.org/publications/pdf/Alberts_Power.pdf.

32. National Institutes of Health. 2006. NIH roadmap for medical research. http://nihroadmap.nih.gov.

33. Bammer, G. 2004. *Proposal for the ANU/CSIRO Institute for Research Integration.* Flyer. Canberra: Australian National Univ. and CSIRO Australia.

34. Gladwell, M. 2000. *The tipping point.* Boston: Little, Brown.

35. ISI Web of Knowledge. 2006. Web of Science. http://www.isinet.com.

36. Global Links. 2006. Sharing surplus, saving lives. http://globallinks.org.

37. Leaf, C., and D. Burke. 2004. Why we're losing the war on cancer [and how to win it]. *Fortune* 149 (6): 76–90.

38. Midgley, G. 2000. *Systemic intervention: Philosophy, methodology and practice.* Contemporary Systems Thinking series. London: Springer.

39. Brownson, R. C., E. A. Baker, T. L. Leet, and K. N. Gillespie, eds. 2002. *Evidence-based public health.* Oxford: Oxford Univ. Press.

40. Community-Campus Partnerships for Health. 2007. http://www.ccph.info.

Initiative on the Study and Implementation of Systems: A Project History

ISIS is interested in creating a generic approach to public health [by] using tobacco control as an example. Our goals include alignment of the relevant network toward policies and practices that work; alignment of each organization toward policies and practices that work; [and] uncovering and agreeing on high-leverage public health policies and practices that work.

This statement from the original 2003 summit meeting that kicked off the Initiative on the Study and Implementation of Systems (ISIS) project summarizes the broad goals of the project: to use systems thinking approaches and theory to address previously intractable issues, to improve the health outcomes associated with tobacco control and, by corollary, to improve all of public health. These goals were not conceived in isolation but were rather a direct response to both the growth of systems methods in recent years and the complexity of today's tobacco control environment. The ideas presented had their roots in trends affecting not only tobacco control but also many areas of human endeavor in the early 21st century.[1–3]

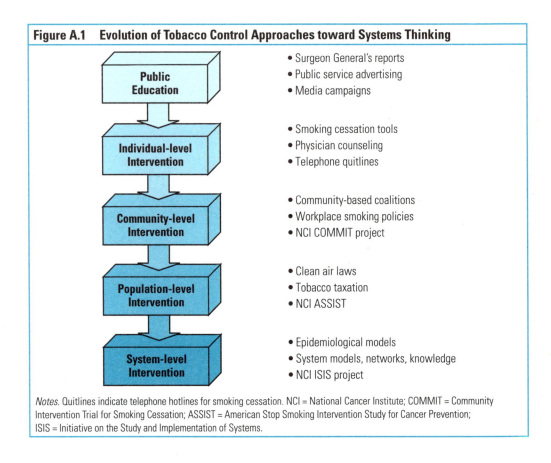

Figure A.1   Evolution of Tobacco Control Approaches toward Systems Thinking

Public Education
- Surgeon General's reports
- Public service advertising
- Media campaigns

Individual-level Intervention
- Smoking cessation tools
- Physician counseling
- Telephone quitlines

Community-level Intervention
- Community-based coalitions
- Workplace smoking policies
- NCI COMMIT project

Population-level Intervention
- Clean air laws
- Tobacco taxation
- NCI ASSIST

System-level Intervention
- Epidemiological models
- System models, networks, knowledge
- NCI ISIS project

Notes. Quitlines indicate telephone hotlines for smoking cessation. NCI = National Cancer Institute; COMMIT = Community Intervention Trial for Smoking Cessation; ASSIST = American Stop Smoking Intervention Study for Cancer Prevention; ISIS = Initiative on the Study and Implementation of Systems.

The numerous approaches that fall under the rubric of "systems thinking" jointly represent a formal effort to deal with the natural complexities of life, as well as a natural evolution of problem-solving abilities. The underlying premise of this project was that the state of tobacco control was ripe for the integration of systems thinking, for four key reasons:

1. Tobacco control efforts encompass numerous disparate communities of interest with frequent duplication of effort.

2. Tobacco control efforts lack organized methods for dissemination and collaboration.

3. Tobacco control activities engender competitive responses from a well-financed and highly organized tobacco industry that has well-integrated dissemination and networking strategies.

4. Specific tobacco control efforts often lack effectiveness on key outcomes such as cessation of tobacco use and morbidity and mortality.

Systems thinking encompasses a set of approaches and methodologies that facilitate understanding of the behavior of a system in terms of both the totality of the components and their dynamic interaction around the knowledge/content. It also reflects a natural evolution in the approach to control of tobacco use (figure A.1).

Since the 1964 Surgeon General's report on smoking and health[4] and resulting public awareness of the risks of tobacco use, early tobacco control efforts were aimed at the individual, through measures such as education, patient counseling, and smoking cessation services.[5] Subsequent initiatives, such as the Community Intervention Trial for Smoking Cessation (COMMIT),[6] underscored the importance of community-level coalitions and smoking policies and demonstrated their effectiveness by using a randomized community trial model. By 1991, the American Stop Smoking Intervention Study for Cancer Prevention (ASSIST)[7] and other efforts, such as the privately funded SmokeLess States program,[8] examined the impact of upstream population-level interventions, such as legislation, taxation, media advocacy, and state-level tobacco control infrastructures. Later, in 1993, the Initiatives to Mobilize for the Prevention and Control of Tobacco Use (IMPACT) led by the Centers for Disease Control and Prevention (CDC) also funded the 33 states not funded by ASSIST, to implement similar interventions.[9] The ASSIST, SmokeLess States, and IMPACT programs were particularly significant in that they marked a period in which fundamental social attitudes toward the acceptability of tobacco use were beginning to undergo a permanent change.[10]

In the wake of such initiatives, it was clear to key researchers at the National Cancer Institute (NCI) and elsewhere that further gains in the reduction of tobacco use hinged on addressing the issues of tobacco use from a systems perspective by using science to address the complex web of forces and counterforces underlying the root causes of the prevalence of tobacco use and tobacco product consumption. This realization mirrored gains from adoption of systems approaches in other areas, such as business,[2] defense,[3] and social policy.[11] As one of few public health areas that had a major industry actively opposing its efforts, together with a complex landscape of social, political, and economic factors, tobacco control seemed to be an ideal context for systems thinking.

To meet this challenge, experts in systems thinking disciplines and stakeholders from the tobacco control and public health communities were recruited to participate in the ISIS project as a transdisciplinary team with funding from NCI. After a series of summit meetings to define the scope and goals of the initiative and funding for specific research efforts, this project ultimately took shape as both a study and a proof-of-concept model for future systems efforts in tobacco control.

The origins of ISIS date back to the summer of 2001, with a series of informal discussions between two key figures in tobacco control who were attending a conference on the National Blueprint for Adult Tobacco-Use Cessation—Scott Leischow, then chief of NCI's Tobacco Control Research Branch, and Allan Best, a senior scientist at Vancouver Coastal Health Research Institute and professor at the University of British Columbia. They were concerned that the systems models in fields such as business and defense were not being more widely applied in public health.

At this conference, Best's presentation, "Building Collaboration: Cautions from the Trenches," set forth his view of core needs for dissemination of evidence-based practice. These included a system for interagency coordination, identification of needs, development of networks and sites, and acquisition of major funding. In examining the issues of dissemination, he sketched the beginnings of a systems view of the world, a topic of interest to Leischow as well. This interest, combined with a shared concern about the state of dissemination, led to discussions that gave birth to the ISIS project. Perhaps more important, this shared interest had deep roots, going back decades, and coinciding with a similarly evolving view among researchers who had worked with community health systems.

Best's interest in a systems view of the world dates back to his doctoral work in psychology, which involved the roles of context and social ecology in effective psychotherapy versus a world that "simply compared therapy A with therapy B." His service as the principal investigator for the first Canadian site of COMMIT preceded eight years in the private sector as a consultant and director of organizational health. In these positions, he learned firsthand the challenges of integrating practices found in the research literature with the real-world needs of practitioners. Similarly, as an academic at the University of Arizona, Tucson, prior to coming to NCI, Leischow noted the strong parallel between the emerging systems theories of researchers such as Peter Checkland of Lancaster University in the United Kingdom and his own work in developing tobacco cessation programs involving multiple stakeholders in Arizona. He was especially struck by the lack of coordinated systems thinking in tobacco control initiatives at that time. For both Best and Leischow, the meeting on the National Blueprint for Adult Tobacco-Use Cessation provided the opportunity to pursue important changes in outcomes for the field of tobacco control.

These discussions were trendsetting on two fronts. First, they engendered a realization that the study of tobacco control at a systems level might lead to improved outcomes. Second, they were an important evolutionary step in the trajectory of integrating research and practice. Subsequent to his arrival at NCI, Leischow and colleagues noted three fundamental disconnects in the discovery, development, and delivery "system": (1) too little discussion between government organizations about disseminating results from funded research to the appropriate programs, (2) the existence of organizational and informational "silos," and (3) insufficient communication between organizations. The ISIS project became a logical extension in efforts to build bridges among tobacco control stakeholder organizations and reflects a broader move toward evidence-based tobacco control practices compared with previous efforts.

The concept of evidence-based practice had steadily grown among the public health community, particularly since the advent of meta-analyses of research data, such as the Cochrane Collaboration in medicine, related initiatives in public health, and their extension to dissemination efforts such as CDC's *Guide to Community Preventive Services*.[12] However, it was clear that evidence-based practices still often sat unused on shelves. These early discussions among Best and Leischow and their colleagues initially examined how systems approaches might help dissemination of evidence-based practice in tobacco control. Over time, they evolved to consider the broader question of why gaps remain between the research of scientists and the needs of practitioners.

Ultimately, NCI determined that systems thinking in tobacco control was sufficiently important to warrant development of an NCI-funded initiative for more in-depth study. Consequently, NCI funded a formal effort that became the ISIS project and issued a contract to the Battelle Centers for Public Health Research and Evaluation, under the direction of Pamela Clark, a noted expert in tobacco control research who had been a major contractor for the evaluation of ASSIST and the Global Tobacco Research Network (GTRN). With a strong voice in the profession and expertise ranging from technical areas such as the biochemistry of smoking to social research in tobacco control, Clark was a key coordinator of what quickly became a broad multidisciplinary project. From there, the effort progressed to a literature review and identification of the members of the ISIS innovation team by Best's colleagues in Vancouver, British Columbia. Project coordinator Gregg Moor, who contacted experts ranging from industry leaders to academic specialists, spearheaded that effort. These activities culminated in an initial planning meeting in late 2002, in San Francisco, California, as a joint meeting with the evolving GTRN to explore a research effort with five modest goals:

1. Pinpoint key perspectives and literature that might contribute to transdisciplinary integration

2. Identify, evaluate, and synthesize seminal documents from key literature

3. Facilitate development of ongoing structures and processes for effective transdisciplinary collaboration

4. Develop a conceptual framework that maps key concepts for future development

5. Produce a mid- to long-term plan for further development of strategic thinking and strategy

Best characterized a subsequent meeting in May 2003, in Denver, Colorado, as a "first date" during which systems and tobacco control experts began to discuss a collaborative research initiative. In June 2003, a summit meeting was held in Washington, DC, featuring an open discussion among key tobacco control stakeholders and a facilitated workshop session with systems expert and consultant Rick Karash, which led to the evolution of an action plan and agenda. These summits served as necessary points of dialogue for establishing the scope of the ISIS project and the range of expertise required.

At the meeting in Washington, DC, it became clear that the problem at hand—using systems thinking to improve tobacco control and public health—required a focus that went far beyond simple system dynamics models. George Richardson, University at Albany, State University of New York, a key expert on system dynamics, had discussed the interaction between systems simulation and network analysis in his Denver presentation. He joined many others in arguing for broadening the focus of ISIS from its base of system dynamics. These early summits were designed with a focus on systems, but by the end of the first Washington, DC, summit, the consensus was that systems and network methods had an important synergy and that network methods should be included in the ISIS project.

After this meeting in Washington, DC, Noshir Contractor of the University of Illinois at Urbana-Champaign, a noted expert in network theory, and Keith Provan, University of Arizona, who had successfully applied network methods to other public health issues, became part of the core ISIS team. After the next ISIS summit meeting in Scottsdale, Arizona, in late

2003, the scope of the ISIS project grew once again to encompass both issues of knowledge management and the broader aspects of large-scale organizational change, aligned with Best's original vision of "managing a federation of systems." Once again, the core team expanded to include knowledge-management expert Francis Lau, University of Victoria, British Columbia, and Ramkrishnan Tenkasi, Benedictine University, Lisle, Illinois.

At the next ISIS summit, in the Washington, DC, area in January 2004, key stakeholders from NCI, CDC, and major tobacco control organizations and advocacy groups met to hear formal presentations on the core technology areas of ISIS. Richardson showed the evolution of a system dynamics simulation of tobacco control efforts, including the simulation of prevalence of tobacco use and cigarette consumption across a 40-year "chain" of aging smokers. Contractor and Provan discussed methods for network analysis and their applicability to public health, and Lau shared findings from his recent work on the use of knowledge-management approaches in the health care profession.

This meeting in Washington, DC, referred to as the Bolger Summit, named after the conference center in which it took place, was an open forum ultimately leading to a fundamental shift in focus for ISIS. After the meeting, a "think piece" developed by William Trochim, Department of Policy Analysis and Management, Cornell University, Ithaca, New York, solidified the ISIS goals around systems thinking for integrating science and practice. This direction evolved to an examination of organization or management of the "systems of systems" inherent to tobacco control and public health. A consensus quickly formed around the think piece. A report presented at a public health conference in Banff, Alberta, Canada, in April 2004,[1] constituted a public statement of its concepts.

This summit and its resulting document also helped to move the focus of ISIS away from a study of the application of four specific methodologies and technologies (system dynamics, network analysis, knowledge management, and systems management) toward a much more synergistic effort to use systems thinking to improve public health outcomes. Gabriele Bammer, Australian National University, Canberra, and Harvard University's Hauser Center for Nonprofit Organizations, Cambridge, Massachusetts, shared a comprehensive view of "integration and implementation sciences." This presentation and the frank discussions from stakeholders in attending the summit helped the group to envision ISIS as the study of a synergistic framework for integrating public health science and practice.

A series of transdisciplinary teams to examine functional areas, such as how researchers and practitioners communicate and work together, anticipate change, and organize themselves with the federation of systems took shape and began working. A follow-up summit in April 2004 in Vancouver solidified the ISIS core group's direction. The original research funded as part of this study moved forward, ultimately leading to publication of this NCI monograph, which is based on the first two years of the four-year project.

Development of this monograph was a systems effort. As the project evolved, the ISIS innovation team chose to depart from the traditional model of chapters contributed by specialists in narrow areas and instead formed a dedicated writing team with the task of integrating "shards" of original research, literature reviews, and content from several broad, transdisciplinary teams of key experts in their fields. This writing team, led by Trochim, included professional science writer Rich Gallagher and research assistants Jennifer Brown and Derek Cabrera. Best's team of project coordinator Moor and assistant Snjezana Huerta-Kralj, at the Vancouver Coastal Health Research Institute, provided logistical support. Timothy Huerta, then a postdoctoral fellow at the Centre for Clinical Epidemiology, Vancouver General Hospital, provided key literature review and synthesis support. Together, this bicoastal, international effort linked the contributions of a diverse group of participants across a high-bandwidth network of teleconferences, meetings, listserv postings, shared drafts, and face-to-face meetings over a two-year period, leading to the completion of a draft monograph.

In February 2005, members of the ISIS core group, meeting in Chicago, Illinois, reflected on their efforts to date and forged a set of conclusions for future needs and directions in applying systems thinking to tobacco control. These conclusions, which form the centerpiece of the closing chapter of this monograph, were put forth as next steps to further explore systems approaches in tobacco control. The conclusions outline the research, policy, and capacity-building efforts that could bring such an environment into reality.

The ideas behind these conclusions evolved considerably throughout the project and will undoubtedly continue to evolve as these recommendations are considered and put into practice by tobacco control stakeholders. The project itself represented a proof-of-concept of a real-life complex adaptive system, in which participants continually learned from one another in working toward a broad consensus that will continue to evolve in future efforts. Within this mosaic, each person had a unique perspective on the meaning of this initiative.

- To some, this project was fundamentally about strategy and how to develop strategic structures and functions to improve health and save lives; how to understand the nature of systems and networks; how to create the networks needed to facilitate this process; and what information is needed to make the system work more effectively.

- To others, the project revolves around the concept of communities of practice, in which stakeholders at multiple levels share collective responsibility for tobacco control strategies and improved outcomes. In this view, people drive the process and the product, so the network comes first—gathering together key stakeholders to reach out and achieve buy-in and bringing people and structures to build a sustainable platform.

- Some felt the key issue within this project was the effect of traditional command-and-control strategies in a tobacco control environment that clearly is a complex adaptive system, requiring a more adaptive and organic strategy.

- Others saw a clear fit between systems modeling approaches and the most frustrating issues in today's tobacco control environment, such as the inability to rationalize gaps and redundancies in surveillance, lessons learned from unintended consequences not being fed back into the system, and lack of true multilevel analyses.

- Most shared the view that the role of efforts like this was to speed up evolution, that systems thinking is going to happen, and that efforts should be directed toward making it happen more effectively and efficiently by promoting public health practice that is more flexible, adaptive, and successful. Evolution is characterized by diversity and selective retention. There is consensus that systems thinking is about making these changes more quickly and more effectively.

At the same time, this very diverse team of experts quickly came to share many goals: a need for connectivity and sharing of information, a commitment to engage stakeholders at all levels, and above all, a desire to address the complexity inherent in public health issues through adaptive and ecological means. The concepts must now be tested in the real world, a broader range of stakeholders must be brought into the discussion, and mechanisms for feedback must be in place to guide this evolution. There are no "cookie cutter" solutions for local communities to begin implementing systems thinking. However, there now is a clear potential direction for the future of tobacco control.

The initial two-years of the ISIS project were necessarily limited by time and resources. Consequently, the project's efforts and this monograph's focus are on tobacco control for the home countries of the project participants, most notably the United States, Canada, and Australia. Given the worldwide challenge of tobacco control, it is clear that the dynamics of tobacco use elsewhere follow their own distinctive evolution. It is fully expected that the results of this study will be generalizable to, and will need to be adapted for, the unique tobacco control contexts of other regions and countries.

This monograph represents the research outcomes and future directions of the first two years of the ISIS project as part of a process that should continue beyond the document. The monograph acts as a current index or snapshot of a dialogue about systems thinking for tobacco control that must evolve beyond what is on the printed page. Social scientist Donald Campbell described this phenomenon somewhat tongue in cheek as "historicist dialectical indexicality." As such, this project has moved from a topical research initiative to a living document that serves as a framework for using systems thinking to improve health outcomes and has evolved much as dynamic systems evolve over time.

In particular, the project has evolved from a study of system dynamics to a broader examination of approaches to integrated systems thinking. It ranges from network analysis and knowledge management to systems organizing and potentially encompassing a number of cutting-edge developments such as syndemics, complex adaptive systems, chaos theory, and complexity theory. It also has evolved from a traditional model that treats many of the methods of systems thinking as separate silos to a model that examines broader questions such as "who we are" and "what we know," which are addressed through joint efforts of transdisciplinary teams. Perhaps most important, the fundamental question has evolved from "how to disseminate evidence-based practices in tobacco control" to the much deeper issue of "how to apply systems thinking to improve health outcomes"—a critical question for the future of all public health efforts.

References

1. Best, A., R. Tenkasi, W. Trochim, F. Lau, B. Holmes, T. Huerta, G. Moor, S. Leischow, and P. Clark. 2006. Systemic transformational change in tobacco control: An overview of the Initiative for the Study and Implementation of Systems (ISIS). In *Innovations in health care: A reality check,* ed. A. L. Casebeer, A. Harrison, and A. L. Mark, 189–205. New York: Palgrave Macmillan.

2. Senge, P. M. 1994. *The fifth discipline: The art and practice of the learning organization.* New York: Currency.

3. Krygiel, A. J. 1999. *Behind the wizard's curtain: An integration environment for a system of systems.* Washington, DC: Institute for National Strategic Studies.

4. U.S. Department of Health, Education, and Welfare. 1964. *Smoking and health: Report of the Advisory Committee to the Surgeon General of the Public Health Service* (PHS publication no. 1103). Washington, DC: U.S. Department of Health, Education, and Welfare, Public Health Service, Center for Disease Control.

5. National Cancer Institute. 1991. *Strategies to control tobacco use in the United States: A blueprint for public health action in the 1990's* (Smoking and tobacco control monograph no. 1, NIH publication no. 92-3316). Bethesda, MD: National Cancer Institute. http://cancercontrol.cancer.gov/tcrb/monographs/1/index.html.

6. National Cancer Institute. 1995. *Community-based interventions for smokers: The COMMIT field experience* (Smoking and tobacco control monograph no. 6, NIH publication no. 95-4028). Bethesda, MD: National Cancer Institute. http://cancercontrol.cancer.gov/tcrb/monographs/6/index.html.

7. National Cancer Institute. 2005. *ASSIST: Shaping the future of tobacco prevention and control* (Tobacco control monograph no. 16, NIH publication no. 05-5645). Bethesda, MD: National Cancer Institute. http://cancercontrol.cancer.gov/tcrb/monographs/16/index.html.

8. SmokeLess States National Tobacco Policy Initiative. 2005. *SmokeLess States: Reducing tobacco use and exposure through policy change.* Princeton: Robert Wood Johnson Foundation. http://www.rwjf.org/portfolios/features/featuredetail.jsp?featureID=1827&type=3&iaid=143&gsa=1.

9. U.S. Department of Health and Human Services. 2000. *Reducing tobacco use: A report of the Surgeon General.* Atlanta: U.S. Department of Health and Human Services, Centers for Disease Control and Prevention, National Center for Chronic Disease Prevention and Health Promotion, Office on Smoking and Health.

10. National Cancer Institute. 2006. *Evaluating ASSIST: A blueprint for understanding state-level tobacco control* (Tobacco control monograph no. 17, NIH publication no. 06-6058). Bethesda, MD: National Cancer Institute. http://cancercontrol.cancer.gov/tcrb/monographs/17/index.html.

11. Zagonel, A. A., J. Rohrbaugh, G. P. Richardson, and D. F. Andersen. 2004. Using simulation models to address "what if" questions about welfare reform. *Journal of Policy Analysis and Management* 23 (4): 890–901.

12. Centers for Disease Control and Prevention. 2005. *Guide to community preventive services.* Atlanta: Department of Health and Human Services, Centers for Disease Control and Prevention, National Center for Health Marketing, Community Guide Branch. http://thecommunityguide.org.

Systems Thinking in Tobacco Control: A Framework for Implementation

The Initiative on the Study and Implementation of Systems (ISIS) was an exploratory effort to apply systems thinking to tobacco control and public health. As such, it examined trends in systems methods and their application through the eyes of a team composed primarily of researchers and leaders in both the tobacco control field and numerous systems thinking disciplines. The conclusions in this monograph outline a broad, general direction for better harnessing a systems revolution that already is under way in this and many other fields.

What does this effort mean to the tobacco control practitioner, the bench scientist, or the community activist? The answer may be "a great deal, in time." This monograph's chapters look ahead to how systems could affect daily life in practice, but the specifics are still unformed and the subject of much investigation to be done in the near future. The real value of this effort lies in setting overall directions for how systems approaches and, more important, their synthesis can benefit tobacco control. This appendix outlines some possible paths for how these directions can be put into action for tobacco control stakeholders.

First, this appendix examines some of the open questions that surround the use of systems approaches by key tobacco control stakeholder groups. It then explores a possible future storyline for how these approaches might affect the work of some of these stakeholders. Next, it discusses some of the core issues in putting systems thinking into practice within tobacco control, together with possible directions for specific stakeholder groups and steps for getting this process started. Finally, it explores key questions that remain for implementing systems approaches in the future.

ISIS did not seek to "build a system." Rather, it sought to foster an ecological process that is ultimately driven by simple rules, which must continue to evolve. In nature, evolution is driven by a process described by Campbell as "blind variation, selective retention." In that process, the more diversity the system has (i.e., the more variation and selective retention it has), the more quickly the system converges on an optimal solution instead of remaining in a static monoculture.[1] Similarly, in systems thinking, more variation (through broader stakeholder groups, systems approaches, and multiple systems) and more selective retention (through improved evaluation and implementation) will accelerate the results of efforts toward tobacco control. Thus, variation and selective retention operate in much the same way that other ecological models do, such as survival and economic competition. The ideas presented in this appendix serve as one possible starting point for simple rules within an ecological framework that could lead to fundamental changes in tobacco control and public health outcomes.

Integrated Systems Thinking: Story Line for the Future

Predicting the future is always fraught with peril: futurists of the 1950s foretold advances such as residential colonies on the moon and personal transportation using jet-propelled backpacks, but they completely missed trends like personal computers and the Internet.[2] At the same time, their visions of a more technological and interconnected future helped to produce today's reality.

The vision of a systems future in tobacco control and in public health more generally is informed by inputs at multiple levels. These inputs range from ongoing trends in practice and methodology, to the increasing complexity and nonlinearity of outstanding issues in tobacco control, and even to the evolution of group thinking among the participants in the ISIS project during its initial two years, which itself can be seen as a systems effort. Like all predictions, the picture of the tobacco control field and public health overall for decades into the future is necessarily hazy, but the overall direction is clear—an integrated systems approach that becomes a natural part of daily practice at all levels of the field. Today's world is a place where increasingly complex issues are understood and managed, where research and practice are tightly linked, and above all, where the possibility of a smoke-free and healthier environment with an attendant decrease in preventable mortality becomes more and more likely.

With this vision in mind, it might be instructive to revisit the real-world questions for tobacco control that are raised in chapter 3 and to examine how the lessons learned from systems thinking might address these questions. The next step is to write a forward-looking scenario of how key tobacco control stakeholders might operate in the systems environment of the near future. First, it is useful to examine some of the questions that initially framed the ISIS study.

Practitioners

Questions relating to systems approaches and practitioners are as follows:

- How can practitioners cope with competition from other organizations for scarce resources?

- How do practitioners communicate the positive achievements of their organizations and still argue that there is a need for continued and/or additional funding?

- How can practitioners maintain trust with clients when changes in funding levels alter the services they are able to provide?

- How can practitioners spend more time in the field and less time with administrative details?

- Where can practitioners find succinct, clear, and practical information on the latest research?

These questions share key threads addressed by the fundamentals of systems thinking: concerns about isolation, access to resources and information, dissemination of results, and perhaps above all, the productive use of human effort. The lessons learned from this project include the following:

- Networks and tacit knowledge resources can provide an infrastructure for discovering the needs, the available resources (e.g., financial) to address them, and the contacts and expertise to support the process of building coalitions. A common data infrastructure also holds the potential to streamline administrative overhead, paperwork, and reporting requirements.

- Explicit knowledge bases can serve as repositories for accumulated data on local outcomes. Tacit knowledge bases can provide a resource for people to access the expertise of individual practitioners. At a more active level, networks serve as a foundation for organizing formal dissemination activities such as conferences, electronic communications, and bulletin boards.

- Data from systems models and their concomitant research results stored in knowledge bases can streamline the planning process and more efficiently keep practitioners abreast of research.

- Perhaps most important, a systems organizing approach of working in a participatory, information-sharing manner with other stakeholders—locally, nationally, and globally—can lead to adaptive changes in the course of both research and practice, focusing practitioners toward efforts that more effectively improve health outcomes.

Researchers

Questions relating to systems approaches and researchers are as follows:

- How can researchers contribute to preventing their research from sitting unread in journals?

- Why don't more people use the science developed by researchers?

- How can researchers access the experiential knowledge of practitioners to be certain they are providing an evidence base for the most important programmatic applications?

- Where can researchers connect with other researchers who have common or complementary interests but who may work in other departments or fields?

- How can researchers streamline the approval and funding processes for their work?

The researchers' questions reflect a sense of responsibility to advance science, coupled with frustration over the funding issues that underpin researchers' work and the dissemination issues that follow it, combined with what may seem to be a structural isolation from the stakeholders they serve. Systems approaches can address these issues in the following ways:

- Adaptive, participatory systems approaches in research can lead to research efforts that engage the very stakeholders the efforts are directed toward. This strategy leads to a more direct path to dissemination and implementation and, perhaps more important, to multidirectional links that push the course of research toward public health outcomes.

- Systems models can provide an evolving, multifactorial basis for research projects, which can help these projects link more directly to the needs of practitioners and other stakeholders.

- Networks and knowledge bases serve as an infrastructure linking researchers to explicit knowledge such as research data, tacit knowledge such as who shares common or complementary research interests, and an infrastructure that in time could be leveraged to streamline research funding and implementation efforts.

Policy Makers

Questions for policy makers are as follows:

- What priorities dictated past resource allocation, and what priorities will be dictated in the future?

- How can policy makers get a better return on investment for research expenditures?

- How can policy makers synthesize all the "silos" of information out there?

- How can policy makers reduce or eliminate duplication of effort among stakeholder organizations?

- How can policy makers convince more professionals to use evidence-based practices?

Policy makers face the need to look ahead and "make decisions at 20,000 feet" that, in turn, must support the objectives of their organizations and of public health outcomes. At a more practical level, they also must make the best use of resources and function effectively in a world of multiple organizations and stakeholders. Systems tools can help in the following ways:

- Systems models can examine the potential multifaceted effects of likely future options to guide policy decisions, resource allocation, and priorities.

- Network and knowledge-based resources can provide access to collaborators and/or funding to efficiently address organizational priorities and break down cross-organizational barriers.

- A common knowledge infrastructure for explicit and tacit knowledge in tobacco control and other public health issues, particularly if linked with existing knowledge resources, can provide a consistent portal for information, as well as a means to disseminate information from organizations.

- Adopting participatory systems-organizing approaches within and outside an organization can tie its efforts more directly to stakeholders and outcomes.

These answers for different stakeholder groups hold promise for each of these groups but share an even more important characteristic—*their similarity.* Moreover, these answers point toward answers to the broader, discipline-wide issues posed in chapter 3 of this monograph. How can a shared vision be built to reduce the prevalence of tobacco use and consumption of tobacco products, link actions (missions) to this vision, learn from each other's knowledge, and ultimately forge a closer integration of research and practice? By linking shared goals, taking action in light of enhanced mutual understanding among stakeholders, and moving each stakeholder group toward a collective vision, participatory action, and common infrastructures, systems approaches do much more than solve individual problems. They move all parties toward an adaptive, collaborative environment that, in turn, holds the key to major changes in the future of tobacco control.

Looking ahead from the lessons learned, it is possible to imagine a future integrated systems environment for tobacco control—not a monolithic system but an accepted environment of tools and procedures, analogous to today's computing environment. Activities of hypothetical stakeholders might include the following:

Researcher. Jessica Smith is a public health scientist studying population-level tobacco control issues.

Practitioner. Michael Washington is a state public health administrator working to reduce the state disease burden due to tobacco use.

Advocate. Stan Rodriguez is a lawyer who, years after becoming a widower due to issues of tobacco use, is actively involved in community antismoking efforts and provides litigation support to regional efforts.

Leader. Barbara Fellows is the chief executive officer of a for-profit hospital chain on the West Coast.

Legislator. State Representative Cheryl Stanton is a legislator who has become a key figure in proposing state legislative action in support of tobacco control.

The findings of this project suggest the vision of an environment in which all of these stakeholders interact in a variety of ways, which are discussed here.

Smith (the researcher) helped to organize an online "town hall" meeting through a central network of stakeholders at many levels of tobacco control to clarify future research priorities. Discussions at the meeting have given her a quantitative and qualitative sense of these priorities. Based on this input, Smith plans to research the relationship between a policy intervention and changes in smoking prevalence and consumption of tobacco products. The policy intervention is a one-cent increase in the federal excise tax on cigarettes to pay for expansion and promotion of national "quitline" services (hotlines for help to stop smoking). Going online to a repository of tobacco control knowledge, she first scans existing research involving quitlines and tobacco health outcomes, and the search convinces her that this proposed increase in excise tax is a promising area for study. Representative Stanton is prepared to support this effort through legislative channels on the basis of the results of the study.

Washington (the practitioner) uses the same network data to link his organization with other state administrators for regular online and onsite meetings, as well as a source of data on current tobacco control trends and practices. As part of the tacit knowledge base in tobacco control, Washington also frequently participates in planning and evaluation of research such as Smith's. He recently used the network to link with global colleagues to collaborate on a peer-reviewed journal article on trends in population-level intervention.

Smith constructs systems models for her research work based on explicit data from tobacco control knowledge bases, as well as feedback and participation from network-based clusters of tobacco control stakeholders, including contacts with collaborative partner organizations, community activists such as Rodriguez, and leading health care professionals like Fellows. These stakeholders assist in developing study designs and evaluation criteria and approaching potential funding sources for the research.

Rodriguez has online access to data that support his advocacy efforts and linkages with advocates in other communities, providing communications and visibility for possible class-action legal challenges and helping him to tap into complementary community resources for building coalitions. More important, the data also provide information on best practices in community activism for tobacco control to help synchronize his efforts with the evidence base of similar advocates in other parts of the country. Conversely, his work influences stakeholders in Smith's research in policy interventions and Representative Stanton's legislative agenda.

Using network data, Fellows linked with colleagues and shared practices, leading to the successful Tobacco Intervention for Patients program her hospital group implemented last year. This year, data from this program are being retrieved from the tobacco control knowledge base for use by researchers in another state as part of an epidemiological study on tobacco control interventions in the health care setting. As a participant in dialogues on research and dissemination efforts, Fellows also is a voice for national efforts at the patient level, in collaboration with stakeholders such as Smith and Washington.

Smith's research studies frequently use an online collaborative group process, and data from this knowledge base are used to help identify simulation models and evaluation methods for her studies. Data from these studies, as well as Smith's own growing expertise, later become part of the tobacco control knowledge base for future research efforts. Network channels are used to actively disseminate the study results among key stakeholders and to publicize them through appropriate industry and publication channels.

The tobacco industry knowledge base provides Representative Stanton with quantitative data on the nation's disease burden and costs associated with tobacco control, as well as access to information she uses to counter tobacco industry lobbying efforts among colleagues. More recently, these data, network information, and tacit knowledge have all enabled her to become active in helping to set the national research agenda in policy-based interventions.

Stories such as these point to a larger environment in which many things depart from business as usual. Local stakeholders have a national or even global reach, clusters of people with common interests or expertise become known to each other, and research becomes more participatory and outcome based, in turn affecting the efforts of practitioners, policy makers, and other stakeholders. Networking, data-driven systems models, and integrated planning, implementation, and evaluation become the norm, leading to an environment in which the actions of any stakeholder ultimately affect the efforts of all stakeholders—a system unto itself. Above all, they create an overall environment for bidirectional linking of research and practice, harnessing both to uncover optimal solutions for complex problems and to change outcomes. However accurate the specifics of predictions such as these are over time, the promise of systems thinking is to create an integrated environment for tobacco control that uses the efforts of all its participants to produce results that could not exist today.

To keep the ideas relatively simple, this example was confined to tobacco control. A more likely future scenario is one in which systems methods are integrated but there also is an integrated approach to public health, so tobacco control is considered in a system that examines factors such as obesity, heart disease, healthy lung function, and stress reduction. Such a scenario is analogous to Milstein's[3] description of syndemics in epidemiology. Thus, Smith might consider a research study on promotion of a lifestyle among adolescents that discourages smoking, excessive drinking, and use of illicit drugs, while encouraging exercise,

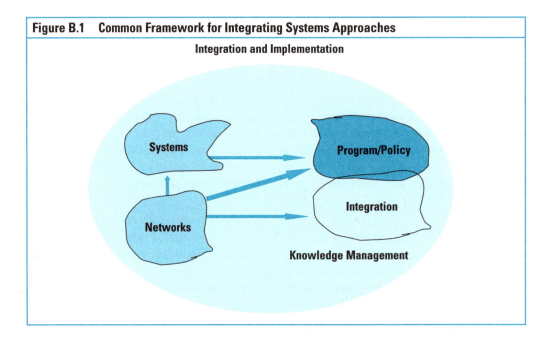

Figure B.1   Common Framework for Integrating Systems Approaches

personal development, and community-based activity and service. Multiple stakeholders would be involved in defining the parameters of well-being.

Putting Systems Thinking into Practice

Moving forward from what is currently known, a desirable near-term goal is engineering a synthesis of methodologies from existing systems approaches to change outcomes. Based on what has been learned and the potential for systems approaches, it may be critical to move past the current "smorgasbord" approach—choosing from among disparate islands of systems approaches—toward further research and development of an integrated environment in which the component pieces work together (figure B.1). Much as early research on computer networks led to the Internet, so must proactive research lead to the systems environment of the future in a way that engages both tobacco stakeholders and the technology field to build an infrastructure that can be applied within tobacco control, public health, and beyond.

Bringing this goal to fruition requires a process that involves tobacco control stakeholders in defining and implementing the future of systems in tobacco control and connecting its vision and missions more effectively to the context of tobacco control. Discussion here centers on a framework for engaging the tobacco control field to move toward an effective systems environment that serves its needs. Systems knowledge is not a "thing." It is an inherently dynamic social process, and the end game of this process is an agenda of research that pushes this social process forward and implements it. At the same time, this effort must engage the public and private sectors, join efforts supporting other disciplines, and lead to a real change in the functioning of the tobacco control stakeholder community, much like the evolution of computing described earlier.

Tobacco control is a diverse field that includes studies of issues such as population surveillance on the prevalence of tobacco use and consumption of tobacco products; research such as developing models to better understand addiction; issues related to practice such as community and clinical interventions and prevention strategies; and policy issues relating to advertising, promotion, pricing, and use of tobacco products. It is a field with a great deal of ongoing activity, with little underlying clarity on the global meaning of the activity, the efficient use of resources, and the optimal linkage of the various segments of the field to increase results. Moreover, because there is no tobacco control discipline per se, scientists and practitioners come from diverse disciplines such as medicine, public health, economics, marketing, health education, toxicology, and genetics. This situation creates a substantial degree of disconnection within the loose "system" that constitutes tobacco control.

Herein lies the challenge for integrated, adaptive efforts to change tobacco control outcomes. *Guidance for Comprehensive Cancer Control Planning,* from the Centers for Disease Control and Prevention,[4] states,

> The scope of comprehensive cancer control involves a diverse group of **stakeholders** who must *coordinate their efforts* to implement such a plan....These coordinated efforts usually occur in the context of a formal **collaboration** across multiple disciplines and organizations.[4] (boldface and italics in original)

This guidance does not address the question of how stakeholders apply this excellent advice. From a systems perspective, there are three requirements for tobacco control initiatives:

1. Feedback mechanisms to enable appropriate responses to changing influences on the system

2. Leadership and decision-making capacity to institute appropriate responses

3. A mechanism for synthesis and translation of research findings into practice

A comprehensive approach to applying systems thinking approaches such as systems organizing, system dynamics modeling, network analysis, and knowledge management techniques has the potential to create this kind of adaptive, collaborative environment. These tools, which are used increasingly in public health and bridge a range of systems approaches, may in turn create a cultural shift to help tobacco control agents "do the right thing right."

An integrated approach to systems thinking can help bring these models together to form a comprehensive strategy for prevention and cessation of tobacco use. Systems thinking also can increase the impact of the tobacco control strategy. Both scientists and practitioners will contribute to and benefit from an integrated approach to identifying how tobacco control could operate in a more systemic way and suggesting steps to create the infrastructure and processes that could make this new mind-set work.

Framework for Large-Scale Change toward Systems Thinking

Between the research efforts outlined in this monograph and its recommendations lies a process of engaging tobacco control stakeholders to strategize and prepare for the form a systems environment should take. Here, broad guidelines for moving forward from theory to practice are examined, and the use of lessons learned to make changes in the real-world practice of tobacco control is explored.

Public health planning has typically proceeded incrementally and in a disjointed fashion, constrained by time pressures and limited guidance. Now that the view of organizations is far more organic than the previous industrialized view of organizations as silos, there is a shift away from these silos toward a systems strategy for organizing an approach to national priorities. International evidence about effective change management can inform the approach to the special case of tobacco control. The main driver of this project will be a synthesis of lessons about large-scale organizational change in public health that can be learned from knowledge management, network theory, and systems theory. This synthesis will help organizations look in depth at their processes and services, to plan change more confidently, and to implement improvements year after year.

A systems thinking approach addresses root-cause issues such as the following:

- What are the systemic leverage points at all levels?

- How should collaborative tobacco control networks be organized?

- How can research and practice be engaged more productively?

- How can tacit knowledge be captured more effectively?

Figure B.2   Integrated Approach that Benefits Scientists and Practitioners

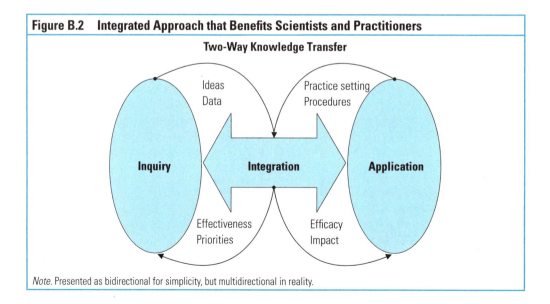

Note. Presented as bidirectional for simplicity, but multidirectional in reality.

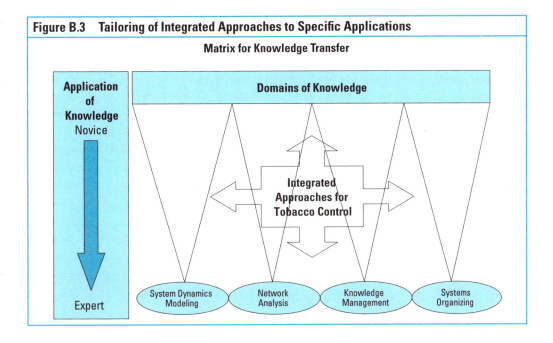

Figure B.3   Tailoring of Integrated Approaches to Specific Applications

With specific and evidence-based tools, tobacco control planning can develop an integrated approach in each agency and community. This integrated approach will be based on the notion of adapting to specific circumstances from various knowledge domains (figures B.2 and B.3).

The process of developing an integrated approach could be broken down into steps such as the following:

1. Identifying an overall vision based on systems thinking and key targets for delivery, according to local priorities

2. Identifying relevant local actions (missions) that are aligned with the vision

3. Analyzing how to develop capacity through a local network or alliance and the specific responsibilities of each health care, social care, or educational organization

4. Creating models for comprehensive planning options that can show different agents in the tobacco control networks where they are and how their missions align to address a common vision

5. Establishing meaningful indicators for monitoring progress and managing performance across whole systems, enabling system learning and adaptation

6. Improving communications and accountability to demonstrate progress

Scope and Objectives: Audacious Vision and Focused Goals

A possible vision for systems thinking is to encourage evolution of self-organizing adaptive networks or federations of systems that can improve effectiveness within the field of tobacco control. Resulting from collaborative development of a coherent integrated framework for tobacco control, this vision could ultimately lead to a significant decrease in use of tobacco products and a reduced toll of disease and death. With use of the systems thinking approach, the framework could establish a cohesive vision at national, state, and local levels, and could provide explicit targets for policy makers and others working in the field of tobacco control. The approach would not attempt to impose a single approach from all agents in the tobacco control system but would instead provide the context for different agents to contribute according to their strengths and abilities. The added power of the project would come from the enduring relationships across the network of experts involved in developing the framework. Through its specific objectives to achieve the overarching goal, a possible next phase could include the following accomplishments:

1. Distill broad priorities for the next 5 to 10 or 20 years through a process, including consultations and workshops, that builds on respectful appreciation and mutual understanding of different perspectives from diverse segments of the tobacco control field

2. Foster a sense of cohesion in the field among key opinion leaders by synthesizing and fostering alignment among their planning activities

3. Develop an articulated tobacco control framework that links priorities and strategies, providing a foundation reference for stakeholders (e.g., researchers and funding sources)

4. Disseminate the framework with advice for strategic implementation, such as critical success factors and guidelines for implementation in diverse settings

The principal outputs of this project could include the following:

- Consultation forums with key stakeholders

- Increased understanding among stakeholders of different perspectives on the problem of tobacco control, the advantages and disadvantages of different approaches, and differences and similarities in visions of desirable future approaches and outcomes

- A series of reports providing guidance to apply concepts such as systems organizing, network analysis, systems theory, and knowledge management to tobacco control at the research, policy, and practice levels

- Planning tools and templates to assist planners in applying the integrated systems thinking framework to local situations and priorities

- Recommendations for pilot projects to apply the systems thinking framework

- An evaluation framework for comprehensive assessment of systems approaches

Bringing the concepts of systems thinking into practice involves specific changes for each of the principal stakeholder groups in tobacco control. The conclusions presented in this monograph represent a possible first step toward making that systems future happen. At the same time, translating these steps into practice requires implementation of new practices at each stakeholder level, and the task of working out specific details remains the next phase of this process. Table B.1 presents one possible vision for putting these conclusions into practice for researchers, practitioners, advocates, and leaders.

The future does not fit neatly into little boxes. Many of these implementation objectives, such as creating learning environments and working across disciplines, apply to groups of multiple stakeholders. Other objectives are global efforts that transcend specific groups, such as the development, use, and maintenance of knowledge infrastructures. Nevertheless, charts such as these illustrate a broader point: implementation of a systems environment revolves around changing the "simple rules" by which each of these stakeholder groups operates in daily practice.

Systems thinking has the potential to become a unified discipline that is crosscutting in terms of other disciplines and fields of endeavor, perhaps by analogy to fields such as statistics that operate at three distinct levels. First, statistics represents an academic field of study unto itself, in which theory and methods of statistics are developed and advanced. Second, other fields (e.g., biology, psychology, sociology, and geography) incorporate statistical training into their core methodologies and have staff and research programs with a strong quantitative orientation. Third, statistics serves as a core competency throughout the fields of research and practice, with an expectation that a large proportion of research staff and students, as well as practitioners, will have at least a basic level of statistical competence.

Like statistics, some elements of systems thinking already are embedded in other significant research areas. For example, many researchers who study environmental issues incorporate integrated assessment, other systems approaches, and participatory approaches into their

Table B.1   Steps for Implementation of Conclusions in Specific Stakeholder Groups

Step	Researchers	Practitioners	Advocates	Leaders
Develop and apply systems methods and processes	Move from logic models to systems models	Use participatory approaches for planning and evaluation	Adopt ecological view of impact of advocacy efforts	Encourage systems thinking and systems processes
Build and maintain network relationships	Link with collaborators within and across disciplines	Build global communities of practice	Harness national and global efforts	Study and leverage network dynamics
Build system and knowledge capacity	Use and add to evidence base	Adapt and incorporate best practices	Share efforts, successes, and processes	Create knowledge infrastructures and break down "silos"
Encourage transformation to systems culture	Engage practitioners and other stakeholders in planning and evaluation	Create learning environment	Foster shared purpose with other stakeholders	Facilitate evolution of vision and paradigm

Integration and Implementation Science: A New Academic Field

In proposing the synthesizing field of Integration and Implementation Sciences discussed in chapter 3, Bammer[a] has gone so far as to propose a full department-level academic field of study for the implementation of systems methods to build the kinds of shared understanding and individual competence that exist in established fields such as statistics. This position supports the view of a unified, integrated approach to systems thinking as a fundamental discipline underlying areas of public health such as tobacco control, in much the same way that fields such as epidemiology and informatics became integrated with public health in years past (see figure below). Like statistics, a "home" department would concentrate on the development of theory and methods, which can be applied in a wide range of areas. These areas can range from specific topics like tobacco control to health more generally, as well as environment and security. A second level of activity would be in sectors in which practice-based research is used to test and develop theory and methods, which in turn are fed back to and assessed by the home department. The third level of activity focuses more on application, with less interest in the development of new theory and methods.

The proposal for a structured academic field or discipline seeks to learn from the troubled history of systems thinking. Institutional barriers stymied attempts to introduce systems thinking in the 1960s and 1970s, and thus avoided a disciplinary focus. This proposal seeks to adopt and take advantage of existing institutional structures to create a new academic field of study, producing graduates prepared for the implementation of systems thinking approaches in specific fields such as public health.

Overview of Integration and Implementation Sciences

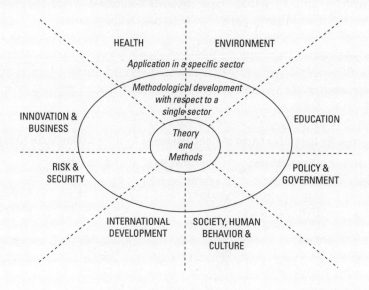

Note. This overview shows how a specific home discipline would relate to key sectors of activity.

[a]From Bammer, G. 2005. Integration and implementation sciences: Building a new specialization. *Ecology and Society* 10 (2): 6. http://www.ecologyandsociety.org/vol10/iss2/art6.

teaching and research. Public health efforts often have a strong orientation to participation and implementation. However, incorporation of systems thinking is largely idiosyncratic, without a "core curriculum" of best practices. The field of systems thinking still is growing and defining itself, as opposed to having well-defined core methods in the way that probability serves as a nucleus for statistics.

A process such as the one proposed here for getting started in systems thinking may serve as an important step to prepare for planning an integrated systems environment for tobacco control. More important, engaging tobacco control stakeholders in the planning for such an environment could build a participatory framework for systems methods in the future. Finally, it can help to focus these systems efforts toward real-world health outcomes in tobacco control, as seen through the shared vision of the organizations and people working to deliver these outcomes.

Implementing Systems Thinking in Tobacco Control: Open Questions and Next Steps

Systems approaches, by their nature, involve creating the capacity to solve more complex problems across a broader network of stakeholders. Implementing such approaches in tobacco control will require key decisions, on the part of these stakeholders, to create this capacity. Four critical open issues remain as the tobacco control community moves forward with the process of integrating systems approaches and engaging stakeholders in the conclusions of this monograph.

1. **Who will construct the infrastructure of systems for tobacco control?** Who will take primary responsibility for moving an integrated systems environment forward? Will the effort be specific to tobacco control needs or leverage more generalized systems efforts in the broader domain?

2. **Will this systems environment be open or proprietary?** To use an analogy from computer science, will this environment be managed by a few, to serve a broad market, as Windows or America Online are, or by a "committee" of stakeholders, as Linux or the Internet are? What will its mechanisms for change be over time?

3. **Will this system be in the public domain?** Do the interests of tobacco control and public health require that ownership and management of those issues rest in the public sector, or can private interests provide more competitive technology and growth?

4. **How does the field of tobacco control get where it wants to go?** What is the role of ISIS in providing incentives for the movement down the road, in a way that is valuable? How does tobacco control begin and sustain the process leading to this systems environment?

A concerted effort to synthesize these systems approaches may hold the potential to answer the field's key questions: What factors lead to prevalence of tobacco use and consumption of tobacco products and their related morbidity and mortality? Can good science be placed into the hands of practitioners within days or weeks instead of years? Can tobacco control stakeholders be linked to work more closely together toward common goals? Perhaps most important, how can the underlying mission to substantially improve health outcomes be fulfilled? Creation of a synthesis of systems approaches holds the promise of a new process that, in turn, holds the answers to these questions.

Based on observations by participants in ISIS and recommendations from key informants, several procedural "next steps" can potentially assist in moving such an implementation process forward, as well as clarify the implications of systems thinking for tobacco control stakeholders:

1. **Identify emergent visions and missions (actions).** All agencies conduct regular planning exercises, so this recommendation is helpful in grounding theory with application. Structured processes for identifying collective vision can enable emergent thinking from many stakeholders. Identifying existing strengths and successes can point to system adaptations that can improve results rapidly. The language of systems thinking must be made accessible to all stakeholders. These processes also would allow for respectful appreciation of differences in perspectives.

2. **Connect system processes overall—focus on the "glue."** Addressing this recommendation begins with a broader and deeper awareness of tobacco control as a "system." The systems perspective focuses on "context" as well as "content." A first step would be to group and classify agencies based on their strategic roles and functions. Description and transformation in the relationships within the tobacco control community are needed. Therefore, the first "adhesive" process should be for agencies at various levels and in various groupings to redesign strategy individually and collectively. This process would create a setting to address the context of tobacco control, specifically its strengths, weaknesses, opportunities, and threats. Such a process should be inclusive to the extent that is realistic. The tobacco control stakeholder community then should consciously encourage the development of "long bond" connections in the network that bring together people and organizations with distinctly different capabilities and strengths. These connections increase both the adaptability and sustainability of the effort.

3. **Recognize that context counts, especially in large organizations, so help practitioners to identify and share tacit knowledge.** This recommendation also requires the full combination of systems thinking approaches. Identification is not only a knowledge management problem, because no one could cope with full disclosure of all tacit knowledge. System dynamics modeling and network analysis must be used to help determine which interventions are relevant (1) to strategic priorities, (2) for efficient use of resources (e.g., stakeholders' time), and (3) for applicability. Systems thinking approaches can help in optimally shaping what is needed from this exchange of tacit knowledge. After this shaping process, initiation

of forums for exchange is a relatively easy task. The approach of knowledge management would again be used to help decide who needs to know what and how.

4. **Help all stakeholders bring their thoughts together on dimensions of the system, not just describing the current system but developing characteristics of the future system.** This key tenet of systems thinking and organizational change also dovetails with the recommendations voiced by many informants throughout this project. The importance of participatory approaches in planning systems strategies for the future should be emphasized. In addition, a vision should be set forth for a forum in which stakeholders would use systems thinking to project the paths of tobacco control and the tobacco industry over the next 5 and 10 years.

The Newtonian view of the world, a world of simple causes and effects, appears to be giving way to a more complex environment that more closely mirrors the behavior of the real world. This evolution of systems is a process of autonomous agents following rules and, in the fashion of Darwinism, ultimately leads to more optimal results. One lesson learned from the science of ecology is that evolution occurs more rapidly with more variations. This conclusion leads to perhaps the central argument for implementation of a systems approach: creation of a participatory environment having multiple stakeholders with interaction across multiple levels and capable of modeling and solving problems of complex phenomena. Such an approach could lead to substantial improvement in the state of public health.

References

1. Campbell, D. T. 1974. Evolutionary epistemology. In *The philosophy of Karl R. Popper,* Open Court vol. 14, 413–63. La Salle, IL: P. A. Schilpp II.

2. Winters, R. 2003. What's always next? Predictions are dicey. Past prognosticators vowed that these innovations would change our lives. A sampling of the future that wasn't. *Time,* September 8. http://www.time.com/time/magazine/article/0,9171,1005620,00.html.

3. Milstein, B. 2002. Syndemic overview: When is it appropriate or inappropriate to use a syndemic orientation? Atlanta, GA: Centers for Disease Control and Prevention, National Center for Chronic Disease Prevention and Health Promotion, Syndemics Prevention Network. http://www.cdc.gov/syndemics/overview-uses.htm.

4. Centers for Disease Control and Prevention. 2006. Guidance for comprehensive cancer control planning. Vol. 1: Guidelines. http://www.cdc.gov/cancer/ncccp/cccpdf/Guidance-Guidelines.pdf.

Index

A

accuracy, 82, 82*f*
action, 7, 77–79, 82, 96
    case study, 85
    collective, 152–153
    in VSAL model, 65, 66*f*, 67, 95
action planning
    in concept mapping, 102–103
    for research utilization, 89, 91–92, 91*f*
active agents, 77–78
adaptation
    of collective vision, 70
    in loosely coupled systems, 75
    in planning, 71
adaptive agents, 45
adaptive organizations, 62, 73–74
administrative work, 52
adolescents
    smoking prevalence among, 15–16
    in system dynamics models, 126, 127*f*, 128–129
advertising, tobacco industry, 13, 16–17, 232
    in causal maps, 119*f*, 120
advocates, participation of, 3*f*, 271, 271*t*
age factors, in system dynamics models, 126, 127*f*, 128–129, 133–134, 134*f*
Agency for Healthcare Research and Quality, 200
agenda setting, 50, 194
agent(s)
    active, 77–78
    adaptive, 45
    in learning organizations, 79
    and missions, 77–78
    network models based on, 179
    participatory, 77–78
agent-centered principle, 68–69
alignment, 116
Amazon.com, 239
American Cancer Society (ACS), 174, 200–201
American College of Surgeons Commission on Cancer, 200
American Legacy Foundation, 27, 169
American Medical Association, 24

American Stop Smoking Intervention Study for Cancer Prevention (ASSIST), 17, 22–24, 228–229, 233–234, 251
    models, 23, 23*f*–24*f*
    monograph on, 245–246
    strength of tobacco control measure, 48, 94–95, 118, 229, 242, 245–246
analysis
    consensus, 102
    cultural, 43–44
    data, 99–100, 167–168
    network (*See* network analysis)
    in systems approaches, 230–231, 231*t*
antitobacco constituencies, in causal maps, 121, 121*f*
appreciative inquiry summit methodology, 73
approval process, streamlining of, 53
architecture workspace, 205
assessment
    needs, 71
    participatory methods for, 50
ASSIST project. *See* American Stop Smoking Intervention Study for Cancer Prevention (ASSIST)
attractor, 46
audience, for knowledge translation, 191
autonomy, networks and, 157
autopoiesis, 46
awareness of health risks, in causal maps, 120–122, 120*f*–121*f*

B

Battelle Centers for Public Health Research and Evaluation, 92, 253
behavior
determined by structure, 116
models of, 45
network, 8, 152–154, 181
organizational, 63, 188
as system, 111–113, 116
tobacco use (*See* smoking behavior)
behavioral management, 63
Behavioral Risk Factor Surveillance System, 201
best practice. *See* evidence-based practice
Best Practices for Comprehensive Tobacco Control Programs (CDC), 169
"better before worse" scenario, 115–116

Note: Page numbers with *t* indicate tables; page numbers with *f* indicate figures.

J

K